MEDICAL EDUCATION: RESPONSES TO A CHALLENGE

MINORITIES AND THE DISADVANTAGED: DEVELOPMENT AND REPRESENTATION IN THE HEALTH PROFESSIONS

Editors:
WILLIAM E. CADBURY, Jr., Ph.D.
CHARLOTTE M. CADBURY, LL.D.
Haverford, Pennsylvania

Associate Editors:
ANNA CHERRIE EPPS, Ph.D.
JOSEPH C. PISANO, Ph.D.
MEdREP, Tulane Medical Center,
New Orleans, Louisiana

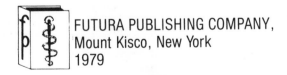
FUTURA PUBLISHING COMPANY,
Mount Kisco, New York
1979

The Conference-Workshops on Medical Education presented by the Medical Education Reinforcement and Enrichment Program of Tulane University Medical Center, sponsored by the Robert Wood Johnson Foundation, formed the basis for this publication.

Cover design after "Students Aspire", sculpture by Elizabeth Catlett for the Lewis K. Downing Hall of Engineering, Howard University, Washington, D.C.—made possible by a grant from Exxon Education Foundation. Courtesy of Howard University.

This publication is made possible by a grant awarded to Tulane Medical Center—Medical Education Reinforcement and Enrichment Program (MEdREP) by the Maurice Falk Medical Fund, Pittsburgh, Pennsylvania, 1978-1979.

*This book is dedicated to
all students, faculty, administrators and friends of MEdREP
at the undergraduate, professional and philanthropic levels*

List of Contributors

Althea Alexander, Research Associate, Division of Research in Medical Education and Director, Office of Minority Affairs, School of Medicine, University of Southern California, Los Angeles, California

Alonzo C. Atencio, Ph.D., Assistant Professor of Biochemistry and Assistant Dean for Student Affairs, School of Medicine, University of New Mexico, Albuquerque, New Mexico

Lezli Baskerville, Faculty Research Assistant, Howard University School of Law, Washington, D.C.

Maxine E. Bleich, Program Director, Josiah Macy, Jr. Foundation, New York, New York

Charlotte M. Cadbury, LL.D., retired Staff Associate and Coordinator of Special Programs, National Medical Fellowships, Inc., New York, New York

William E. Cadbury, Jr., Ph.D., Professor of Chemistry, Emeritus, Haverford College, Haverford, Pennsylvania, and former Executive Director of National Medical Fellowships, Inc., New York, New York

J W Carmichael, Jr., Ph.D., Professor of Chemistry and Pre-Health Advisor, Xavier University of Louisiana, New Orleans, Louisiana

James D. Dexter, M.D., Associate Professor of Neurology, School of Medicine, University of Missouri, Columbia, Missouri

Paul R. Elliott, Ph.D., Professor of Biological Science and Assistant Vice President, Florida State University, Tallahassee, Florida

Anna Cherrie Epps, Ph.D., Professor of Medicine and Director, Medical Education Reinforcement and Enrichment Program, Tulane University Medical Center, New Orleans, Louisiana, and Vice-Chairperson (1978-1979) and Chairperson-Elect (1979-1980), Minority Affairs Section, Group on Student Affairs, Association of American Medical Colleges, Washington, D.C.

Therman Evans, M.D., National Health Director for Operation PUSH, Health Manpower Development Corporation, Washington, D.C.

Alfred Fisher, M.Ed., Vice President for Administrative Affairs, National Medical Association, Washington, D.C.

Frances D. French, Director of Academic Services, The University of Michigan Medical School, Ann Arbor, Michigan

Christine Grant, M.B.A., Program Officer, Robert Wood Johnson Foundation, Princeton, New Jersey

Laia Hanau, M.A. (in Ed.), Study Skills and Writing Consultant and author of *The Study Game: How To Play and Win,* Lexington, Kentucky

Charles S. Ireland, Jr., M.S.W., Assistant to the Dean, Temple University, Health Sciences Center, School of Medicine, Philadelphia, Pennsylvania

Eleanor L. Ison-Franklin, Ph.D., Professor of Physiology and Associate Dean for Academic Affairs, College of Medicine, Howard University, Washington, D.C.

Barbara M. Jarecky, Coordinator, Academic Support Services, Health Career Opportunity Office, University of Kentucky, Lexington, Kentucky

Judith W. Krupka, Ph.D., Associate Professor and Associate Dean for Student Affairs, College of Human Medicine, Michigan State University, East Lansing, Michigan

Walter F. Leavell, M.D., Associate Professor of Medicine and Vice Dean, College of Medicine, University of Cincinnati, Cincinnati, Ohio, and Chairman, Minority Affairs Section, Group on Student Affairs, Association of American Medical Colleges, Washington, D.C.

Richard P. McGinnis, Ph.D., Professor of Chemistry and Premedical Advisor, Tougaloo College, Tougaloo, Mississippi

Joseph C. Pisano, Ph.D., Associate Professor of Physiology and Associate Director, Medical Education Reinforcement and Enrichment Program, Tulane University Medical Center, New Orleans, Louisiana

Dario O. Prieto, Director, Office of Minority Affairs, Association of American Medical Colleges, Washington, D.C.

Herbert O. Reid, LL.D., Charles Hamilton Houston Distinguished Professor of Law, School of Law, Howard University, Washington, D.C.

Norma E. Wagoner, Ph.D., Assistant Professor of Anatomy and Associate Dean, Student Services and Educational Resources, College of Medicine, University of Cincinnati, Ohio

Miriam S. Willey, Ph.D., Assistant Professor and Director, Office of Medical Education, College of Medicine, Howard University, Washington, D.C.

Preface

For those of us who are concerned with the current status and eventual destiny of the economically and educationally disadvantaged of our society, the assurances of equality and opportunity in education for all citizens of this nation are paramount. Our system of government must maintain these assurances and protect the educational rights and privileges of our youth, particularly in the pursuit of health career goals.

One of our nation's most outstanding statesmen and minority leaders has stated that "science and scientific endeavor will be enriched by the full participation of a broader group of people," and that "the participation of citizens from all segments of society will ensure a more equitable and compassionate distribution of the fruits of science and the application of technology."

America was built on the idea of risk and trust; rational man accepted and recognized the value of taking chances and trusting his fellow man. As a result, this country has led the world in so many fields, and yet this profound and moving people for many years showed little progress and interest in such vital areas as health manpower until the health manpower crisis occurred, in the late 1960's. The profound effects of this crisis were evidenced where health care needs were not being met, and the uneven distribution of health personnel and the underrepresentation of minorities in the health care delivery system, particularly in the inner city and rural areas where the economically, educationally and socially disadvantaged reside, were recognized.

vii

Today, moreover, all of America is concerned and involved with health care delivery and it will probably continue its interest for many years to come. The changes we make today in the educational sphere, whether it be at the elementary, secondary, or higher educational levels, must indeed impact the trends of future progress. This progress depends on the challenges of today's innovations, produced by changes in educational approach which will be expressed in our educational institutions of tomorrow throughout this nation and the world.

Despite rational man's achievements of the past and recent years, there is still a demonstrated need to improve the status of underrepresented minorities and the economically and educationally disadvantaged in the fields of medicine, medical education, and science. The concerned individuals who have so diligently worked to achieve this end, and who have so graciously accepted our invitation to further contribute of their time and effort toward this volume, are to be applauded for their continuing contributions to insure educational equality and opportunity by making this publication possible. It is our desire to provide, in concert with these contributing educational leaders, a profound resource and a sound base for the broad spectra of educational institutions both nationally and internationally, to reflect the changes which challenge our future in education and the health care field.

This publication contains the expressed concerns and ultimate strategies considered necessary to succeed in meeting the challenges of change in medical education today, to achieve the goals of yesterday, and to insure inclusion of those underrepresented segments of our society in the fields of medicine and science tomorrow. It is our wish to provide the premedical and medical education communities, the architects and guardians of our health care policies, and all other interested persons, with some insight into the proven constructive and established program and educational processes necessary for the continued growth of minorities and the disadvantaged as participants in the graduate and professional educational pathways in the fields of medicine and science.

These selected topics are directed to the interested and concerned professionals, educators and students in the premedical and medical education fields, the public and private sectors of our nation, particularly as they relate to the health care policies of our future, the philanthropic organizations, foundations, and federal agencies whose initiatives give thrust and momentum to the goals and objectives to increase the underrepresentation of minorities and disadvantaged groups in the health professions and the health care delivery system, and those project and program directors who are, have been and will be committed to and involved in efforts to insure equality and opportunity in the health professions fields for all mankind.

Anna Cherrie Epps, Ph.D.
Director of MEdREP and
Professor of Medicine

Joseph C. Pisano, Ph.D.
Associate Director of MEdREP and
Associate Professor of Physiology

Tulane University Medical Center
School of Medicine
New Orleans, Louisiana

Acknowledgments

We wish to express our deepest appreciation for the sustained and prior support of the United States Department of Health, Education and Welfare, Public Health Service, Health Resources Administration, Office of Health Resources Opportunity; the Robert Wood Johnson Foundation; the J. Aron Charitable Foundation, Inc.; the Gulf Oil Foundation; the Exxon Education Foundation; the Maurice Falk Medical Fund; and the Josiah Macy, Jr. Foundation; the National Urban Coalition; and the Alfred P. Sloan Foundation; for without their support, the Medical Education Reinforcement and Enrichment Program (MEdREP) would not have been able to evolve to its present stage.

Our sincerest gratitude is extended to both the Maurice Falk Medical Fund and the Robert Wood Johnson Foundation for their support and assistance in making this publication a reality. Our special thanks to the Maurice Falk Medical Fund for recognizing the importance and timeliness of a publication of such selected topics and their sincere expression of faith in mankind.

To the Robert Wood Johnson Foundation, our heartfelt thanks for its many constructive efforts and innovative approaches designed to ultimately eliminate the underrepresentation of minorities and the disadvantaged in the fields of science and health care delivery, and for its continued support of project models, such as Tulane University Medical Center's Medical Education Reinforcement and Enrichment Program (MEdREP). In addition, our sincerest appreciation to the Robert Wood Johnson Foundation for its support over the last several years of our Conference-Workshops in Medical Education. These conferences provided the optimum milieu for information exchange among colleagues and an assembly of experts in the field, making possible the evolution of this publication and the further identification of the problems and values, as well as the demonstrated need for continued provision of basic information and program designs for success in meeting the challenges of tomorrow in the educational world of medicine and science.

We who are responsible for the direction of the Medical Education Reinforcement and Enrichment Program of the Tulane University Medical Center at New Orleans, Louisiana, are indebted to the many who have contributed to and attended our Conference-Workshops in the past. Foremost among those to whom we are truly indebted are the many contributing authors, as listed: Ms. Bonnie Riess, whose time, efforts and organization provided a basis for this publication; Dr. John J. Walsh, Chancellor and Vice-President for Health Affairs, Tulane Medical Center, Tulane University, New Orleans, Louisiana; Mr. Jack Aron, Past Chairman, Tulane Medical Center, Board of Governors; Dr. Robert Sparks, Past Dean, Tulane University, School of Medicine; Dr. Herbert Longenecker, Past President, Tulane University; and to the past and present membership of the Tulane Medical Center's Board of Governors and University Board of Visitors. We are especially grateful to our present Dean of the School of Medicine, Dr. James Hamlin, and to the President of Tulane University, Dr. Sheldon Hackney, for their continued interest and support of the program efforts. We owe special thanks to Mr. Philip Hallen, President of the Maurice Falk Medical Fund; to Ms. Maxine Bleich, Program Director, Josiah Macy, Jr. Foundation; to Ms. Christine Grant, Program Officer, Robert Wood Johnson Foundation; and to Dr. Clay Simpson, Associate Administrator for HEW-Health Resources Administration and Director of Health Resources Opportunity Program, Office of Health Resources Opportunity, for their unfailing faith, understanding and support of programs for the underrepresented in the fields of medicine and science.

We are especially grateful to our authors for their literary contributions; to Dr. and Mrs. William Cadbury, Editors, for the massive editorial responsibility they have undertaken and their exceptional response to the challenge; to Mrs. Jeanne Allender,

Editorial Assistant, for her sustained contributions and administrative assistance to both the Directors and Editors of this project; to Miss Kathryn I. Holten, In-House Editorial Staff Assistant, for journalistic and editorial contributions, as well as editorial and administrative assistance to the project Directors; to Ms. Linda Schexnaydre, for staff library research and assistance to the authors; and to Mr. Steven Korn, Chairman of the Board of Futura Publishing Company, for his interest and assistance in making this publication possible.

Last but not least, our thanks to the many consultants and participants who made our Medical Education Conference-Workshops a tremendous success. This volume attests to the success of the past Conference-Workshops, but more importantly focuses on the future in medical education. This publication addresses some of the methodologies and strategies considered necessary for maintaining the inclusion, growth and continued participation of minorities and the disadvantaged in the mainstream of American Medical Education and the health care delivery in our nation.

Anna Cherrie Epps, Ph.D.
Director of MEdREP and
Professor of Medicine

Joseph C. Pisano, Ph.D.
Associate Director of MEdREP and
Associate Professor of Physiology

Tulane University Medical Center
School of Medicine
New Orleans, Louisiana

Introduction

William E. Cadbury, Jr.

The serious under-representation in medicine of certain minority groups—Blacks, Mexican-Americans, American Indians, and Mainland Puerto Ricans—is too well known to require elaboration. Until recently, very few members of any of these groups were enrolled at any medical schools except Howard and Meharry. For these schools to expand their enrollments very much would have been impossible, given limitations in their resources. Increasing opportunities for minorities in medicine depended at first on the willingness of the medical schools whose doors had been closed to open them, and of those whose doors had been open a little to open them wider. Only then would increasing the pool of qualified minority applicants be effective.

In 1968, first-year minority enrollment, which never before had much exceeded 200, jumped suddenly to 292. By 1974, this number had grown to 1,473, but since then there has been no appreciable change. What was it that made such rapid progress possible? Why did it stop? And what can be done to promote resumption?

In this book, an attempt will be made to suggest answers to these questions. The book had its origin in a series of conferences, or workshops, held in the years 1975 to 1978 in connection with Tulane Medical Center's Medical Education Reinforcement and Enrichment Program, directed by Dr. Anna Cherrie Epps. She selected the authors for the various chapters, all of whom had been

William E. Cadbury, Jr., Ph.D., formerly Executive Director of National Medical Fellowships, Inc., is Professor of Chemistry, Emeritus, at Haverford College, Haverford, Pennsylvania.

participants in one or more of these conferences. What they say here is in many cases an updating of material presented there. The conferences provided an opportunity for the exchange of information and ideas among people in a position to make things happen.

The value of this kind of sharing was very well expressed by Jerry Lewis, President of National Medical Fellowships, Inc., in a letter in July 1978, to Christine Grant, of the Robert Wood Johnson Foundation, reviewing two of these workshops. He says:

> As you know, the purposes of the workshops were to: (1) provide accurate and updated information, and (2) improve communication between medical schools and undergraduate advisors, and students in relation to minorities in medicine.
>
> Although a number of smaller efforts have been made to address the above problems, most of these have occurred at the level of program operation rather than program planning at the regional or national level. I believe that if there is to be any significant improvement in the recruitment, admissions, and retention processes of minorities, minorities and others concerned with the problems must play a greater role in shaping the thought and directions which will provide the real know-how in implementing workable and successful programs at the premedical and medical school levels.
>
> . . . these conferences . . . have successfully identified the many facets of health care policy, planning and financing relevant to minorities, and have helped to clarify and review the issues in the light of some positive statements of principle. These conferences have also developed an analytical basis from which to work for modified or alternative solutions concerning financial aid packages and enlightened and legal admissions programs for minorities.
>
> To accomplish the above, Dr. Epps assembled the most knowledgeable and respected administrators, educators and providers from both government and private sectors. These individuals . . . are the leaders in the fields of medical education, health care delivery, government manpower programs, and planning. During the general sessions, these leaders provided useful, updated information; during the special sessions, they joined other program participants in the development of strategy. . . .
>
> After reflecting on the Bakke Supreme Court decision, I now believe more than ever that this forum should continue. Judging

from the audience and participants' reactions, the conferences have been an unqualified success. The remarks, discussions, and recommendations were informative, insightful, and gave many premedical and medical school educators something to build on.

With the Bakke decision behind us, the most important and positive thing we can all do over the next twelve months is to develop clear and unbroken lines of communication between medical schools, premedical advisors and students on ways to share vital and successful experiences.

This book is an attempt to extend these "clear and unbroken lines of communication" to an audience much wider than the necessarily limited number of participants in the workshops.

The increase in minority enrollment which began in 1968 did not occur just by accident. Major social forces were partly responsible, helped along by some decisions made deliberately to bring about this change. It may be useful to identify some of the operating factors, and to try to understand why progress stopped so soon and to see what can be done to cause it to resume.

The Civil Rights Movement, which had produced major advances in many fields, had failed by the mid-1960's to make much impression on the medical profession. There had been some advances in opportunities for Black physicians to practice in other than all-Black hospitals, and there had been some changes in the practice of segregating patients by race. But until 1968 there was no significant increase in the number of Black medical students— and so, of course, there was no increase in the number of Black physicians until at least 1972.

One agency, National Medical Fellowships, Inc., had been providing financial aid for two decades for Black students with superior academic qualifications. In addition to assisting a few students at Howard and Meharry, this program gave some impetus to opening up some of the traditionally White medical schools, but the numbers of students involved were never very large. There was little or no general recognition that under-representation of Blacks in medicine was a problem, still less was there concern about under-representation of other minorities.

One of the most important factors in making progress possible was the decision of the federal government to provide financial aid to medical students. Beginning about 1965, federal funds were made available to the medical schools for scholarships and loans to their students, so as to make it possible for low-income students to attend medical school.

There is no evidence that the problems of minorities had anything to do with the initiation of this progam. But the fact that large-scale financial aid was available was important where efforts were made to enroll minority students. There would have been little point in recruiting and granting admission to them if they could not afford to attend.

Unfortunately, the magnitude of federal support never reached the level anticipated. Non-governmental funds took up the slack for a time, but now with rising costs, private agencies cannot meet the need. Since it is clear that the federal government has no intention of resuming large-scale support of needy medical students, financial problems constitute one of the major obstacles to a resumption of progress.

As early as the mid-sixties there were a few modest efforts at improving opportunities for minorities in medicine. For example, the Zale Foundation offered scholarships to Black Texas residents who could gain admission to the Texas medical schools. The University of California at San Francisco began in 1966 to seek out students at some of the Black colleges in the South. What has since become the Harvard Health Careers Summer Program began, in the summer of 1966, as part of the Intensive Summer Studies Program of Harvard, Yale, and Columbia.

In January of 1966 the Rockefeller Foundation made a generous grant to Haverford College for the Post-Baccalaureate Fellowship Program. This money was to be used mostly for students preparing themselves to enter graduate programs in preparation for careers in college teaching, but part of the grant was to support a director for the program, who was expected to obtain from other sources funds for students with other objectives. As is described more fully in Chapter 17, in the fall of 1966 the Josiah Macy, Jr. Foundation decided to award substantial funds for students in this program to improve their preparation for medical school.

The first of several Macy conferences was held in June of 1967. Its purpose was suggested in the Preface of the published conference report: "Mindful of the need for more physicians, and the need for more Negro physicians, the Macy Foundation, with the cooperation of National Medical Fellowships, Inc., gathered together from all parts of the country forty-two Negro and white representatives of the medical profession, of academic medicine, of government, of churches and of philanthropic organizations to break through the ignorance and lack of communication."*

This conference was of special importance because it gave to a number of concerned people a chance, which few of them had had before, to share ideas about opportunities for Blacks to participate in medicine. Given the climate of the time, it was not hard for these people to disseminate this concern among their colleagues; the ripples from this conference spread widely. People who had not realized that there was a problem now became aware of it, and this included many who were responsible for admissions at the medical schools.

It is interesting to note that at this first Macy Conference the Association of American Medical Colleges (AAMC) was not represented. As is made clear in Chapter 3 of this book, it was not long before the AAMC began to play an important role, including co-sponsorship of several later Macy Conferences. With the establishment of the Committee on Medical Education of Minority Group Students in 1968, the Association for the first time took notice officially of the need for change in the attitudes of the medical profession toward minorities. Perhaps even more important was the publication in 1970 of what has become known as the Nelson Task Force Report, also mentioned in Chapter 3 and elsewhere.

Developments in the provision of financial aid were of crucial importance in efforts on behalf of minorities. Given the economic status of many minority families, financial assistance was essential.

The number of first-year minority medical students, 292 in 1968, took a big jump, to 501, in 1969. It was in that summer that the first indications appeared that federal funds could not be counted on to provide the assistance needed if low-income students were not to be excluded from medical school for financial reasons. At some of the medical schools which had accepted a number of low-income minority students for the fall of 1969, there was grave concern whether sufficient financial aid could be provided to enable them

---

* Cogan, L.: *Negroes for Medicine: Report of a Macy Conference.* Baltimore: Johns Hopkins Press, 1968, p. ix.

to matriculate. Responding to this concern, several foundations late in the summer made emergency funds available, through National Medical Fellowships, Inc., for distribution that Fall.

Before 1969, NMF's awards had been based on academic achievement or promise. In that year, NMF began to reconsider this policy, and in 1970 they stated that henceforth, with very few exceptions, their awards would be based on need. At the same time, they announced that other under-represented minority groups—Mexican-Americans, American Indians, and Mainland Puerto Ricans—would be eligible for assistance on the same basis as Blacks.

Another important development at this time was the decision in 1969 by the Alfred P. Sloan Foundation to devote a substantial proportion of their resources for the next five years to increase opportunities for minorities in medicine. Many other foundations, and other donors, joined the Sloan Foundation in providing financial aid to minority students through NMF. In addition to helping in this program, the Robert Wood Johnson Foundation began, in 1972, a large-scale program of financial aid administered through the medical schools (see Chapter 22 and Chapter 3.)

Since Howard and Meharry can accept only a limited number of students and since most other schools, before 1968, accepted very few Blacks, if any, Black school children and young Black men and women in college had been given little encouragement to seek places in medicine. The pool of available Black candidates was very small; of other minorities it was smaller still. As it became apparent that the medical schools would accept many more minority students than they ever had before, increasing the size of the pool became essential.

If recruitment is to be successful, not only must minority students be made to see that careers in medicine are not out of the question for them, but provision must be made for improving their education in grammar school, high school, and college. We do not attempt here to mention all of the efforts, successful and otherwise, which were made in these years. Several examples are given in the chapters which follow.

Mention should be made at this point of one program not touched on elsewhere in this book: Project 75. This was an ambitious recruitment program, financed largely by federal funds, and administered by the National Medical Association. The name—Project 75—came from the recommendation of the Nelson Task Force that medical schools should strive to achieve an enrollment of 12 percent minority students by the year 1975. Project 75 opened a number of regional offices, where information about minority opportunities was made available, as well as counseling, tutoring, and practical advice for minority students. The program brought the idea of medicine to a great many young men and women who might not have considered that profession seriously for themselves.

Medical students played an important part in recruitment, both informally and through their organizations. A few chapters of the Student American Medical Association (now known as the American Medical Students Association) helped to recruit minority students; some chapters brought pressure to bear on their medical schools; some did both. At a good many schools, new chapters of the Student National Medical Association (SNMA) were established when the number of their minority students became large enough. These chapters have been very important, not only in recruitment but also in providing support services in medical schools for minority students. A publication of SNMA, "So You Want to Be a Doctor. . .," revised from time to time, is distributed widely as part of SNMA's recruitment program.

The scholarly demands of medical education are enormous. Only students of superior ability can learn what must be learned in order to succeed in medical school. Given the inadequacies of the early education of many minority students, even the potentially best of them may have trouble meeting the demands placed on them in a very competitive college or in medical school.

Recognition of this fact has led to the establishment of special programs to supplement the regular offerings of schools and colleges. Several of these are described in some detail later on. These programs have been effective in both admissions and retention. It seems clear that without them, some of the minority students who entered medical school could not have done so, and some of them would have had more difficulty than they did in succeeding when they got there. However, much of the credit for success must be given to the students themselves, who showed great courage, stamina, and strength of character in reaching their goals.

There were numerous obstacles as well as aids along the way, and for each individual attaining the M.D. degree it was a major triumph.

Academic support in medical school takes many forms, ranging from the informal conversation after class between teacher and student, through more or less organized tutorial programs, to special decelerated curricula. Some of these methods of support are available to all students; some have been initiated particularly to help students with gaps in their preparation.

Unlike law schools, or more especially graduate schools of arts and sciences, where fewer than half of those who begin doctoral programs eventually earn their degrees, medical schools expect practically all of the students they admit to become physicians. A number of years ago, the success rate in medical school for all students was a little over 90 percent; now it is well over 95 percent. Among minority students, many of whom have suffered from inferior early education, the success rate in recent years is a little lower than for other students, but still as high as or higher than the rate for all students a decade ago.

When the expansion of opportunities for minorities in medicine began, nobody really knew whether or not the early handicaps suffered by minority students could be overcome in medical school. It is clear by this time that they can be, and have been, overcome. There is good reason to think that reinforcement and enrichment programs have been an important factor in this success. Capable minority students, with courage and persistence, have accepted the opportunities offered to them.

The nature of the verdict on the outcome of more than a decade of effort depends on the point of view of the judge, whether optimistic—the glass is half full—or pessimistic—the glass is half empty. The optimist sees that the vast majority of minority medical students receive the M.D. degree; the pessimist sees that some of these students fail to do so. Noting that there was a many-fold increase in minority enrollment from 1960 to 1974, after which progress stopped, the optimist could say: "Look at the progress we have made, and then we have held our own in a bad time; think what could have been done if we had been wiser, had tried harder, and had had more money." Noting the same facts, the pessimist could say: "Progress was made when progress was easy; since then, there is little to show for all our efforts."

Progress began when it did largely because then, and only then, there was widespread recognition that the under-representation of minorities in medicine and the resulting inadequacy in health care constituted a problem. Progress was accelerated by official recognition of the need for change—especially the Nelson Task Force Report and the AAMC Statement on Medical Education of Minority Group Students (see Chapter 3). Progress would have been nearly impossible without provision for financial and academic assistance: financial aid provided through Federal funds and guarantees, and through scholarships and loans through private agencies and the medical schools themselves; academic assistance through academic year and summer reinforcement programs.

The goal for 1975 which was proposed in 1970 was not reached. Since 1975, instead of progresss, there has been a slight decline. This progress is evident in the fact that more minority physicians are being graduated today than ever before. However, since the increase in minority admissions did not begin until 1968, and it takes so long for physicians to complete their training, the effect of the added minority doctors is only now beginning to be felt. It is not yet possible to say for sure to what extent the problem of maldistribution of physicians will be solved by increasing the heterogeneity of the physician population. The evidence available suggests that, as anticipated, minority physicians are more likely to practice among minority populations. Since it takes even longer for a physician to complete training for a permanent academic career than for most areas of practice, there has to date been little change in the representation of minorities in tenured positions on medical school faculties.

Dr. James L. Curtis, in a forthcoming book, will present the results of studies he has made on the geographic and specialty distribution of training programs chosen by recent minority medical school graduates. He finds that Black medical graduates are attracted to first-year graduate programs in states with large urban Black populations, and that other minority graduates, whose numbers are much smaller, are choosing programs in states where their population groups tend to live. Since location of training often has a strong influence on location of practice, these findings are suggestive of the way in which increasing the numbers of minority physicians may affect the distribution of medical care.

His data on types of programs chosen suggest that minority

medical graduates choose about the same kinds of progams as are selected by others. (He notes one exception: obstetrics-gynecology is chosen much more often by Blacks than by other minorities or by non-minorities.) In the past, Black physicians were much less likely than White physicians to be board-specialized. Present-day minority graduates are entering specialty training programs at about the same rate as others.

If the factors mentioned promoted progress, what caused it to stop? And what can be done to get it started again?

The number of minority students entering medical school depends on the number of applicants and on the proportion of that number which is accepted. When progress began, the proportion accepted was high, and the number of applicants—the size of the pool—grew rapidly as it became clear that new opportunities for careers in medicine were opening up. Later, the proportion of minority applicants who were accepted declined to about the same level as the proportion of all applicants, and the pool stopped growing. Must we assume that there is a limit to the possible size of the pool—that there is a maximum number of young people from the under-represented groups who can be made interested in medical careers? Must we assume that that limit has been reached? Must we also assume that the proportion of applicants accepted cannot be increased? Progress will resume only if one or more of these assumptions is not correct. Much of this book is concerned, directly or indirectly, with these problems.

The 22 chapters which follow, all written by different authors, reflect as many different points of view, and so give interest to the book. They contain some repetition, a good deal of overlap, and some outright contradictions.

The first three chapters are general in nature. The first deals with recruitment; the second with opportunities in medicine; the third with the actions of organized medical education to meet the problem. Most of the rest of the book deals rather directly with education.

Although the education of a doctor is a continuous, life-long process, we are concerned here especially with those parts of the process which affect the accessibility of the profession to members of minority groups. The undergraduate college years are especially important. In Chapters 4 and 5, premedical advising is discussed—in chapter 4 from the point of view of the undergraduate advisor himself, in Chapter 5 from that of the medical school. Four chapters, 6 through 9, are on special help available—special programs for undergraduates both in the undergraduate and the medical school environment—and study and test-taking skills.

Before the undergraduate can become a medical student, the high hurdle of acceptance to medical school must be overcome. Chapters 10 through 13 discuss this process, with special emphasis on admissions problems which may be faced by minority students. Another major obstacle—financing medical education—is treated in Chapter 14.

Once admitted to medical school, the student must adjust to a radically new environment—an adjustment especially difficult for those minority students entering predominantly White medical schools after having attended traditionally Black colleges. The next six chapters deal with the interface between college and medical school, and include descriptions of several programs which have been developed especially to help minority students to make this adjustment.

The final two chapters look to the future. Chapter 21 deals with possible consequences of the Bakke decision; the last chapter is concerned with the impact of foundations on these problems.

The book is not intended to be complete. There are important programs which have not been mentioned. It is hoped that the information included, and the expression of opinions and the description of experiences of the authors will provide an understanding of some of the efforts of the last few years and suggest some constructive approaches to old problems not yet solved and new ones which will develop.

Contents

Medical Education, Health Care Delivery,
and Responses

CHAPTER 1

Identification and Recruitment of Minorities into the Medical Professions

Therman E. Evans

The first question important to the identification and recruitment of minorities into the medical professions is, why is it necessary? The response speaks to the health and medical needs existing in certain communities, and, who is best suited and/or committed to address them.

A 1977 Congressional Budget Office report on the health differentials between white and nonwhite Americans concluded:

> The health of nonwhites is not as good as that of whites, yet nonwhites get less—and possibly less effective—health care than whites do . . . . Nonwhites still experience nearly 50% more bed disability days, 70% higher infant mortality and a life expectancy six years shorter than that of whites. Nonwhites are more likely than whites to suffer from a number of specific conditions known to be improved by health care, which may indicate failure to receive needed prevention or treatment.[1]

Therman E. Evans, M.D., is National Health Director for Operation PUSH, Health Manpower Development Corporation, Washington, D.C.

[1]U.S. Congress, Congressional Budget Office, Health Differentials Between White and Nonwhite Americans (1977), p. XI.

The health deficits in minority communities are attributable to many things. Included are poverty, racism and discrimination, language and cultural barriers. For example, few health and welfare agencies have multicultural and multilingual staffs who could more effectively meet the problems which minorities present.

Inner cities and rural areas are tremendously lacking in competent, sensitive medical expertise. Poor people in general and poor Black, Chicano, Puerto Rican, and Native American people specifically, have long suffered from being low on this nation's medical priority listing. Medical and health problems that have been greatly reduced in affluent groups, continue to flourish amongst poor people. A significant part of the reason for this is the difficulty in getting medical science centers to turn out general practice specialists, and the difficulty in getting physicians, whatever their specialty, to locate in areas of shortage. If reached, these two goals (production of general practice specialists and location in shortage areas) would do more than present policies towards alleviating some of the medical problems faced by twenty to twenty-five percent of the public. The question is, how are these goals best achieved?

There is significant evidence indicating that the race of the physician is important to achieving the above goals. First of all, it is known that Black doctors tend to set up practice along the residential migratory patterns of Black people. This point is supported by Drs. Thompson, Haynes, and Cornely, whose studies were published in the *Journal of the American Medical Association* in 1974, 1967, and 1942 respectively. In addition, a more recent survey by Dr. Lawrence Lezotte examined the location of Black physicians in Michigan. The survey reached two conclusions. The first was that Black physicians are significantly more likely to be located in areas with high concentrations of Blacks. The second was: "Black physicians are significantly more likely to be located in areas with lower median incomes."[2] Further, according to a publication of the National Planning Association, *Looking Ahead,* significant evidence exists supporting the greater likelihood that minority physicians will serve in shortage areas. The publication included an article entitled, "Minority Physician Practice Patterns and Access to Health Care Services," in which the authors say, "some care

[2] Lawrence Lezotte: Locaton of Black Physicians in Michigan, A Summary Report. Paper presented at AAMC Minority Affairs Session, November 1976.

obviously must be exercised in generalizing from the experience of Howard and Meharry graduates to all minority graduates. However, the available evidence does support the contention that minority physicians are more likely to practice in areas with large underserved, low-income urban populations. An increased supply of these physicians can therefore be viewed as contributing to eliminating the existing geographic maldistribution of physicians."[3] In an unpublished staff analysis of medical school alumni data, entitled "Minority Physicians Engaged in Primary Patient Care," the AAMC compared graduates from minority medical colleges with graduates of all U.S. medical schools. The analysis indicated the following: (1) "Minority medical school graduates have a greater proportion of living physicians who practice in primary care specialties than do graduates of other schools. (2) Minority medical school graduates have a greater proportion of alumni since 1960 who practice in primary care specialties than do graduates of other schools."[4] Finally, the National Center for Health Statistics, in its recently completed National Ambulatory Medical Care Survey, examined the issue of whether or not Black physicians serve Black patients. The survey (published summer of 1977) indicated that of all the visits made to Black doctors, 86.95 percent were made by Black people, 10.54 percent were made by Whites, and 2.51 percent by "others."[5] Further, in a brief for the Lawyers' Committee on Civil Rights as *amicus curiae* to the Regents of the University of California v. Bakke, it was stated,

Race is, in fact, an important factor in choosing what kind of practice to pursue, in what location, and for the custom of what kinds of clients. Further, doctors perform important functions in determining priorities and modes for the delivery of health services. . . . In all the varieties of judgments that need to be made in such matters, it is certainly not irrational to believe that racial diversity is desirable, indeed essential. Nor is it inconsistent with known facts to think that clients to be served by the

---

[3] M. Koleda and S. Craig: Minority Physicians Practice Patterns and Access to Health Care Services. *Looking Ahead.* 11, 1-6, 1976.

[4] Minority Physicians Engaged in Primary Patient Care. Unpublished staff analysis by AAMC utilizing data from medical school alumni published by the American Medical Association.

[5] National Center for Health Statistics: National Ambulatory Medical Care Survey. Washington, D.C.: Department of Health, Education and Welfare, 1977.

professions, particularly the poor, the underrepresented, and the disadvantaged, deserve the choice of the opportunity of consulting with racially identifiable doctors or lawyers they believe will best understand and sympathize with their problems; it is certain that race has, in fact, played an enormously important role in their own lives.

Certainly it cannot be said definitely that Native American, Chicano, Puerto Rican, and Black medical professionals will all establish their practices on reservations, in barrios, or in poor inner city neighborhoods. What can be said, however, is the likelihood of this occurring is much greater with professionals who are products of these areas than with professionals who have never been exposed to this sociology.

The importance of identifying and recruiting minorities into the medical professions extends beyond the greater likelihood they will address unmet health needs in disadvantaged communities. It is important because it is a chance to take advantage of, and/or develop the great leadership abilities and other talents lying in wait in these areas. This, in turn, restricts the numbers of positive role models for minority youths. Clearly, the training of minorities in the medical and health professions has broader implications than just the production of more medical professionals who are minorities. Unmet health needs are more likely to be addressed, multicultural, multiracial shaping of institutions more consistent with this pluralistic society is more likely to occur, and more people and families are more likely to break out of the educational, philosophical, economical, and spiritual poverty cycles.

When trying to identify and recruit minorities into the medical professions, there are certain myths and mistakes that can and should be avoided. For example, it is important not to allow the myth of "having to be a genius to be a doctor" move you to make the mistake of informing, encouraging, and motivating towards medicine only those students with very high averages and test scores. Though a generally accepted rule should be, "the higher your scores and averages, the better your chances of admission," there are other very important points to remember.

The standardized test scores of Black students, on the average, are lower than those of White students. This is true for the Scholastic Aptitude Test (SAT), the Medical College Admission Test (MCAT), the Dental Aptitude Test (DAT), the Law School

Admission Test (LSAT), and for Part I of the National Board of Medical Examiners examination. The admission of minority students with average lower test scores, regardless of its socioeconomic implications, has resulted in the charge that professional schools have "discriminated" against "better qualified" majority students in their efforts to gain entrance to these institutions. Implicit in this charge is the issue of "lowering standards" to favor admission of certain racial groups.

What does one's performance on these standardized examinations mean? Will a high standardized test score result in a "good physician"? Are standards being "lowered" to admit Black students? Is discrimination against majority students a real issue in this regard? It is appropriate to examine each of these questions and others.

Standardized examinations in whatever area they are administered foster the "myth of measurability." Their existence suggests that one's academic or intellectual ability can be equated to a number, thus removing the subjectivity and, therefore, the difficulty from determining who is intellectually superior. If my score is higher than yours, then, obviously, I am your intellectual superior, or I know more about the subject matter than you. If my group—economic, racial, or otherwise—generally scores higher than yours, then, obviously, your group is inferior. Of course, no one likes the thought of, let alone the practice of, allowing "intellectual inferiors" to fill training or professional positions that could have been filled by "smarter" or "brighter" people. What do standardized tests tell us? Perhaps a better question is: what don't they tell us? The response to this question is consistent throughout the literature. These tests do not indicate a student's ability to learn, they do not indicate a teacher's ability to teach, they do not indicate whether or not one will do well in his or her chosen profession and they do not predict success in life. With all they do not do, standardized tests still are administered religiously by various educational training institutions. The score results, equated—though incorrectly—in most instances to academic achievement, and/or intellectual ability, are utilized to select out applicants for entrance. Herein lies one of the reasons for their continued use—an easily identifiable method of selecting out applicants. It is important, however, to note that tests, standardized and otherwise, will always be with us. Therefore, it behooves those involved to be aware and, as much as possible, to be prepared—especially in test taking.

The process of selecting students for admission to a medical school class has been related to the question of whether or not standards are being "lowered" to admit Black students. We must be careful not to fall into this intellectually insolvent trap. There is, and should be, only one standard to be equitably applied to all. That standard is the production of a physician qualified to handle the medical and health problems of this society. No other standard matters in the face of this one. The routes taken to reach this standard may vary. Some may take five, six, or seven years after high school, while others may take eight, nine, ten, and more years. The important thing is that more of our focus must be output rather than input.

One of the very serious problems with the selection process for professional training institutions is the emphasis placed on input criteria. This means "merit." Those who have the highest grades and the highest aptitude test scores are those who should be admitted. This is the public position that medical schools and other professional training institutions have assumed for years. It is, of course, not complete truth. In fact, it is somewhat hypocritical since as Kirp and Yudof, in a November 1974 *Change Report,* say,

> Colleges have never relied exclusively upon objective criteria such as test scores or grades in selecting students. If the traditional admissions process can be described as meritocratic, its under-standing of merit has not been governed by simple "probability of success" formulae. Special treatment is routinely accorded to people with particular talents (someone who writes plays or knows how to pass a football), to the offspring of alumni and professors, and to those who make a student body geographically diverse by the simple expedient of residing in some God-forsaken corner of the republic. Each of these kinds, and numerous others, is deliberately favored by admissions officers over students whose paper records are better, but who appear for some reason to be less eye-catching. The persuasiveness of the rationales advanced for such preferences differs, as does the candor with which these policies get publicized. But the fact of preference is quite the same in each case, and that fact has gone largely unchallenged.

Though counselors, teachers, recruiters, administrators, and others involved with large numbers of minority students on a frequent basis should be aware of the above points, it still must be reemphasized that the higher the test scores and grade point averages, the better are the chances for admission.

IDENTIFICATION AND RECRUITMENT

Ideally, students with a potential in science, in math, should be identified as early as possible. This means as far down as elementary and junior high school. However, lacking any precise instrumentation to accurately identify what does, or does not represent a "potential" in the sciences, it is necessary—and also fair—to implement ways and means to expose as many children as possible to scientific career directions.

Systematically this can be achieved through securing public school commitments to:

1. Emphasize in the early grades (K-6) teaching science and math in a way that shows their importance to everyday life.
2. Expose children (K-6) through visitations and hands-on demonstrations to institutions, instruments, and individuals alike: hospitals, clinics, laboratories, offices, microscopes, stethoscopes, telescopes, physicians, physical therapists, dentists, technologists, and others. This should be done on an intensely regular basis serving as the focus of the didactic information delivered in the regular curriculum. It should not be adjunct.
3. The above processes should be continued through junior and senior high school. In these grades, students can be farmed out to actually work for a year or a semester in the various medical career settings. In addition, local elementary and secondary schools can work with local medical professional students or undergraduate premedical professional student organizations to establish big brother and sister relationships designed to give children real life connections to the future of themselves.

The public schools do not represent the only system that can be utilized in this effort.

Religious institutions, which remain extremely stable and viable in many minority communities, should be utilized. Churches represent large, organized, weekly collections of adults and youths that can be utilized in innovative, inoffensive ways to inform, identify, and recruit minority students into medical careers.

Religious institutions can be utilized in the following ways:

1. The ministers (Baptists, Pentecostal, Methodists, etc.) of various churches in a city or circumscribed community can be convened to be counseled on the importance of medical careers, the potential of medical careers, and how they can, and/or should enhance the involvement of their congregations' youth.
2. Churches can sponsor career clubs.
3. Churches can utilize their members—preferably—or non-members who are medical professionals to deliver messages through their religious services.
4. Churches can sponsor health fairs and/or health career fairs designed to gain maximum exposure for their community youth to good information.

Other than established educational and religious institutions, any outlet that works in reaching unreached youths about medical careers is acceptable.

Viable mechanisms that should be considered are:

1. Disc jockeys—radio announcers on rock-and-soul stations have more access to the ears and minds of our youths than most teachers. Therefore, they should be utilized in spreading brief messages of information.
2. Coaches and athletes are also strong role models that have tremendous leadership recognition in minority communities and could be tapped for this purpose.

The Applicant Pool

It is extremely important that the applicant pool size continue to expand. Obviously, it is from the pool that the entrants will come. The larger the applicant pool, the greater the range of selection; and, therefore, the greater the likelihood of increased admissions. Although this is not a foolproof direct relationship, a larger number of minority students with an interest in pursuing medical careers should be desired over a smaller number.

Presently there are between 45,000 and 55,000 applicants to more than 120 medical schools for the 15,000 plus first-year positions. The total number of Black applicants has never reached 4,000 or less than 1/10 the total number of applicants.

Minority admissions into medical career training programs in recent years have leveled, and in some instances have begun to decline. This is partially due to the current sociopolitical climate and the economic climate. In the midst of a definite conservative shift and an unfortunate economic climate, the admission of minorities into training for the medical professions has fallen to a lower priority. This point only adds to the importance of generating larger numbers of even more qualified applicants from minority groups. This means that a greater effort must be expended at earlier points in the educational pathway (as previously mentioned). It also means time and effort must be spent generating and searching for minority students with science potential at later points in the educational pipeline. For example, students who are majoring in engineering, math, statistics, economics, or business administration, ought to be sought out and challenged with the possibility of pursuing a medical career. Further, graduate students in scientific and non-scientific areas represent potential candidates for admission to training in the medical professions. Many of these students are extremely talented intellectually, but have no interest in any of the medical professions. This is where identification and recruitment come in.

THE MESSAGE IS THE METHOD

What is said to young people is important. How it is said can be even more important. Who says it is also important.

In my experience with young people and recruitment activities across the country, the message brought, how, and by whom have much to do with their receptivity. The intellects, attitudes, and interets of minority students can be stimulated in positive directions provided the messenger knows what to say and how to say it to whomever it has to be said.

The tremendous health and medical needs existing in minority communities is always a good place to start. From a discussion of the "needs" one can proceed to incorporate how the student listening can contribute to their solution—a health career. It is always important to first talk about real life problems with which the students are familiar, either from a community, family, or personal perspective. For example, from a discussion of health problems like lead poisoning, cirrhosis/alcoholism, high blood pressure, or infant mortality utilizing specific examples, it is easy to go into what needs to be, and can be done to alleviate these serious conditions. Following this, of course, is how the individual can participate. This is where all the health/medical careers and their spheres of operation are expounded.

Who the messenger is, is less important than what the message is and how it is said. I think it helps to have a role model from the particular profession being discussed. However, one of the reasons so much weight is placed on having members of the profession serve as the panel discussants is that there are so few people who know how to effectively reach young people. Non-members of the profession who can effectively communicate with youths will do very well with getting the message across. Members of the profession who can effectively communicate with youths will do even better.

CONCLUSION

Generally our students must be provided information, inspiration, and academic and economic means to reach a destination. It is important that they are motivated early. This motivation must be sustained through frequent exposure to positive role models and to situations that will require their attention in the future.

In addition to inspiration and motivation, the basics of academics must be attained. None of us can go wrong by continuing the thrust to assist minority students in pushing for academic excellence. Unless our students are firmly grounded in study skills, and other basics of academics, higher educational achievement opportunity in medical and other careers will continue to escape them.

CHAPTER 2

The Varied Roles of Physicians in Society

Alfred F. Fisher

Physicians have historically been accorded a place of importance within American society. Black physicians can now be found in a variety of roles which are of particular significance, in light of the limited involvement of Black Americans within the key economic, professional, political, religious, and social aspects of the mainstream of American life.

The desire to be of special help to fellow humans, coupled with a quest for financial independence and prestige, have been the primary motivating forces for numerous Blacks who have entered the medical profession; therefore it is not surprising that the varied roles of Blacks in medicine are broad and diverse. Medical careers which interface with non-medical interests are not an uncommon occurrence and situations in which individual physicians are not involved in the direct delivery of medical services, but are engaged in formulating and effecting public health policy, as well as managing health services, are frequently observed in an important segment of the 9,300 American physicians who are Black.

Black medical pioneers such as Daniel Hale Williams, the nation's first heart transplant surgeon, and Charles R. Drew, the father of

Alfred F. Fisher, M.Ed., is Executive Vice President for Administrative Affairs with the National Medical Association, Inc., Washington, D.C.

blood banking, are reasonably well known, but lesser known Black physicians have had and continue to have significant impact on all avenues of American life.

In the field of higher education and specifically medical education, there is now a cadre of Black physicians holding key administrative positions, and without their dedication, keen perceptions, and influence, the significant increase in the overall numbers of Black physicians would not have been possible. Among these are Lloyd C. Elam, M.D., President of Meharry Medical College; Carleton P. Alexis, M.D., Vice President for Health Affairs, Howard University; Louis Sullivan, M.D., Dean, Morehouse School of Medicine; Marion Mann, M.D., Dean, Howard University College of Medicine; Ralph Cazort, M.D., Dean, Meharry Medical College; C. W. Johnson, M.D., Dean of the Graduate School, Meharry Medical College; James L. Curtis, M.D., Associate Dean, Cornell University Medical School; Alvin F. Poussaint, M.D., Harvard University Medical School; James Comer, M.D., Yale University Medical School; Walter F. Leavell, M.D., Vice Dean, University of Cincinnati Medical School; Middleton Lambright, M.D., Assistant Dean for Minority Affairs, the Medical University of South Carolina; Thomas R. Georges, M.D., Associate Vice President, Temple University Health Sciences Center (currently on loan to the Agency for International Development, Office of Health Affairs); Vivian W. Pinn, M.D., Assistant Dean, Tufts University Medical School; Bernard Challenor, M.D., College of Physicians and Surgeons, Columbia University; Anthony Clemendor, M.D., Associate Dean, New York Medical College; Helen O. Dickens, M.D., Associate Dean for Minority Affairs, University of Pennsylvania Medical School; Roland T. Smoot, M.D., Johns Hopkins University Medical School; Claude Organ, M.D., Creighton University Medical School; Robert C. Stepto, M.D., formerly Chairman of the Board of Directors, National Medical Fellowships, Professor and Chairman, Department of Obstetrics and Gynecology, Chicago Medical School.

Other Black physicians have served as role models and effectively represented the medical profession through membership on the governing bodies of higher education institutions. Among such individuals are Emerson C. Walden, M.D., University of Maryland, Member of the Board of Regents; Frank S. Royal, M.D., Member of the Board of Overseers, University of Virginia; Robert E.

Dawson, M.D., Member of the Board of Trustees, Meharry Medical College; Alma R. George, M.D., Member of the Board of Trustees, Meharry Medical College; Jesse B. Barber, M.D., Member of the Board of Trustees, Howard University; Edward C. Mazique, M.D., Member of the Board of Trustees, Morehouse College; Arthur H. Hoyte, M.D., Assistant Dean, Georgetown University School of Medicine and Health Advisor to the Mayor of Washington, D.C.

Politics is such a vital part of American life that it is not too surprising that Black physicians are also represented therein. John Rosemond, M.D., currently serves as Chairman of the City Council of Columbus, Ohio; Paul P. Boswell, M.D., is a senior legislator in the State of Illinois. The first successful Cleveland, Ohio mayoral campaign of Carl Stokes was coordinated by the late Kenneth B. Clement, M.D., a prominent surgeon. Therman E. Evans, M.D., a young and dynamic pediatrician, was elected to membership on the District of Columbia Board of Education in 1974 and became its Chairman in 1975. Dr. Evans is currently Assistant Health Services Director with Connecticut General Life Insurance Company.

Consistent with the notion of a personal responsibility to society through involvement in public service, a number of Black physicians have distinguished themselves through service in high level positions. James G. Haughton, M.D., President of the Cook County Health and Hospitals Governing Commission, also happens to be the highest paid public official in the State of Illinois. John L. S. Hollomon, Jr., M.D., Member of the Board of Regents, State of New York, and Chairman of the Board of Trustees, Virginia Union University, headed the billion dollar New York City Health and Hospitals Corporation (1974-1977), which operated 21 health facilities and employed 45,000 individuals. Norma Goodwin, M.D., served the New York City Health and Hospitals Corporation as Senior Vice President for Ambulatory Care.

James R. Cowan, M.D., served as Commissioner of Health for the State of New Jersey until President Gerald Ford appointed him Assistant Secretary of Defense for Health, a position which placed him in charge of all health facilities and personnel related to U.S. Armed Forces Health Services. Upon leaving the Department of Defense, Dr. Cowan subsequently became a Senior Vice President with Blue Cross of Greater New York and moved from there to his current position as President of the United Hospital Fund of

Newark. In 1978 Virginia's Governor, John Dalton, appointed Jean L. Harris, M.D., Commissioner of Health. Dr. Harris is the first Black graduate of the University of Virginia Medical School. Harold W. Jordan, M.D., is State Commissioner of Mental Health in Tennessee.

Thomas R. Georges, M.D., served as Secretary of Health and Welfare for the State of Pennsylvania during the Scranton Administration. Earl Caldwell, M.D., is presently Commissioner of Health for the City of Gary, Indiana. E. Frank Ellis, M.D., Commissioner of Health for the City of Cleveland, Ohio during Carl Stokes' administration, now serves as the Regional Health Administrator for DHEW Region IX in Chicago, Illinois. H. McDonald Rimple, M.D., Director of the National Health Service Corps at its inception, now serves as the Regional Health Administrator for DHEW Region III in Philadelphia, Pennsylvania.

G. Texiera Hunter, M.D., co-developer of health services for the Head Start Program of the Office of Economic Opportunity (OEO), moved from that position to become the first Black DHEW Regional Health Administrator and served in DHEW Region I (New England) for approximately four years. Dr. Hunter is currently Professor and Chairman of the Department of Community Health and Family Practice at Howard University College of Medicine.

June Jackson Christmas, M.D., President of the American Public Health Association, is also Commissioner of Mental Health in the City of New York and a member of the Board of Directors, New York Health and Hospitals Corporation. Dr. Christmas served as principal health advisor to the Carter transition team and was in contention for a cabinet level appointment as Secretary of the Department of Health, Education and Welfare.

George I. Lythcott, M.D., formerly Vice Chancellor for Health at the University of Wisconsin, is the highest level Black in the Federal Health establishment. Dr. Lythcott whose personal fame is derived from activities in international health, now manages the Health Services Administration with a budget in excess of a half billion dollars.

The sphere of influence in public health planning and policy by Black physicians in elective or appointive positions is not to be taken lightly. The late Arthur C. Logan, M.D., a renowned supporter of the Civil Rights Movement and a "mover and shaker" in New York City served on the Board of Directors of the New York City Health and Hospitals Corporation from its inception in 1971 until his death in 1974. Dr. Logan was an advocate for the hopes and aspirations of Black physicians and patients in the New York City health care systems. Vernal G. Cave, M.D., the first Black board-certified dermatologist and syphologist in the State of New York, headed the Division of Venereal Diseases of the New York City Health Department for more than 20 years and currently serves on the Board of Directors of the New York City Health and Hospitals Corporation. Julius W. Hill, M.D., a prominent Los Angeles orthopaedist, is a Director of the Los Angeles County Hospitals Authority. Paul B. Cornely, M.D., a well-known health consultant and former head of the United Mine Workers Health Services, was the first Black President of the American Public Health Association.

Black physicians have a presence in high level positions within key health and health-related organizations. Jean Spurlock, M.D., is Executive Director of the American Psychiatric Association. Effie O. Ellis, M.D., formerly Special Assistant to the Director of the American Medical Association, is now a consultant to that organization. William E. Matory, M.D., is a governor of the American College of Surgeons. LaSalle D. Lefall, M.D., Chairman and Professor of Surgery at the Howard University College of Medicine, a renowned oncologist, is President of the American Cancer Society. Charles S. Ireland, M.D., is Director of Howard University Hospital (formerly Freedman's Hospital). William O. Mays, M.D., is Chairman of the Board of Directors of Michigan HMO Plans, a prepaid health services organization. Dr. Mays is also a member of the Democratic National Committee and an advisor to Mayor Coleman Young of Detroit.

Charles D. Watts, M.D., is Vice President and Medical Director of the North Carolina Mutual Life Insurance Company, the nation's largest Black business. W. Montague Cobb, M.D., Ph.D., D.Sc., Professor Emeritus of Anatomy at Howard University College of Medicine, past president of the National Medical Association, Inc., and Editor Emeritus of the *Journal of the National Medical Association,* has been at the forefront of the national efforts to assure that Blacks have equal access to health care and the professional career opportunities within the health fields. Dr. Cobb is the current President of the National Association for the Advancement of Colored People (NAACP).

The rewards of medical practice generally afford most physicians with an array of opportunities for meaningful participation in the nation's economic life. The result of this particular situation is Black physicians who are bank directors, corporate directors, radio and TV station owners, medical facilities directors and owners, shopping center and real estate development owners, professional sports team owners, private foundation directors, and participants in all other spheres of national life where entrepreneurial and investment opportunities are found.

Corporate or industrial medicine is a new career area in which Blacks have made modest gains. Charles C. Bookert, M.D., Past President of the National Medical Association, is on the staff of Westinghouse Corporation in Pittsburgh, Pennsylvania. Bezelle Thomas, M.D., is the Medical Director for IBM operations in the Washington, D.C. area. Robert Rhodes, M.D., is the Associate Medical Director for General Motors' Hydramatic Division in Ypsilanti, Michigan. W. Alexander Miles, M.D., is a consultant in radiology to several New York based corporations.

The aforementioned examples of Black physicians in varied roles and the diversity of these roles might cause one to hypothesize that the highest level of personal and professional preparation will readily result in an onslaught of career opportunities with unlimited diversity. However, to understand the modern day successes of Black physicians and view them in their proper perspective, one must be cognizant of the struggle of Blacks as related to careers in medicine. Black physicians continue to be an integral part of the longstanding minority struggle for full participation in the American mainstream. The Black M.D.'s economic base often conveys the aura of success and no major problems, while in reality equal access to each and every facet of the medical profession may elude him/her because of medical practice restrictions and the subtleties of racism in American medical institutions.

As a general observation, a very substantial number of Black physicians are neither board-certified nor board-eligible in any medical specialty; consequently, they are not accorded full hospital privileges and are often limited to practicing medicine in their offices or in other ambulatory care settings.

At the beginning of this century, there were eight (8) Black medical schools and more than thirty Black hospitals. Adverse financial circumstances and the Flexner Report of 1910 eliminated all but two of the medical schools, Howard University College of Medicine and Meharry Medical College, and continuous financial problems and hospital integration eliminated more than three-quarters of the Black hospitals. One should not overlook the fact that the Black medical schools and the Black hospitals provided the base from which a substantial number of Black physicians acquired their education and training, thereby enabling them to address the health needs of the Black community.

The first half of this century was characterized by a segregated health care system which exists in part today. The NAACP conjointly with the National Medical Association and the National Urban League have done much to change this situation and are largely responsible for the access to health services which minorities enjoy today. Over the past decade, much time and effort have been focused on increasing the number of minority physicians from those segments of the national populace which have traditionally been underrepresented within the medical profession, i.e., Blacks, Hispanics, Native Americans, and women. The steady flow of Federal dollars which began in 1968 resulted in an array of other groups becoming actively involved with minority health professions development. Among these groups were the Association of American Medical Colleges, the National Urban Coalition, the American Foundation for Negro Affairs (AFNA), Delta Sigma Theta Sorority, the National Council of Negro Women, and the National Scholarship Service and Fund for Negro Students.

The strategic role of Black physicians in this process is often overlooked as the accolades are being distributed to those responsible for the progress to date. Prior to the efforts of private foundations and the federal government in minority recruitment and retention which began in the late sixties, the National Medical Association's Council on Talent Recruitment and the National Medical Fellowships, Inc. were the principal organizations engaged in this endeavor.

AAMC data for the years 1975-1979 reveal a declining medical school enrollment by minorities at a time when the overall enrollment is still rising. This situation has far-reaching implications and points to a major role for each minority physician, that being the identification, motivation, and development of at least one additional minority physician. The individual minority physician's involvement in things other than medical care must always be respected as a personal right. However, the social responsibility for assuring accessible, available, and continuous quality health care to one's fellow humans must always be of paramount importance among minority physicians and should undergird their individual career choices. Health needs in minority communities are greatest and resources therein are always limited. All things being considered, perhaps the most important role for minority physicians now and in the foreseeable future is the provision of high quality health services directed toward the population from whence they come and advocacy for health service programs which address the divergent needs of all Americans.

CHAPTER 3

The Role of the Association of American Medical Colleges in Minorities in Medicine: A National Perspective

Dario O. Prieto

ASSOCIATION OF AMERICAN MEDICAL COLLEGES

Organization

Founded in 1876, the Association of American Medical Colleges (AAMC) is an educational entity which has as its purpose the advancement of medical education and a working relationship with all other programs that are important to the nation's health. Its membership includes all of the U.S. and Canadian medical schools and over 400 of the country's major teaching hospitals, as well as 60 major academic and professional societies with over 100,000 members. In addition, its governing body includes an Executive Committee and Council, a Council of Deans, a Council of Teaching Hospitals, a Council of Academic Societies and an Organization of Student Representatives.

Dario O. Prieto is Director, Office of Minority Affairs, Association of American Medical Colleges, Washington, D.C.

Programs

As an educational association representative of members having similar purposes, the primary role of the AAMC is to assist those members by providing services at the national level which will facilitate the accomplishment of their mission. Such activities may include collecting data and conducting studies on issues of major concern, evaluating the quality of educational programs through the accreditation process, providing consultation and technical assistance to institutions as needs are identified, synthesizing the opinions of an informed membership for consideration at the national level, and improving communication among those concerned with medical education and the nation's health. Other activities of the Association reflect the expressed concerns and priorities of the officers and governing bodies.[1]

In addition to major issues concerning the academic medical center, biomedical research, health services, financing of medical schools, educational activities and specifically students' issues as they affect racial minorities in medical education are of great concern to the AAMC.

EARLY EFFORTS

The fact is well known that prior to 1968 medicine and the other health professions were viewed by many as an opportunity to be pursued only by upper and middle-class males. More specifically, women and those from ethnic minority and disadvantaged backgrounds were outside the mainstream of medical education.

Professional education before 1968 had not assumed the goal of providing equal opportunity to heterogeneous groups to assure that the racial and ethnic makeup of the classroom would more accurately reflect the demographic character of the U.S. population.[2]

In April 1968, the assassination of the great civil rights leader,

---

[1] *Issues, Policies, Programs of the Association of American Medical Colleges.* Washington, D.C.: Association of American Medical Colleges, 1974.

[2] Prieto, D. O.: Minorities in Medical Schools, 1968-78. *J. Med. Educ.* 53:694-695, 1978.

Dr. Martin Luther King, Jr., proved to be the spur for partially galvanizing administrators and faculty of medical schools to greater action in the recruitment and admittance of minorities.

At the same time that the Josiah Macy, Jr. Foundation was pioneering in efforts to improve Blacks' preparation for medical school admission through the establishment of the Post-Baccalaureate Premedical Fellowship Program under the leadership of Dr. William E. Cadbury, the AAMC at its Annual Meeting in 1966 presented a report entitled "Minorities, Manpower, and Medicine".[3] This was the first time that the serious problems caused by the underrepresentation of minorities in medicine had been posed publicly by a major national education association. This report, as well as the conferences sponsored by the Macy Foundation revolving around the "Negroes for Medicine"[4] study, helped bring to the attention of the movers and shakers in medicine the need to increase the number of Blacks and other minorities in medical education and to find ways to increase the number of qualified applicants in the pool.

Based on the Hutchins report[3] and the societal mood of the time, the Executive Council of the AAMC began to encourage positive action on the part of the medical schools to increase opportunities for minorities to pursue a medical career.

In 1969, the AAMC co-sponsored a series of Macy conferences. The first, held in Atlanta, brought together presidents of traditionally Black colleges and representatives from medical education and centered on "Preparation for Medical Education in the Traditionally Negro College: Recruitment-Guidance-Curriculum".[5] The second, held in Ft. Lauderdale, dealt with "Liberal Arts Education and Admission to Medical School". The purpose of the second conference was to bring together premedical advisors from undergraduate colleges in the deep South and medical school admissions officers to discuss ways in which the number of medical school minority applicants and enrollees could be increased.

---

[3] Hutchins, E. B., Reitman, J. B., and Klaub, D.: Minorities, Manpower, and Medicine. *J. Med. Educ.*, 42:809-821, 1967.

[4] Cogan, L.: *Negroes for Medicine: Report of a Macy Conference.* Baltimore, Maryland: Johns Hopkins Press, 1968.

[5] Josiah Macy, Jr. Foundation: *Preparation for Medical Education in the Traditionally Negro College: Recruitment, Guidance, Curriculum–Addresses Presented at a Macy Conference.*

GROUP ON STUDENT AFFAIRS

The part of the Association of American Medical Colleges which has most direct involvement with students and which has been in the forefront of the Association's efforts to increase opportunities for minorities in medicine, is the Group on Student Affairs (GSA). Membership in the GSA is made up of Deans of Students, Admissions Directors, Financial Aid Officers, Officers of Minority Affairs, and other members of medical school administrative staffs who have special responsibility for students.

The GSA is divided into four regions: Northeast, Central, Southeast, and Western. Each region holds an annual meeting, attended not only by GSA members but in many cases by premedical advisors and representatives of foundations. Much like the early Macy conferences and the Medical Education Reinforcement and Enrichment Program (MedREP) conferences originated by Dr. Anna Epps at Tulane Medical School, they provide an excellent opportunity for the development and exchange of ideas related to minority affairs issues and programs at U.S. medical schools.

At the AAMC Annual Meeting in 1968, the Group on Student Affairs of the Association presented a report addressing the need for massive scholarships for minority students heading for a career in medicine as well as the need for the AAMC to examine the former Medical College Admission Test (MCAT) as a selection device in admissions.

GSA-Committee on the Medical Education of Minority Group Students

In addition, in 1968 the Group on Student Affairs established a Committee on the Medical Education of Minority Group Students. This Committee served a crucial pioneering function in ensuring that minorities had a voice in medical education and provided a channel whereby these issues could be brought to the attention of the Association. Those who have served as Chairman of this Committee are Drs. Roy Jarecky, Associate Dean for Administration, University of Kentucky College of Medicine; Paul Elliott, Associate Vice President and Director, Division of Academic Support Systems, Florida State University; John Watson, Associate

Dean for Admissions, University of California, San Francisco, School of Medicine; John Wellington, Associate Dean for Clinical Affairs, University of Hawaii John A. Burns School of Medicine; and Walter Leavell, Vice Dean, University of Cincinnati College of Medicine.

AAMC'S SPONSORSHIP OF MINORITY PROGRAMS TO ASSIST MEDICAL SCHOOLS' RECRUITMENT

Office of Economic Opportunity

The AAMC's interest and attention to the issues of minorities in medicine were heightened in 1969 when the Association obtained grants from the U.S. Office of Economic Opportunity (OEO) for the establishment of an Office of Minority Affairs within the organization. Funds from this grant also permitted the AAMC to support and administer a number of programs designed to correct the underrepresentation of minorities in medicine and other health professional schools.

In the interest of testing a variety of approaches to providing the best possible method to increase the minority applicant pool and to increase the enrollment and retention of students from these groups, the AAMC through the OEO grant supported 58 projects at various institutions across the country. Although the majority of the programs were conceived and funded at medical schools, programs were also sponsored for other health professions institutions, non-profit organizations, university consortia, and community organizations. Target population groups included Black Americans, Mexican Americans, American Indians, Mainland Puerto Ricans, and disadvantaged Caucasians.

A total of $1.5 million was funded by OEO and administered by the AAMC between 1969 and 1973. Site visits were undertaken in 1970 and continued throughout the time AAMC provided support for these projects. Evaluations of the projects' progress and information on programs that appeared to be meeting their objectives later provided valuable suggestions to other schools, which became interested in setting up similar programs in a nationwide effort to increase their numbers of underrepresented minorities. Some of these programs were described in an AAMC publication entitled "33 Programs to Increase Educational Opportunity for Minorities in the Health Professions".[6]

AAMC's interest, support, and leadership provided to the medical schools during the pioneering days when the predominantly White medical schools began their drive to attract minorities appear to have had a great positive impact. As a result of these efforts, those of philanthropic organizations, and federal support, minority enrollments increased rapidly. By 1974-75 the representation of minorities had risen to 10 percent of the total entering class as opposed to little more than 2 percent before 1968-69, when most of these students were enrolled at Howard and Meharry.

A second major impact of AAMC's influence as a result of these efforts is reflected in the fact that by 1975-76 many medical schools had developed programs to recruit and retain minorities. Even after funds became scarce, most of these programs were continued.

Thirdly, between 1970 and the present, after the AAMC adopted a policy statement on minorities in medicine, a great number of the medical schools instituted admissions programs which provided alternate selection processes in efforts to admit more minority students to vary the class composition. This development later led to a series of concerns confronting medical schools with litigation which threatened the progress of their affirmative action programs.

In 1969 the OEO grant, in addition to assisting the AAMC in establishing the Office of Minority Affairs, afforded the basis for current minority programs. These include a clearinghouse operation which provides information to premedical advisors and counselors at undergraduate colleges, organizations and agencies, as well as to minority students wishing to learn about opportunities to pursue medical careers.

Minority Student Opportunities in United States Medical Schools

The first issue of the publication, *Minority Student Opportunities in United States Medical Schools (MSOUSMS),*[7] was initially sponsored

---

[6] Manly, H. F.: *33 Programs to Increase Educational Opportunity for Minorities in the Health Professions.* Washington, D.C.: Association of American Medical Colleges, 1971.

[7] Johnson, D. G. (ed.): *Minority Student Opportunities in United States Medical Schools, 1969-1970.* Evanston, Illinois: Association of American Medical Colleges, 1969.

by the AAMC in 1969 and underwritten by the OEO grant. Since its first publication, a new edition of *MSOUSMS* is published every other year. This communication provided the minority student with up-to-date information and descriptions of programs at U.S. medical schools which were designed to provide opportunities for racial groups underrepresented in medical education. The narrative descriptions of *MSOUSMS,* usually pronounced "mouse mouse", cover five topic areas: recruitment, admissions, academic aid programs, student financial assistance. In addition, other pertinent information includes statistical data depicting minority student enrollments, the number of applicants, and the number of students accepted by each medical school.

The usefulness of *MSOUSMS* has been demonstrated over the years to both the minority applicants and to the professionals who advise them. In particular, it is of prime importance to the minority students because it provides them with a reasonable assessment and comparison of the many programs available. This information offers the applicant yet another tool with which to make decisions concerning the schools to which he or she should apply.

Medical Minority Applicant Registry

Along the same line, as with the initiation of *MSOUSMS,* the Medical Minority Applicant Registry (Med-MAR) was introduced as an additional tool to assist minorities interested in pursuing a medical career. A program of the AAMC, Med-MAR was created to identify minority group applicants. The purpose is to identify the minority students in the applicant pool and to provide admissions officers at all U.S. medical schools with the biographical data and MCAT scores of these students.

Students have been able to voluntarily participate in Med-MAR by identifying themselves as belonging to a minority group on a questionnaire completed at the time they take the Medical College Admission Test (MCAT). This registry identifies approximately 3,000 minority students every year and is circulated to medical schools twice a year after each MCAT administration. Medical schools interested in assuring themselves of a substantial number of minority applicants usually correspond directly with the students and request more detailed application material from them. This service is without cost to minority applicants participating in Med-MAR.

Medical School Admission Requirements

Medical School Admission Requirements is another AAMC publication which offers pertinent information to all students. Revised annually, this publication contains the most current information on premedical preparation and admission to medical school. As a source of information, it helps students aspiring to a medical career to approach their goals realistically and provides the premedical advisor with a most practical source for giving students sound advice. It devotes one whole chapter to information of special interest for minority students. Reprints of this chapter are available at no cost to all students upon request from the Office of Minority Affairs.

In 1970, the AAMC was assuming a leading role as a major national association in efforts to provide more access to the medical profession to groups who were underrepresented and who had been traditionally excluded from participation in medical education. Two events contributing to minorities in medicine which took place as a result of AAMC's role in minorities in medicine and as an educational association were: (1) the establishment of a task force to investigate the underrepresentation of minorities in medicine and to formulate recommendations and ways to alleviate the situation and (2) the adoption of the AAMC Statement on Medical Education of Minority Group Students.

AAMC 1970 Minority Task Force Report

The 1970 "AAMC Task Force Report to the Inter-Association Committee on Expanding Educational Opportunities in Medicine for Blacks and Other Minority Students", chaired by Dr. Bernard W. Nelson and funded by the Alfred P. Sloan Foundation, was endorsed by the AAMC, the American Medical Association, the American Hospital Association, and the National Medical Association. In its landmark report, the task force recommended as a short-term goal that "U.S. medical schools increase the representation of minorities in the M.D. degree programs from 2.8 percent in 1970-71 to 12 percent in 1975-76."[8] In 1970 data for minority matriculants were available only for those who identified themselves as Black. If other underrepresented minorities such as American Indian, Mexican American, and Mainland Puerto Rican had been taken into account, a more comprehensive goal would probably have been set at a total minority representation of 17 percent by 1975-76. Nonetheless, this report spurred a vigorous and intensive nationwide effort by the medical schools to attract and recruit minority students to their medical education programs.

Recognizing the importance of financial assistance in the efforts to increase opportunities for minorities in medicine, the Task Force Report included a recommendation that "a single national organization, such as the National Medical Fellowships (NMF) perhaps augmented by a standing committee composed of representatives of concerned public and private institutions, be responsible for coordination, solicitation, and distribution of financial aid to minority students." Aided by this official recognition of its importance, NMF was able in the next few years to obtain the funds needed to provide large-scale assistance to students from racial ethnic minorities underrepresented in medical education.

AAMC Statement on the Medical Education of Minority Group Students

The Group on Student Affairs (GSA), consisting as it does of those individuals most directly involved with students, was the first entity within the AAMC to express an active concern for increase in opportunities for minorities in medicine. Aided by its own GSA Committee on the Medical Education of Minority Group Students, a statement on the medical education of minority group students was prepared, approved by the GSA, and presented to the AAMC Executive Council for approval at the 1970 Annual Meeting of the Association.

---

[8] Nelson, B. W. (Chairman): *Report of the Association of American Medical Colleges Task Force to the Inter-Association Committee on Expanding Educational Opportunities in Medicine for Blacks and Other Minority Students.* Washington, D.C.: Association of American Medical Colleges, 1970.

The Statement on the Medical Education of Minority Group Students was adopted as an official AAMC Policy Statement on December 6, 1970 by the Executive Council of the Association of American Medical Colleges. This statement was a significant public commitment on the part of the AAMC and its governing constituent, and it is proper to insert it here because it represents an endorsement by the deans of all U.S. medical schools:

> The AAMC and its constituent members are directing earnest attention and effort toward the goal of increasing minority opportunities in medical service, teaching, and research. A detailed description of these goals is contained in the "Report of the AAMC Task Force to the Inter-Association Committee on Expanding Educational Opportunities in Medicine for Blacks and Other Minority Students" that was approved by the AAMC Executive Council on May 7, 1970.
>
> Medical schools, working with cooperating preprofessional colleges, are urged to help increase minority student awareness of the opportunities for professional education and the specific preparation necessary for medical school. Minority students, thus motivated, prepared, and recruited, should be provided encouragement to complete their course of study.
>
> In order to provide the most conducive educational milieu, medical schools are urged to identify a faculty member or administrator who can be specifically charged with responsibility for minority student affairs. This individual should work closely with the AAMC Group on Student Affairs (GSA) and should represent the medical school in GSA minority affairs activities. An individual from a minority group may be particularly effective in this position.
>
> In developing new and modifying existing educational programs, medical school faculties should be aware that minority students, while not always as well prepared in the traditional sciences basic to medicine, bring to the profession special talents and views which are unique and needed. Educational programming for all medical students should be sufficiently flexible to allow individual rates of progress and individualized special instruction. With such programming, the opportunity for minority student success will be maximized.
>
> The AAMC-AMA Liaison Committee on Medical Education is strongly encouraged to review critically the degree of individual

opportunity provided in medical school curricula. The Liaison Committee is also urged to include in its membership (and on its accreditation teams where possible) individuals with special knowledge and experience in the education of minority group students.

Financial assistance for minority students must be maximized and medical schools are urged to pursue actively the expansion of minority student support funds at the local, state, and federal levels. The Association is making known to the American public and to the Federal Government these needs for increased financial aid for minority students.[9]

AAMC-SNMA Study

In 1971, the AAMC, in conjunction with the Student National Medical Association (SNMA), formulated and sponsored the first indepth study to examine the characteristics of the successful and unsuccessful minority applicants to U.S. medical schools. The three-year study utilized AAMC data for the years 1970-71 through 1972-73 and made comparisons with the assumptions, conclusions, and predictions of the 1970 AAMC Task Force Report.

In general the AAMC-SNMA study documented the progress and efforts made by medical schools in compensating for the dire underrepresentation of minorities in their student bodies in the past and stated that: "It is essential that the medical schools reaffirm their commitment to minority peoples, perhaps through a renewed affirmative action goal which goes even further than that of the original Task Force. Such a goal should not only reflect the 12 percent Black American population but also the approximately 6 percent American Indian, Mexican American, and Mainland Puerto Rican population."[10]

By the time of this report, the Association had already implemented several of the items recommended by the 1970 Task Force, including the establishment of the Office of Minority

---

[9] Groo, V. E. (ed.): *Medical School Admission Requirements*, 29th ed., Washington, D.C.: Association of American Medical Colleges, 1978, p. 47.

[10] Johnson, D. G., Smith, V. C., and Tarnoff, S. L.: Recruitment and Progress of Minority Medical School Entrants 1970-72. *J. Med. Educ.*, 50:713-755, 1975.

Affairs, which has provided various services. The implementation of other new projects designed to help medical schools admit and successfully educate more students from racial minority groups also took place.

AAMC Survey

In 1972, 91 M.D.-degree-granting schools responded to an AAMC Survey which focused on the minority affairs needs of U.S. medical schools. The analysis of this survey gave the Office of Minority Affairs the impetus to develop a proposal for regional workshops for the purpose of assisting medical schools to strengthen their minority programs specifically as they related to admissions policies, procedures, and problems inhibiting the recruitment, selection, and retention of minority students.

Simulated Minority Admissions Exercise

In May 1973, the AAMC sought and secured support from the Grant Foundation to sponsor such workshops. The workshops were designed to focus on topic areas such as recruitment, admissions, and retention. Experts introduced and led the discussions on successful methods and models in each area.

An example of a successful program which evolved from these workshops and which is currently in demand is the *Simulated Minority Admissions Exercise (SMAE)*.[11] Introduced initially to involve admissions committee members in highlighting positive minority-oriented variables through a live practical experience, it later evolved as a tool to demonstrate how such variables could be utilized by simulating the role of admissions officers.

The *SMAE* demonstrates how educational techniques, such as simulation, active individual involvement, peer teaching, group discussion, and decision-making processes can be applied to the somewhat perplexing area of minority admissions. The developers of the *SMAE* are student-personnel-oriented medical educators

---

[11] Prieto, D., et al.: *Simulated Minority Admissions Exercise*. Washington, D.C.: Association of American Medical Colleges, 1978.

who, like most admissions officers, are struggling to find new and perhaps more appropriate approaches to minority admissions. The *SMAE* is intended to provide learning experiences as bases for attitudinal change in managing the admissions enterprise.

The *SMAE* simulates 10 minority applicants, only six of whom can be admitted to medical school. The participants work in groups of five or six members, functioning as admissions committees in a specified medical or health professional school setting. The purpose of the *SMAE* is to demonstrate how certain critical noncognitive data might be identified in application material and then further elicited from a personal interview with the applicant. This encourages the admissions process to respond to current societal demands for a wider sociocultural mix of health care providers. The central objective of the *SMAE* is to help medical schools select potentially successful minority applicants and to improve their retention by ensuring that they enter medical school under positive circumstances with improved chances of success.[12]

Through this technique of the *SMAE,* admissions committees can enhance the successful prediction of minority student performance by weighing certain noncognitive information or variables such as positive self-concept, realistic self-appraisal, understanding racism, preference of long-range goals to short-term, availability of strong support person or persons, successful leadership experience, demonstrated community service, demonstrated medical interest as well as other academic variables.[13]

It is the belief of the authors of the *SMAE* and of legal-minded individuals that this process provides medical school admissions committees with a legal rationale for broadening and making their admissions criteria more flexible to accommodate the variety of students, to provide more classroom diversity, and to train physicians to serve the nation's heterogeneous population. Since its development, the SMAE has been used successfully with over 27 medical school admissions committees in addition to other groups such as premedical advisors and other health professional schools. Normally, the participants from medical schools include admissions officers, medical school faculty, deans, department chairper-

---

[12] Prieto, ibid.

[13] Sedlacek, W. E. and Brooks, G. C., Jr. *Racism in American Education: A Model for Change.* Chicago: Nelson-Hall, 1976.

sons, minority affairs officers, premedical advisors, and medical students. The *SMAE* has a built-in evaluation of the responses from the various participants to constantly monitor the value of the exercise. Thus far, over 900 individuals have participated, and all evaluation responses have produced extremely high ratings for this technique.

Loan and Scholarship Program for Minorities

To supplement other sources of financial aid, the Association, at the request of the Robert Wood Johnson Foundation, began in 1972 the administration of a $10 million student aid program. Under this program, the country's American Indian, Black American, Mexican American, and U.S. Mainland Puerto Rican medical students became eligible for scholarship and loan awards from the nation's 108 participating medical schools and seven schools of osteopathy. Other eligibles for these funds included women and students from rural backgrounds. In announcing the grant, Dr. David E. Rogers, president of the foundation, cited as one of the reasons for choosing the focus on these groups "evidence indicating that student physicians with such background characteristics are the most likely to choose practice locations in underserved areas upon completion of their professional training." The only stipulation to the schools was that the grants be restricted to the categories of students covered by the program and that the funds be expended within a 4-year period, which started with the 1972-73 fiscal year. The program was extended in 1976-77 for one more year with an additional grant of $2.5 million.

ADMISSIONS

National statistics suggest that by 1973, medical schools' efforts to increase the numbers of minority group students were initially quite successful. In the years from 1968-69 to 1973-74, the number of underrepresented minorities in the freshman class rose from 292 (2.9 percent of the entering class) to 1,301 (9.2 percent of the entering class).[14] Unfortunately, it was during this period in the

---

[14] Groo, V. E. *Medical School Admission Requirements, 1978-79,* 28th ed., Washington, D.C.: Association of American Medical Colleges, 1977.

history of medical education that legal issues surfaced and began to pose a threat to the continued progress and existence of the affirmative action programs heretofore developed by the country's medical schools.

The first case attracting national attention as regards the legality of the affirmative action or special admissions programs for minorities was the law school case which reached the Supreme Court of the State of Washington in 1973, better known as the *DeFunis* case. The University of Washington's minority admissions program was declared constitutional, and in August 1974, when the case was appealed to the U.S. Supreme Court, the court chose not to make a decision by declaring the case moot. The nondecision in the *DeFunis* case left medical school admissions committees without guidance in the troubled area of special programs.

Three months later, on November 25, 1974, a similar case based on the same argument came up in California in *Bakke vs. Regents of the University of California*. An important difference between this case and the *DeFunis* case was that this one involved a medical school applicant (to University of California, Davis). This case contributed further to the degree of uncertainty which was already facing medical schools in regard to the future of affirmative admissions programs.

In mid-1978, the U.S. Supreme Court rendered its decision in the *Bakke* case, thereby partially removing the cloud of uncertainty in special admissions programs. However, the decision by the U.S. Supreme Court was split and left both sides of the argument claiming victory. In general, on the one hand the Supreme Court ruled that a quota system was a specific instance of reverse discrimination, and on the other it ruled that certain types of affirmative action programs employed by medical schools were constitutional and that the use of race as a factor used to fulfill certain state compelling interests was legal.

AAMC's Amicus Curiae Briefs

During this period of legal confrontations by the medical schools, the AAMC took a strong position in favor of special admissions programs for minorities. In both the *DeFunis* case and the *Bakke* case, the AAMC submitted "amicus curiae" briefs at the state and U.S. Supreme Court levels in support of affirmative action. The underlying theme of the AAMC's briefs was "that the purpose of medical schools—to educate qualified individuals who will best serve the country's compelling need for medically trained professionals—will be significantly advanced by special admissions programs for minorities."[15]

Total enrollments of underrepresented racial minority groups peaked in 1974-75 when they reached 10 percent of the entering class. However, a decline to 9.1 percent in 1975-76 became of major concern to the Association and to some of its affiliates.

GSA-Minority Affairs Section

The AAMC Committee on the Medical Education of Minority Group Students under the chairmanship of Dr. Walter Leavell was one of the groups which became concerned with these enrollment trends. In addition, the Committee expressed a strong desire to have more interaction with other committees and groups within the Association. In efforts to become more involved and to provide more input to the AAMC on issues of significant concern to minorities, the Committee in 1975 presented a position paper to the Association recommending the organization of a new group on minority concerns.

In November 1976, in response to a recommendation by the AAMC Committee on Governance and Structure, the AAMC Executive Council approved the Minority Affairs Section (MAS) of the Group on Student Affairs. The formation of this new group on minority concerns eliminated the Committee on Medical Education of Minority Group Students, and a new administrative committee to represent this Section came into being as the Group on Student Affairs-Minority Affairs Section (GSA-MAS) Coordinating Committee.

The Minority Affairs Section (MAS) provides the opportunity for greater participation in AAMC activities by minority affairs directors and individuals concerned with minority student affairs from the country's medical schools. This is made possible by

---

[15] Association of American Medical Colleges. (In the Supreme Court of the United States.) The Regents of the University of California, Petitioner versus Allan Bakke, Respondent. Brief of the Association of American Medical Colleges, Amicus Curiae. Washington, D.C.: Association of American Medical Colleges, 1976.

ensuring that all MAS members become members of the Group on Student Affairs. Each medical school appoints a representative to the new Minority Affairs Section, which has as its purpose five major objectives as follows: (1) to serve in a recognized advisory and resource capacity to all elements of the AAMC on issues of minority concern; (2) to provide a means by which minority constituent views on matters of interest to the Association may find expression; (3) to provide input into AAMC statements, papers or reports which present themselves as the minority viewpoint; (4) to assist and facilitate in the development and implementation of methodologies that will enhance the recruitment, enrollment, retention, and postgraduate education of minority medical students; and (5) to provide a means for the interchange of ideas and perceptions among minority educators and administrators and others concerned with medical education through approved AAMC channels.

The Minority Affairs Section, modeled after the GSA, selected national and regional officers in 1976 and held its first annual plenary session in that year.

Medical College Admission Test

In April 1977, the AAMC introduced the New Medical College Admission Test (MCAT) to replace the former version. Its development took advantage of all available approaches for assuring that performance on the test depended on the variables to be measured and not on incidental differences in culture or race. These approaches took cognizance of the findings from the related literature and were especially sensitive to problems in test areas commonly questioned. In addition, the AAMC took steps to ensure appropriate involvement of minority educators and professionals in various committees associated with the development of the New MCAT.

The New MCAT makes an effort to eliminate cultural biases inherent in the old MCAT. Another facet of the New MCAT which was expected to aid minority students was the reduced emphasis on "speed" as an important factor by allowing students more time to complete the examination items.

A third innovation presented by the New MCAT recognized as a potential benefit to minority students is the separation of the former MCAT science section into separate areas of biology, chemistry, and physics tests. This allows advisors, counselors, and admissions committees to assess students' strengths and weaknesses in a particular area and to recommend a plan for students to improve their skills accordingly. Whether the New MCAT will indeed be an important factor in expanding the number of suitable minority applicants remains to be seen at this point. Studies to establish findings of this sort will require much time.[16] The chapter by Paul Elliott elsewhere in this book provides more detailed information on the New MCAT.

AAMC 1978 MINORITY TASK FORCE

Growing concern on the part of the AAMC in regard to the rising cost of medical education and a declining trend in minority admissions (two major issues affecting both majority and minority students) led to the establishment of two major task forces in February 1976.

The AAMC Task Force on Student Financing grew out of the alarming situation that escalating costs of medical education would limit the opportunity to study medicine to only the more financially capable. In addition, as stated by this Task Force Report:

> More recently, public policy has reflected a shift in national priorities from expanding the number of health professionals to remedying their geographic and specialty maldistribution. Consequently, the nature of Federal financial assistance has shifted largely to scholarships which require a service commitment and loans which may be forgiven in part for practice in primary care. The most recent health manpower legislation embodies these concepts in its two major programs related to student financing, the National Health Service Corps and the Health Education Assistance Loans. This trend has had a major and often disturbing impact on students whose personal career goals are not compatible with the constraints imposed by Federal financial assistance but who, in the face of rising costs and diminishing

---

[16] Prieto, D. O.: The Expansion of Opportunities in the United States for Minorities to Become Physicians. Unpublished manuscript, Washington, D.C., 1978.

private resources, are otherwise unable to finance a medical education.[17]

Declining financial aid and grant support both from the federal government and philanthropic organizations to fund special programs to motivate, recruit, and graduate minority students in the health professions became a critical issue with the Association. The AAMC feared that the declining trend of these activities would inevitably lead to reduction in the size of the minority applicant pool and that the final result would be a reduced number of minority admissions and a consequent lower number of trained minority physicians.[18]

These were the second and combined set of issues which led to the establishment by the AAMC of the 1978 Task Force on Minority Student Opportunities in Medicine.

Both the Task Force on Student Financing and the 1978 Task Force on Minority Student Opportunities in Medicine Reports concluded with significant findings and made major recommendations to U.S. medical schools, to federal, state, and local governments, and to the private philanthropic sector on how best to assist in the alleviation of the problems currently facing minorities in medical education.

AAMC'S CONTINUED INVOLVEMENT IN MINORITIES IN MEDICINE AND THE FUTURE OUTLOOK

In the years 1968-69 to 1974-75, the number of underrepresented minorities (Black American, Mexican American, American Indian, Mainland Puerto Rican) rose in first-year classes from 292 to 1,473. However, despite the efforts of the medical schools and the encouraging early statistics, it has become evident that major problems in recruitment and retention of minority students have

---

[17] Nelson, B. W. (Chairman): *Report of the Association of American Medical Colleges Task Force on Student Financing.* Washington, D.C.: Association of American Medical Colleges, 1978.

[18] Elliott, P. R. (Chairman): *Report of the Association of American Medical Colleges Task Force on Minority Student Opportunities in Medicine.* Washington, D.C.: Association of American Medical Colleges, 1978.

developed and are persisting.[19] By 1976-77, a declining trend in first-year admissions of minority students became evident when the number dropped from 1,473 in the previous year to 1,400. A more alarming factor may be that there has been no substantial increase in the minority applicant pool since 1973, when it leveled off at slightly over 3,000 per year.

AAMC statistics for 1978-79 indicate that first-year minority enrollments have suffered yet another decline to 1,446 (8.7 percent) from 1,450 (8.9 percent) for the previous year. Furthermore, no indication of an increase in the size of minority applicant pools can be foreseen in the near future.

The AAMC has attributed a number of barriers to the declining trend in minority medical schools enrollments over recent years. Among these are the lack of financial aid to medical students, especially in light of rising tuition costs, legal issues, premedical advising and counseling, retention, and academic adjustment of minority students. Most recently, the shift in federal programs from awarding loans and scholarships on a financial need basis to awarding them to any student regardless of financial status will have an adverse effect on minorities and other economically disadvantaged students because a large percentage of these students tend to come from low-income families.

For these reasons, the AAMC has consistently taken strong positions in support of affirmative action programs, not only in filing amicus curiae briefs on their behalf but also in supporting legislation favorable to these programs and in seeking higher appropriations for existing programs such as the Health Career Opportunity Program provided for in Public Law 94-484.

In anticipation of the effect that the shift in federal programs would have on minorities and other low-income individuals, the AAMC worked vigorously in an effort to change the regulations of the legislation affecting scholarships for First Year Students of Exceptional Financial Need. Recognizing also that the minority applicant pool requires a dramatic increase, the AAMC supported legislation designed to establish special health education programs in biomedical sciences for minorities at the high school level which was designated Public Law 95-561.

---

[19] Association of American Medical Colleges: *Medical Education: Institutions, Characteristics, and Programs—A Background Paper*. Washington, D.C.: Association of American Medical Colleges, 1977.

The Association of American Medical Colleges will strengthen and will continue its firm commitment to minorities in medicine and to affirmative programs. As new health manpower legislation evolves, the AAMC will support those items which are of concern to minorities as well as all other legislation promising to affect minorities in medicine in an affirmative manner.

Finally, as the goals and recommendations of its Task Force on Minority Student Opportunities in Medicine will be reviewed biennially, the efforts and commitment of the AAMC and its member schools in this area will be more visible and measurable. "This commitment to affirmative action programs for the recruitment, admission, and retention of minority students must become a part of each institution's continuing philosophy and objectives."[20]

---

[20] Elliott, P. R. (Chairman): *Report of the Association of American Medical Colleges Task Force on Minority Student Opportunities in Medicine.*

Undergraduate Advising, Summer Programs, and Study and Test-Taking Skills

CHAPTER 4

The Organization and Function of a Pre-Health Professions Office in an Undergraduate School

JW Carmichael

Most colleges and universities in the United States now have pre-health advisors to provide assistance to students in the time-consuming and competitive task of preparing for and gaining admission into health professional school. Such individuals are generally very concerned that those students who gain acceptance into professional school possess the intellectual ability to understand the scientific principles upon which modern medicine is based, the physical ability to master the needed technical skills, the motivation to complete the grueling period of training, and the interpersonal skills needed to contribute when placed in the nation's health care delivery system. However, most premedical programs focus narrowly on these goals and fail to perform to their fullest potential. This lack of breadth works to the detriment of that portion of the American populace who have traditionally been excluded from the mainstream of the nation's development.

JW Carmichael, Ph.D., is Professor of Chemistry and Pre-Health Advisor, Xavier University of Louisiana, New Orleans, Louisiana.

This chapter attempts to provide insight into pre-professional education in a manner designed to be of assistance when organizing pre-health professional programs which will be of benefit to minority or disadvantaged students. It is based largely upon my experiences as pre-health advisor at a small historically Black institution, Xavier University of Louisiana, which placed fifty-five students into health professional schools in 1977-78. Although "pre-health" is used in this context to mean the pre-professional education of students interested in medicine, osteopathic medicine, dentistry, veterinary medicine, optometry, podiatry, and pharmacy, most examples were chosen from medicine as a representative health profession.

RATIONALE FOR OPERATION OF
A PRE-HEALTH PROGRAM

All pre-health advisors are acutely aware that approximately two-thirds of the applicants to medical school are rejected each year, that many of those who are not accepted have all of the qualifications needed to become good physicians, and that the competition for admission into other health professional schools is also very stiff. Therefore, all pre-health programs are organized so as to eliminate those pre-health students who lack the ability, motivation, or personal characteristics desired in the competent health professional. Unfortunately, however, personnel in many pre-health offices allow the need to eliminate the unqualified to obscure the equally important need to train qualified applicants who will work to ensure that *all* Americans receive adequate health care. In so doing, they fail to accept the responsibility of providing access to health careers for those individuals, minority or disadvantaged students, who are most likely to have experienced directly the consequences of inequitable health care and, consequently, are more likely to be willing to work to remove them. It is, therefore, proposed that a pre-health program should be organized so as *both* to eliminate the unqualified students *and* to encourage qualified minority and disadvantaged students. A rationale for the organization of such a program includes:

—The *first* prerequisite for a successful pre-health program is an advisor (or advisors) whose *primary* commitment is to the pre-health student.

—Although it may be possible to determine the general features of a good pre-health program (as is attempted in this chapter), specific details must be tailored to fit the institution in which the program is located.

—Pre-health advising is a continuous process beginning with recruitment into undergraduate school, continuing with retention, and ultimately culminating (from the point of view of the advisor) with placement in professional school.

—The pre-health advisor must establish close working relationships with the students to be served, undergraduate faculty (especially in biology and chemistry), and representatives from professional schools.

—Premedical programs, regardless of their structure, are often under suspicion by faculty in a liberal arts college because they are "pre-professional" and by faculty in the sciences especially because they remove students who might otherwise pursue graduate degrees. The successful advisor must strive continuously to dispel these doubts if a successful program is to be established.

—In spite of the popular misconception, students are human too. The successful premedical program must, therefore, place the human element foremost by considering qualified students *as individuals*.

The remainder of this chapter is organized around and reflects a belief in this rationale. Specific examples from my home institution are intended merely to illustrate ways of implementing a general idea and should certainly not be considered the only method of doing so.

Recruiting students into the undergraduate institution, counseling the premedical student, guiding academic preparation, and assisting in gaining admission are clearly interrelated stages of a continuous process. However, it is easier to discuss the features of a successful pre-health program if they are treated as separate components. Therefore, this separation is effected in the following discussion.

RECRUITING THE PRE-HEALTH STUDENT

Very few pre-health advisors are actively involved in recruitment into pre-health programs. They perceive (correctly) that there is an overabundance of applicants to health professional schools, they have insufficient time to accomplish all that needs to be done, and justifiably they are concerned that students who lack the motivation to choose a health profession without recruitment may not have the perseverance to complete professional training. Although reasonable as far as it goes, this approach is unacceptable because it fails to recognize the pre-health advisor's responsibility to increase the number of applicants who, after professional school, are likely to provide health care to minority and disadvantaged populaces. Specifically, it does not recognize that minority and disadvantaged students are less likely than majority students to be aware of the opportunities in the health professions or to consider the possibility of personally striving to become a health professional. Thus, whereas recruitment may not be necessary for majority students from conventional backgrounds, it is very important for minority and disadvantaged students if they are to have reasonable access to health careers.

A good recruitment program should not be limited to college students already interested in the sciences, but should also focus on those with demonstrated potential in other college majors, as well as students at the pre-college level. Examples of activities which have proven to be effective at Xavier include: (a) the publicized willingness of the pre-health advisor to visit local high schools to discuss career opportunities in the health sciences, (b) development of a special "CheMagic Show" which can be taken to science classes at local high schools as a means of stimulating interest in careers in science, (c) development of a Science Rally which provides the opportunity for high school students to visit the University's science departments and obtain first-hand some perspective of career opportunities, (d) development of special summer programs to stimulate interest in natural and health sciences and to provide the academic reinforcement needed to be competitive, (e) publication of a weekly Pre-Health Newsletter for circulation on Xavier's campus (500 copies/issue on a campus of 1600), and extensive publicity for speakers from professional schools, acceptances into professional school, etc. Such activities have resulted in a 100% increase in the number of minority pre-health students at Xavier in the past four years. There are now more than 400 in the pre-health programs.

COUNSELING THE PRE-HEALTH STUDENT

In the present context, "counseling" is intended to include those activities which keep pre-health students informed of extracurricular activities of interest, provide opportunities for them to gain a perspective of the various health professions, and develop or maintain motivation for a career in a health profession. Curricular counseling is discussed in the following section.

It is important that all applicants to professional school be aware of the scope and magnitude of their endeavor, the relationship of their intended career to that of others in the total health care system, what they can expect from life as a professional in their chosen area, etc., and all pre-health programs attempt to provide this information. However, many fail to realize that minority and disadvantaged students are unlikely to have had prior exposure to a variety of professionals, often have no one in their family or circle of friends to whom they can direct specific questions, and must put much more effort into obtaining this information than does the traditional pre-health student. Some pre-health programs therefore fail to develop an organizational structure for counseling which is adequate for the nontraditional student. A program which attempts to correct this inequity must, at the very least, do the following:

—Establish contact with the pre-health student as soon as possible, preferably before arrival on campus.
—Provide informative and/or motivational materials on a regular, continuing basis to pre-health students as a group.
—Provide the opportunity for interaction on an individual basis as an integral part of the program.
—Contain a formalized, systematic method of obtaining input from pre-health students.

Each of these is discussed in more detail in the following portions of this section.

The transition from high school to college is likely to be more traumatic for a student unfamiliar with the mainstream of American life than for one from a more traditional background. Therefore, it is extremely important that the pre-health advisor establish contact with minority and disadvantaged students as early as possible if many are to have an equitable opportunity to perform in a manner which would indicate that they should be encouraged to remain in the program. At Xavier, a workable procedure for accomplishing early contact is begun in January of each year when the University's Admissions Office begins to publish lists of students accepted for the following fall. Those students who have indicated an interest in a pre-health field receive a letter of congratulations from the pre-health advisor, information about the spectrum of pre-health programs at the University, and an open invitation to communicate if they have questions or problems. Second contact is made via a short presentation to all entering students at Freshman Orientation. This presentation emphasizes the opportunities available, outlines the general requirements for admission to health professional schools, and specifies the location of the Pre-Health Office. At this time also, "interest" cards, which ask for the student's name and local address, are distributed and collected.

During the first week of the semester, all who completed the cards collected at the initial session are contacted by mail and invited to drop by the Pre-Health Office to pick up a free copy of Xavier's own Pre-Health Handbook. The latter was prepared by members of Xavier's chapter of Alpha Epsilon Delta (the National Premedical Honor Society) and is organized around a series of questions pertinent to the freshman pre-health student. Its practical, student-oriented approach to pre-health is an excellent general orientation to Xavier's program. The mailing and subsequent visits to the Pre-Health Office to obtain the Handbook provide a way of checking the accuracy of the names and addresses, get the entering pre-health students into the Office before they become involved in too many other campus activities, and establish a good basis for future visits and communication.

Early initial contact must be coordinated with and lead into continuing contact in a systematic fashion if a pre-health program is to serve all students effectively. At Xavier, contact with the entire pool of pre-health students is accomplished primarily through the publication of a weekly two-page Pre-Health Newsletter which is distributed widely on campus, and through a series of well-publicized meetings at which pre-health students may discuss specific areas of concern, meet guest speakers from professional schools, plan future activities, etc. Contact with subgroups is maintained by direct mailings from the list of pre-health students obtained by cumulative collection of the interest cards. For example, a scheduled visit by a representative from the University of Alabama School of Dentistry would not only be publicized by distribution of posters in areas on campus where pre-health students are likely to congregate, but also by a direct mailing to all students who have indicated an interest in dentistry or who had listed Alabama as their state of residence.

Group or subgroup contact as described above provides a gross structure for effective counseling of pre-health students. However, these activities must be integrated with ample interaction with students on an individual basis if a pre-health program is to operate properly. Individual interaction is, of course, especially important to the minority or disadvantaged student who may have no one else to whom he or she can turn to discuss what a particular career choice may mean in one's personal life, the pros and cons of one profession as compared to another, realistic discussion of the rigors of professional school, etc. In such interaction, a good pre-health advisor must be willing and able to recognize students who lack the academic ability, the motivation, or the personal traits to become a health professional and must be willing to "bite the bullet" and tell the students so before they waste too much time pursuing unrealistic goals. However, at the same time, the good pre-health advisor must also be willing and able to distinguish characteristics which merely reflect differences in cultural background or economic status from those which would limit the ability of the individual to provide competent health care. The critical factor for the pre-health advisor who has had little exposure to minority or disadvantaged students is the willingness to admit that the general perceptions by which one judges traditional pre-health students may not be adequate when encountering nontraditional ones. For example, it is my observation that students who have suffered earlier educational handicaps, which is often the case with Xavier students, are *most likely* to have the ability to complete professional school successfully than are students who *appear* to be about equally competent, but who have not had those handicaps. At the same time, however, the educationally handicapped student is *less likely* to have the self-confidence to actually pursue a career in the health professions. This would suggest that pre-health advisors who wish to serve minority or disadvantaged students should place more emphasis on efforts to retain the qualified students than on efforts to eliminate those who are unqualified.

Finally, although often overlooked or underrated, a successful pre-health program must include a systematic, formal mechanism for obtaining input from students from a variety of majors, levels of development, backgrounds, potential areas of interest, etc. At Xavier, this input is secured via two structures. The first is our chapter of Alpha Epsilon Delta, the National Premedical Honor Society. This group consists of junior and senior pre-health students with high academic averages. The chapter is an excellent asset to the pre-health program because its members developed the Handbook which is distributed to all entering freshmen (as mentioned previously), host a number of speakers on campus, conduct yearly recognition ceremonies for outstanding pre-health freshmen and science faculty, systematically attempt to acquaint all students with the scope of the health professions, publish a weekly Pre-Health Newsletter, etc. The second component from which the Pre-Health Office at Xavier receives student input is the Student Pre-Health Advisory Committee (SPAC) which consists of five students chosen from a number of levels of development and representing various academic majors. This Committee is an integral component of the pre-health program and was designed purposely to provide a broader spectrum of student input than is possible from the highly selective honor society. Generally, the SPAC serves to coordinate the activities of the various groups from which pre-health students are drawn, of which Alpha Epsilon Delta is one.

ACADEMIC PREPARATION FOR HEALTH PROFESSIONAL SCHOOL

In today's world, the competent health professional must know an awesome volume of scientific facts, principles, and theories, as well as how and when to apply them. Because the scientific rigor of professional school is well known, most individuals seeking admission into professional school not only complete the minimum science requirements for admission, but also choose to major in some biological or chemical science in undergraduate school. Many people decry this fact and suggest that more matriculants into health professional schools from humanities and social science majors would provide a humanizing influence on the health care delivery system. There is no reason why a student cannot choose as major any subject offered, but whatever the major, the number of science courses taken and the student's performance in them must be adequate to indicate that the student can meet the demands of medical school.

Most pre-health advisors have a genuine concern that applicants to professional school be academically prepared when taking the examinations for admission (such as the Medical College Admission Test, MCAT) and that, if accepted, they successfully complete the rigorous professional school curriculum. However, many advisors do not recognize the role that they should play in such preparation and thus fail to provide the guidance needed by those students who do not come from backgrounds in which one learns to be aware of and operate within the unwritten rules of the system. Some general guidelines for establishing a pre-health program which does provide this assistance are itemized below and then followed by more detailed discussion of each point.

—The pre-health advisor must maintain good relations with other departments, especially biology and chemistry.
—The pre-health advisor must have a definite mechanism for providing advice, official or otherwise, concerning academic offerings.
—It is essential to remember that staying in professional school is as important as getting in *and* to plan academic preparation accordingly.

At most institutions, there is no "pre-health major" separate from traditional academic departments. In my opinion, this is to the benefit of the students because those who complete traditional degree programs have wider career options than those who are in programs aimed solely at professional school. Further, such an arrangement is probably good for the health care delivery system since it provides students who have a broader perspective on life than would be likely in programs which are strictly pre-professional in nature. However, attempting to provide adequate advising in the area of academic preparation for health professional school to students with official academic advisors in some other unit of an institution can be a very frustrating experience. The best solution appears to be for the pre-health advisor to establish and maintain good working relations with all of the departments, especially those in which pre-health students are likely to be seeking a major: biology and chemistry. This not only makes it possible to gain assistance in distributing information to students, but also provides a mechanism for gaining input from academic departments in planning pre-health activities, for representing (occasionally, don't push your luck) the pre-health perspective when departments are planning curriculum changes, and for publicizing career options. Establishing and maintaining these relations is undoubtedly the most difficult task for the pre-health advisor. A pre-health advisor who is not from either biology or chemistry has little chance of gaining good rapport with the departments or exerting influence on them, whereas one who is from one of the two departments is likely to function poorly because of an inability to clearly distinguish between duty to the pre-health program versus that to the department. I believe that this, more than any other aspect of a successful pre-health program, must be developed with the individual institution in mind. At Xavier, a viable program has been developed by appointing a pre-health advisor who is a member of one of the departments (Chemistry) *but* who clearly recognizes the necessity for representing pre-health (rather than Chemistry). Official input from the various academic departments at the University and assistance in coordinating activities originated by the Pre-Health Office with those from departments is provided by a Faculty Pre-Health Advisory Committee composed of faculty from the departments most directly concerned with pre-health.

The mechanisms by which colleges and universities provide academic advising vary widely. In most schools it is unlikely that the pre-health office has full control over the courses in which students enroll. However, it is important that the advisor have input when pre-health students consider what courses to take, when they should be taken, what electives to choose, what to do if they have a low grade in a major course in midsemester, how to space academic requirements so as to demonstrate ability without becoming over-extended, how to adjust course loads for non-academic commitments, etc. In addition, pre-health advisors who attempt to serve minority or disadvantaged students should be aware of and be able to provide advice concerning the various summer programs which offer academic and/or motivational reinforcement.

The Pre-Health Office increases its chance of adequately providing this assistance without generating undue friction if it provides information both to official academic advisors and to pre-health students simultaneously. Items of a general nature can easily be distributed both to official advisors via the contacts in departments recommended above and to pre-health students through the communication mechanisms discussed when considering counseling. Problems of an individual nature will likely require that the pre-health advisor interact directly both with the student and with his or her academic advisor if they are to be solved in a reasonable fashion. Whatever the specific mechanism by which this is accomplished, it is important for the pre-health advisor to treat each case individually and to realize that advice given a low-income nontraditional student might differ from that given an upper-income traditional one. For example, while it is important that pre-health students be exposed to actual working conditions in the health care system and most pre-health advisors would unhesitatingly advise traditional students to undertake volunteer work in a hospital or clinic while taking a full academic load, it would be unreasonable to make the same suggestion to a low-income student who must work twenty hours per week merely to live and attend school. At Xavier, the task of keeping academic advisors and pre-health students aware of both the general guidelines and the specific details of academic preparation for health professional school is an unending series of memos, telephone calls, publications, etc.

Many pre-health programs focus on ensuring that students who apply to health professional school have the minimum science requirements, that they complete them in time to take the admissions exams for professional school, and leave all other choice of academic preparation to the student or the academic advisor. To students with system-savvy this is not detrimental because they recognize the importance of taking related courses which will assist them after admission. However, those with less sophistication often fail to realize that getting into professional school is only half the problem and that the years as a pre-health student should also be used to gain the academic depth needed to maximize the chances of staying in professional school. A good pre-health program should analyze the strengths of the departments on its campus, the expectations of the professional schools to which most pre-health students apply, and the attrition rate of students who have attended such schools in the past so as to know what advanced courses are likely to be most useful *and* should take every opportunity to emphasize their importance.

PLACEMENT IN HEALTH PROFESSIONAL SCHOOL

Placement in a health professional school is the obvious culmination of the process of providing an advising program for pre-health students. Further, in a day when the application process is long and tedious and more applicants are rejected than are accepted, the pre-health advisor can provide valuable assistance to those students who are applying for admission. Five general types of activities in which the pre-health advisor should be involved as a means of facilitating admission of qualified applicants are itemized below and then discussed briefly in the following paragraphs. A good pre-health advisor should assist students applying to professional school by:

—Maintaining good contact with health professional schools.
—Maintaining good contact with other health professional advisors.
—Supplying timely information about the application process to potential applicants.
—Providing support services to applicants.
—Keeping the personal element in the forefront—always.

Very few pre-health advisors have actually attended a health professional school. It is , therefore, extremely easy for advisors to have misconceptions about the application procedure, the selection process, the level of difficulty of professional school, what the professional schools *really* expect (as opposed to what they say they expect), etc. The most effective way of remedying this situation is (a) to recognize that faculty and administrators at professional schools are basically honest, hard-working individuals who have an extremely difficult task to perform and (b) to establish regular contact with a number of individuals from these institutions in order to obtain more detailed information. At Xavier, it has been possible to identify at least one individual from each of the local health professional schools who attends a general planning meeting on campus once per semester and provides assistance as needed during the interim. The general meetings are usually three to four hours in length, are arranged around a definite agenda of topics pertinent to pre-health at Xavier and/or developments at the local institutions, are attended by both faculty and students from Xavier, and are scheduled so as to best fit the convenience of the representatives from professional schools. This contact has been a major factor in the development of Xavier's pre-health program.

A pre-health advisor can also benefit greatly from establishing contacts with counterparts at other institutions, particularly when encountering new or especially difficult problems. One mechanism for meeting individuals with whom such relationships can be established and for keeping abreast of general developments in pre-health education is to join one of the four regional Associations of Advisors for the Health Professions (current information about each may be obtained from the Association of American Medical Colleges). These organizations also publish newsletters, conduct workshops, etc. which are of particular value to the inexperienced pre-health advisor.

Application to most professional schools must be made nine months to a year in advance of the expected date of enrollment. It is, therefore, of critical importance that pre-health students know when to take the admissions exams, when to begin the application process, how many schools to which they should apply, the schools at which they have the best chance of gaining acceptance, etc. The pre-health advisor can assist greatly by widely publicizing pertinent deadlines and making specific suggestions based on past experience and a review of the student's academic record, recommendations, career goals, state of residency, etc. The primary sources of information for this purpose are the publications available from the national offices of the various health professional schools such as the Association of American Medical Colleges (AAMC), the American Association of Colleges of Osteopathic Medicine (AACOM), the American Association of Dental Schools (AADS), etc.

The application procedures for most health professional schools are both time-consuming and tedious. A pre-health office can assist by providing secretarial help for typing, practical advice about what is important to report in "non-academic" portions of the application forms, constantly stressing the importance of meeting deadlines, collecting and transmitting recommendations, and answering an almost infinite array of other practical questions which arise.

Finally, it should be reiterated that *all* activities within a pre-health program should be conducted within a framework which recognizes that each student is an individual and deserves to be treated as such.

SUMMARY

Pre-health advisors at the nation's colleges and universities should encourage toward health careers students who are not only qualified but who will *also* contribute to the equitable delivery of health care in the United States. In attempting to do so, the advisors must recognize that minority and disadvantaged students are more likely to have experienced these inequities and, consequently, are more likely to be willing to work to remove them. At the same time, the pre-health advisor must recognize that minority and disadvantaged students are also more likely to be needlessly eliminated from a pre-health program because of differences in cultural background, economic status, or degree of sophistication. Pre-health advisors should therefore seek to identify and retain those elements of pre-health programs which are *essential* for maintaining quality while implementing other activities specifically designed to encourage minority and disadvantaged students to pursue careers in the health professions. In so doing, pre-health programs will come to embody *quality with equity*.

CHAPTER 5

Premedical Advising:
Principles and Practice

Walter F. Leavell

THE ADVISING SYSTEM

The art of advising is an ancient craft, the practice and principles of which have changed little since Polonius gave his classical advice to his son to "neither a lender nor a borrower be." Although Polonius' advice would seem timeless, we instantly recognize its impracticality in today's world. For to follow this sage advice would exclude most minority students from a medical education, since rapidly increasing medical school expenses mandate extensive borrowing. However, this example does serve to point out some of the pitfalls of advising. An endeavor will be made in this chapter to examine the philosophy, principles, and practices of advising as it pertains to advising minority students at all levels who are interested in pursuing a career in medicine.

From a philosophical perspective, in a model advising system the advisor would have extensive if not comprehensive knowledge in the areas of responsibility for student advising and would enjoy the

Walter F. Leavell, M.D., is Associate Professor of Medicine and Vice Dean, College of Medicine, University of Cincinnati, Cincinnati, Ohio, and Chairman, Minority Affairs Section, Group on Student Affairs, Association of American Medical Colleges, Washington, D.C.

complete confidence of the advisee. The advice would be offered in a timely, concise, clearly understood manner and its merit would be immediately apparent. The advisor would enjoy the assurance that recommendations were faithfully executed and would receive reasonably quick feedback regarding the effectiveness of the advice. On the other hand, the advisee should have immediate access to the advisor at all times to consult on current and future plans, as well as to review the progress made to date. (Ideally, the advisor would serve as a role model and inspire the advisees to achieve their goals.) Implicit in this relationship is mutual respect, cooperation, trust, and credibility.

The schools should provide the fiscal resources for advising as well as the necessary time for accomplishing the set goals and objectives. There should be rewards and incentives to the advisor for maintaining and updating a data base as well as recognition in the professional promotional process in the advisor's primary field. As will be pointed out subsequently, it is a rare situation in which an advisor has advising as a primary function rather than as an add-on responsibility.

In discussing medical education we frequently refer to "The Advising System". However, nomenclature is often deceiving or misleading and in this instance the reference to an advising system is a misnomer, for the word system denotes a defined procedure or method. We are therefore lulled by this descriptive term since it infers an ordered process that students may interface with at some initial point in their educational lives and receive advice and assistance until such time as their educational goals are achieved.

In the United States our educational system is multilayered beginning with the primary grades through secondary school and subsequently college. Since we live in a mobile society, individuals may receive various phases of their education in a variety of institutional and geographical settings. The 1970 AAMC Task Force[1] recommended that a network of regional centers be established to provide factual and personal information about career opportunities in medicine for minority students. Experience has demonstrated the potential difficulty in establishing regional cen-

---

[1] *Report of the AAMC Task Force to the Interassociation Committee on Expanding Educational Opportunities in Medicine for Blacks and Other Minority Students.* Washington, D.C.: Association of American Medical Colleges, April 1970.

ters which would relate both to the minority community and the medical schools of a region. For some professional endeavors a lack of early student contact and continuity of advice presents relatively few problems for the student since subsequent stages of education are not heavily predicated on the preceding stages. For the minority student interested in medicine this clearly is not the case, for the basic education which is a prerequisite for the study of medicine should begin minimally at the high school level. The minority student who enters college without having taken a course in high school biology, chemistry, or physics is academically behind his peer group on the first day of class in these comparable subjects at college irrespective of the level of the individual's intellectual ability. Herein lies the dilemma of the minority student which necessitates costly and after-the-fact educational reinforcement programs at the medical school level to bridge the educational deficits.

Even to the uninitiated it is readily apparent that the successful pursuit of a medical career requires long-range goals and objectives. However, it is difficult for students to aspire to a goal or an objective which they have little information about or contact with individuals in that profession. Sedlacek and Brooks[2] note that in the absence of available role models and due to the fact that the reinforcement system has been relatively random for them, minority students may have difficulty perceiving the relationship between current work and the ultimate practice of their profession. The format of the standardized test such as the SAT and MCAT continues to perpetuate the assumption that each student who takes such an exam has had similar educational exposure and opportunities and that therefore the test results are interpreted as measuring educational ability in absolute rather than relative terms.

Even the student who is fortunate enough to identify a sympathetic and helpful advisor in grade school will likely have to begin the process anew upon entering high school and again on entering college with the loss of the benefit of continuity of program planning and goal setting. Often the advice received at subsequent levels in the educational process is contradictory, as

[2] Sedlacek, W. E., Brooks, G. C., Jr.: *Racism in American Education: A Model for Change.* Chicago: Nelson-Hall, 1976.

evidenced by the recent experience of the parents of twins who were attending a highly competitive liberal arts college and subsequently discovered that the siblings, although sharing the same career objectives and having nearly identical past educational experiences, were receiving contradictory advice from different counselors at the college which in one instance was even contradictory to departmental recommendations in the course area.

While there is a general acknowledgement of this problem, each educational level perceives it as the responsibility of the next level; subsequently it is the minority student who suffers the consequences.

Another example of the fragmentation of the advising system exists throughout the United States where there is a medical school on the same campus with the undergraduate college with premedical emphasis. Frequently, there is no formal relationship or tie between the medical college and its admissions committee and the undergraduate premedical committee. In many instances the communication is informal and consists of the chairman of the medical school admissions committee speaking on an annual basis to the student premedical society. The members of the premedical committee may not have had an opportunity to attend a meeting of the medical school admissions committee, and therefore are likely to have limited insight into its structure and operation. The medical school admissions committee likewise may have little insight into the process that evolves into the recommendations which the admissions committee receives from undergraduate campuses. As frequently as not, medical schools receive letters of recommendations from undergraduate programs that are not very helpful. However, since this is a relatively sensitive issue, rarely is this information provided as feedback to the submitting institution even when it is a local one. Similarly, when an admissions committee has difficulty in interpreting a rating system, the undergraduate school does not receive adequate feedback and therefore continues to use the same system year after year to the relative disadvantage of its students. Therefore, better lines of communication must be established between the undergraduate campus and the medical school.

Many premedical committees evaluate the potential of students for medical school solely on their academic standing. This practice is particularly harmful to minority students and other disadvantaged students, since the medical school admissions committee already has at its disposal the student's academic record and can make their own judgment regarding it. Most medical school admissions committees believe that the noncognitive aspects of an applicant's background are equally important and if this is not taken into account in the premedical evaluation, it is the opinion of many medical educators that the applicant has been done a serious disservice. This is particularly true if the medical school admissions committee is not aware that the overall premedical rating is made on the basis of academic performance alone.

THE RESPONSIBILITY FOR ADVISING THE STUDENT

Ideally one would make contact with students prior to their entering high school since request for mathematics and science courses for the first year of high school is made at the eighth grade level. In addition, the basic educational tools which the student will need to pursue any area of scientific endeavor must also be acquired prior to high school entry. It has been pointed out that people who major in science in college made the decision to do so in primary or secondary school.[3] Grade schools and high schools must offer general education and given the realities of the fiscal problems confronting most school boards cannot provide career tracks or training programs for each profession. However, each school system has the obligation and responsibility to prepare its students to pursue any career they desire and are capable of mastering. Citizens can influence their portion of the educational system through their interaction and participation with PTA's and boards of education, as well as through the political process. In some communities magnet schools may be the answer. However, it must be assumed that it is the responsibility of all those who are interested in increasing the number of minority physicians to provide grade school and high school advisors and students with more information about the profession of medicine. The only exposure students have should not be a one-shot career night at the

---

[3] Shelling, W., and Boruch, R.: *Science in Liberal Arts Colleges.* New York: Columbia University Press, 1972.

close of the senior year of high school. Minority medical students and minority physicians in the community can serve an important function as role models and should be requested to participate in student advising. Without much difficulty medical schools could sponsor science fairs and provide weekend and summer programs which permit interested students to gain experience and insight into the profession of medicine.

On the basis of a study of the City University of New York (CUNY), Marshall[4] concludes that, "attempts to increase minority representation in the medical profession should take the direction of direct intervention at the high schools by both colleges and medical schools." He goes on to say that there is an obvious need for improved secondary education.

The message is a clear one and indicates that each educational level must play an active role and not settle into complacency by blaming the previous level for not adequately preparing the student, while simultaneously lobbying and working for upgrading all aspects of the educational process.

IDENTIFYING THE ADVISOR

Although most advisors are dedicated and are sincerely interested in the students who seek their advice, this frequently is not the criterion which leads to the selection of advisors. Often this responsibility is passed on to the least senior faculty member as an add-on assigned task. The advisor may have no formal training in counseling and have little insight into the professional area about which expert counsel is needed. Not surprisingly then, information provided to students is often outdated, irrelevant, and in some instances, actually harmful.

The neophyte advisors are often at a point in their career where they must maintain their teaching and research activities at a high level if they are to gain tenure, since it is well known that there is relatively little recognition in the academic process for excellence in advising.

Schools at each level of the educational system rarely have

---

[4] Marshall, C. L.: Minority Students for Medicine and the Hazards of High School. *J. Med. Educ.*, 48:134-140, 1973.

full-time career advisors and often this responsibility is a shared committee endeavor. The advantages of having a full-time professional advisor/counselor in a college of arts and sciences was pointed out by Lipman in a letter to the editor of the Journal of Medical Education.[5] It was noted that the impact on the undergraduate campus was almost immediate when a full-time advisor/counselor was established as an administrative position and all of the premedical advisory operation was placed in one office. Fortunately for students, even when the process of selecting the advisor is not a well-planned event, many advisors rise to the occasion and become knowledgeable in most facets of their advising role. There should be professional recognition, incentives and academic reward built into the advising system.

DEFINING THE ROLE OF THE ADVISOR

The task of defining the role of the advisor appears simple at first. However, it becomes less obvious when examined more closely. Often when premedical advisors on a large undergraduate campus are asked to identify or make available information pertaining to minority students who have a potential interest in medical education, the response is "This is not my role." Premedical advisors often perceive their role not as career counselor or recruiter but rather as resource persons for students who have already decided to go into medicine. While this attitude is understandable, since the advisor may be responsible for advising in a variety of areas other than medicine, it often places minority students at a serious disadvantage since they may not have achieved that level of self-confidence to declare their interest in medicine, particularly during the first undergraduate year when they may be counseled by well-meaning individuals that their aspiration cannot be transformed into a reality. Another problem faced by the minority student is that many advisors also perceive their role as being limited to answering questions posed to them. However, for the unsophisticated student the major problem may be that of knowing what questions to ask. A lack of previous information such as may be gained by access to fraternity files may preclude an

---

[5] Lipman, Z. B.: Premedical Advising. *J. Med. Educ.*, 53:787-788, 1978.

awareness of the information frequently available to majority premedical students. It is readily apparent that one cannot ask sophisticated questions about oncology or forensic pathology if one is not aware of even the existence of these professional entities as potential career pathways.

The advisor should be aware of the following:

1. The existence of precollege preparatory programs for minority students.

2. Summer educational enrichment programs which selected students may participate in during the summer while they are undergraduate students.

3. Postbaccalaureate programs and other less formal arrangements for minority students who decide late or otherwise do not have the necessary premedical courses.

4. The S.M.A.E. (Simulated Minority Admissions Exercises).[6] A realistic simulation exercise in which premedical advisors can participate to gain firsthand knowledge and insight into the practical aspects of medical school admission processes, particularly as they relate to minority students.

5. The AAMC Medical Minority Applicant Registry (Med-Mar)* which provides the opportunity for any medical school minority applicant to have basic biographical information sent to the admissions offices of all U.S. medical schools.

THE PREMEDICAL COMMITTEE

The Premed Committee serves as a gatekeeper and in some instances the committee's role is almost exclusively an evaluative one. Student contact is limited to perhaps a one time encounter for the interview which may be probing and in depth. The student academic record is then reviewed and an assessment of motivation is attempted. Subsequently a letter of recommendation is composed and forwarded to the medical schools designated by the applicant or to AMCAS.

---

[6] D'Costa, A., Baghook, P., Elliott, P., Jarecky, R., Leavell, W., Prieto, D., and Sedlacek, W. E.: *Simulated Minority Admissions Exercises Workbook.* Washington, D.C.: Association of American Medical Colleges, 1975.

* Minority students register by self-identification at time the MCAT is taken.

Many premedical committees see their students who request letters of recommendation as falling into one of four groups. The first group consists of those who are fairly well known to them from previous contacts during their undergraduate years. The second group consists of students they felt they were familiar with through casual and intermittent contacts with their office. The third group they may have some superficial knowledge of but have not had any significant direct contact. Then there would be a final group of whom they had no prior knowledge at all so that they must write their letters of recommendation based almost exclusively on the one interview session. The more sophisticated student with regard to the admissions process is likely to be in the first group, establishing an early relationship with the premedical committee. These students are also generally at the epicenter of the university student life. They are likely to be members of the Student Premedical Society which maintains sophisticated files on medical schools and the admissions process and also maintain a close working relationship with premedical committees.

In some instances the premedical society has been given almost exclusive control over volunteer appointments for premedical students by local hospital's volunteer staff since hospital volunteer offices find it more convenient to deal with one individual or organization rather than a large number of individual students. Therefore when the medical admissions committee reviews the minority students' hospital experience it may be lacking not from a lack of interest but rather from a lack of availability.

The minority students, for many complex social economic reasons such as the necessity to work extensively and participation in their own culturally related activities, are more than likely to fall into the final group of students who are unfamiliar to the premedical committee. They therefore tend to receive information late or not at all which in some instances results in a delayed application. They have often previously received insufficient counseling and have arranged their curriculum in inappropriate ways, carrying the wrong sequence of courses or a disproportionate credit hour load. They may approach the MCAT examination without formal preparation while increasing evidence indicates that many students who now sit for the MCAT have taken a formal preparatory course.

In many instances the minority students' inadequate precollege educational background places them in a position of continually having to review and reinforce information that the majority students have as a base, and therefore preplanning may be a luxury since the student is constantly confronted with day-to-day academic survival.

The student is often conditioned by previous bad experiences at the undergraduate institution and may approach the AMCAS application with uncertainty. They are not sure, for example, what the implications are in filling out the extracurricular experience section. They may wonder in listing all their extracurricular activities whether they will be perceived as less than serious students interested in outside affairs rather than academic pursuits, while parenthetically the medical school admissions committee views this as a very desirable noncognitive pursuit. Likewise, minority students are concerned about stating the number of hours worked while in school, often believing that this will highlight their need for financial assistance, perhaps making them a less attractive applicant. This information, however, provides the medical school admissions committee and also the premedical committee with valuable information in accounting for the circumstances under which a student's grades were obtained. For example, a 4.0 average may be discounted significantly if the applicant took a very light course load, did not work, and engaged in relatively few extracurricular activities. On the other hand, a student with a 3.0 average who worked 20 to 30 hours a week and participated in numerous extracurricular activities may be valued more highly on a relative rating scale.

Undergraduate schools are cognizant of and are often asked about the number of students who apply to medical schools who are accepted (acceptance ratio). This ratio may be used inappropriately as a selector indicator by applicants seeking an undergraduate college to attend. This practice lends itself to discouraging applicants who do not have a very high academic average and therefore are viewed as not likely to be accepted by a medical school, thereby adversely affecting the ratio. Unfortunately, minority candidates are sometimes advised on this basis in order to protect the acceptance ratio. Frequently a premedical committee will give a low rating based exculsively on cognitive factors. However, medical school admissions committees take a more comprehensive view of the student's overall application and are helped appreciably by letters of evaluation which state the circumstances under which the student's grades were obtained and an estimate of the potential that the student is perceived to have, based on both the cognitive and noncognitive performance of the student. In some instances this comprehensive evaluative approach utilized by medical school admissions committees may be a mystery to the premedical committee and the acceptance profile of minority students may be almost totally unknown. Many minority students, feeling that they have received relatively little support from their undergraduate institutions, may check the block on the AMCAS application indicating they *do not* wish to have information sent back to their undergraduate school. Thus, a valuable feedback process is closed off to the premedical committee. Many err in assuming that a given minority student was not accepted who may in fact have received several acceptances.

Recommendations:

1. The premedical committee and premedical advisor should make a concerted effort to make entering students aware of the committee's existence, role, and function.
2. Students should be provided in the first week of school with an outline of general medical school requirements and appropriate course sequencing.
3. At the appropriate times, students should be given a list of the important dates such as when to apply for AMCAS application, MCAT exam, submission of letters of recommendation and requests for transcripts.
4. The student should be advised to secure a copy of the AAMC's *The New MCAT Student Manual*[7] at the time of enrollment. This would serve as a reference guide for the student, outlining course requirements. Answering the sample questions will help students to ascertain whether they are obtaining and retaining the expected information in each course.
5. The student at the beginning of the junior year should be made aware of the following publications:
   a. A Complete Preparation for the New MCAT[8]

---

[7] *The New MCAT Student Manual, New Medical College Admission Test.* Washington, D.C.: Association of American Medical Colleges, 1977.

[8] Flowers, J. L., and Wallace, W. D.: *A Complete Preparation for the New MCAT: Health Careers Summer Program.* Washington, D.C.: Howard University, 1978.

b. Medical School Admission Guide for Minority Applicants[9]
6. A formal program should be offered in the first year to assist students to develop appropriate study skills. In addition, since these students tend to perform poorly on standardized tests a formal course should be offered in the development of test taking skills. If this is not feasible the student should then be advised to consider a commercial course.

THE RESPONSIBILITY AND ROLE OF THE MEDICAL SCHOOL

Notwithstanding the responsibilities of society at large and the educational components at different educational levels, it is apparent that the medical school, by virtue of its admissions process, sets an educational standard which may influence curricular patterns at the undergraduate level. Many advisors may never have had an opportunity to attend a medical school admissions committee meeting and therefore are not readily conversant with what medical schools perceive to be important, as, for example, the relative perceived merit of letters of recommendation. Many advisors are not aware of the profile of selected minority students and therefore may be discouraging viable candidates. Medical schools could be helpful in providing advice to premedical advisors, but when discussing this aspect of their responsibility, they frequently indicate that moneys are not available for this valuable endeavor. However, if we are to be successful in increasing the number of minority physicians this is a task that the medical schools themselves must be willing to undertake, for there is no viable alternative for delegation. Many opportunities exist to participate in counseling and advising activities at relatively minimal expense to the medical school. Premedical advisors can be provided opportunities to attend admissions committee meetings; minority medical students are usually enthusiastic about working with minority students at the undergraduate and high school levels. Some medical schools through this mechanism have assisted undergraduate campuses to establish minority premedical societies and have involved themselves in other student interactions. Administrators, advisors, and faculty

---

[9] Leavell, W. F. Medical School Admission Guide for Minority Applicants. Cincinnati, 1979.

from medical schools can serve in an advisory capacity to minority student organizations at a local, state, and national level.

Many medical educators theorize that if the advisory process is successful at the preadmissions level there will be less need for many of the costly reinforcement programs currently supported by the medical schools, and these moneys can then be more appropriately channeled into providing support services at the preadmission level.

Recommendations

1. Premedical advisors should be routinely invited to medical school admissions committee meetings.
2. Undergraduate schools should be given routine feedback regarding their letters of recommendation and other pertinent information pertaining to their process.
3. Workshops including the Simulated Minority Admissions Exercise (S.M.A.E.) should be sponsored for premedical advisors by the medical schools. In addition, information pertaining to interviewing techniques as well as financial aid options should be explored.
4. Minority students at the medical school should be encouraged to work with undergraduate students and programs.
5. Medical schools should consider programs either during the summer or on weekends aimed at providing minority students in proximity to the medical school at the high school level with opportunities to work in laboratories or other types of exposures (including clinical) to the medical school environment.

Advisors should be kept aware of changing emphasis in medical education.

The library of each premedical advisor should include a copy of the AAMC publications: *Medical School Admission Requirements, Minority Students Opportunities in U.S. Medical Schools,* as well as copies of medical school bulletins from the schools to which most students from that school apply. In addition, students who are interviewed for medical school admission as well as those from the undergraduate institution represented by the premedical advisor who are currently enrolled in medical schools should be requested to fill out a questionnaire to provide up-to-date feedback.

Emphasis in the past decade has shifted from the primary focus being on an individual interested in pursuing a scientific research-oriented career to one of clinical specialization and currently to primary care as an example. Students often receive conflicting advice regarding courses such as embryology and biochemistry at the undergraduate level with the indication being that these subject areas are covered in the medical school curriculum but from a different perspective and therefore they should not be taken at the undergraduate level. However, minority students following this advice are sometimes placed at further disadvantage when they discover that in medical microanatomy courses it is assumed that the student has an understanding of embryology. When the same student enters into his freshman biochemistry class he is confronted with the fact that a significant number of his peers have had biochemistry at the undergraduate level and many in fact place out of the course through an examination process prior to enrollment. While the minority student is mastering the material for the first time it may be a review with new emphasis for many other students.

Similarly most medical school bulletins contain the list of minimal prerequisite required courses for admission and it is emphasized that it is highly desirable for students to supplement liberal arts and other educationally broadening courses to this base. While this is excellent advice for a student who has had an adequate science background at the primary and secondary level it must be viewed with caution for a student for whom this is not the case. Considering the fact that 50 percent or more of the individuals accepted to medical school have majored in a scientific area, minority students should be advised to take additional courses in the science area based on the individual's own specific background.

COUNSELING THE UNACCEPTED APPLICANT

Sixty-four percent of applicants who apply for admission to medical school are not accepted on their initial try. Of the 60 percent who reapply, approximately 40 percent are admitted into either an American or foreign medical school.[10] Although it is

---

[10] *Medical School Admission Requirements 1978-79, United States and Canada.* Washington, D.C.: Association of American Medical Colleges.

impossible to discuss the specific reasons why applicants are rejected, one can categorize the major reasons as either low demonstrated cognitive performance, either as reflected by the GPA or MCAT scores, or lack of demonstrated personal and motivational characteristics. Therefore the reapplicant must first engage in an honest self-appraisal process. It can safely be assumed that, if an applicant is invited for an interview, the cognitive values were within acceptable limits and the noncognitive assessment was relatively positive. The interviewed applicant may subsequently be rejected on the basis of not receiving a high enough interview rating, which in itself may reflect a lack of communication skills, personability, or perceived lack of adequate motivation or thoughtfulness and knowledge about a medical career.

It should be appreciated that when a student makes reapplication and the admissions committee reviews the application, little documented change usually has occurred in the records, since few additional course scores would be available. If, however, the student was rejected primarily on the basis of low MCAT scores or if the student's motivation was in question, this period of time is sufficient for corrective measures. Students should not be advised to take a full-time job in a health-related field, since this rarely adds substance to the application unless demonstrated motivation or the question of medical awareness was at issue. Similarly, students should not be advised to take one or two courses in the science areas, for even if they do very well in these courses the question of their ability to carry a full academic load usually arises. The successful reapplicant has almost always taken a significant science course load at the graduate level and done well academically. All students who have low MCAT scores and were not accepted should be advised to retake the MCAT and to give serious consideration to enrolling in a formal preparatory program. In addition, students should be advised to make an appointment to sit down and discuss their application with someone in the Student Affairs Office of the Medical School. They should be counseled not to ask the leading question "Why was I not accepted?" but should ask "What are the strengths and weaknesses of my application and what can I do to strengthen it?" While foreign medical school has been in the past a viable option for the majority student the expense of such an endeavor and also the current advisability of this alternative is seriously in question and therefore minority students should not usually be counseled in this direction.

Finally, students who enter a graduate program should be advised to pursue an area that will lead to a career alternative if they are not subsequently accepted into medical school rather than taking a graduate program solely in order to get into medical school without thought of its subsequent application.

ALTERNATIVE CAREERS

The advisor walks a tenuous line in discussing alternative career paths with individuals interested in becoming physicians. For the advisor is dealing with a group of individuals who have had medicine as a career objective for many years. Although students are advised repeatedly to participate in a broad variety of educational experiences at the undergraduate level, the majority of medical school applicants accepted into medicine have majored in a science area. Students are also aware that certain extracurricular activities are deemed important by medical schools and endeavor to engage in these activities, particularly those in health-related areas to a significant degree. Therefore, inadvertently or indirectly, we have developed a "tracking system" for medical school entrants.

Any discussion of career alternatives by an advisor may be interpreted as discouragement and the important relationship between advisor and advisee may be impaired. The advisee, particularly a minority student, may interpret the well-intended discussion as prognostic, indicating little chance of the student being accepted into medical school or, worse yet, as a discouragement. Considering the fact that a baccalaureate degree may not adequately prepare a student for a lifetime career and therefore a subsequent master's or terminal degree may be required, it is of utmost necessity to explore with the student alternative career paths.

One is occasionally surprised in exploring students' motivation for the study of medicine that, when asked their goals and objectives, they wish to become physicians because they believe that this is the only career option which can accomplish the goals they have set. An individual who may state a wish to become a psychiatrist, when made aware of the discipline of clinical psychology, may realize that this career would meet the goal equally well. However, it should be cautioned that the advisor in exploring realistic alternative careers does not steer or redirect an individual away from medicine since this should be left totally up to individuals to decide for themselves. This still does not negate the fact that all students applying or indicating an interest in medical school should be asked their objectives and what thoughts they have given to alternative careers and what their plans are should they not be accepted into medical schools. Appropriately done in a sensitive manner this will be seen by the student as a positive assistance. Some minority students are advised to seek alternative career paths because of their financial situation and are informed that the study of medicine is an unrealistic goal since it is not within their financial means. Although currently scholarships are limited and the major source of moneys for medical education is student loans with relatively high interest rates, this situation changes dramatically over a relatively short period of time. Currently there is an increase in the number of professional service types of scholarships. In addition, it is a little discussed fact that many medical schools will permit an applicant to delay matriculation for up to one year after being accepted. In this instance a student may wish to work for a year in order to earn money to defray a portion of the educational expenses.

Although most medical schools wish to see as evidence of motivation some work effort in a hospital or heath-related setting, this may be poor counseling for a minority student with minimal financial resources. Better counseling advice perhaps is for the student to take a summer job which offers maximum income potential and gain exposure to the health care field through volunteer effort if this is possible in one's spare time, since the major purpose of this effort is for the student to have a realistic perspective of what being a physician entails rather than for the experience itself. In the event the student, for financial reasons, is unable to obtain this type of experience, this should be called to the attention of the admissions committee so that it does not appear as a lack of motivation. The best advice irrespective of the minority student's financial problem is to be prepared academically and work out the financial problems as they present themselves.

In 1969 Black Americans comprised only 2.75 percent of the medical school student body, while at the same time only 2.2 percent of the practicing physicians in the United States were

Black.[11] By 1978 Blacks comprised 6.1 percent of the total medical school student body enrollment.[10] Even allowing for the fact that there is an increase in the absolute numbers, the impact on the number of practicing minority physicians has been minuscule. Statistical projections indicate that had the goal of the 1970 AAMC Task Force been realized in achieving minority enrollment at the level of 12% of the entering medical school class on a national basis it would have required minimally three decades to achieve proportional minority representation among practicing physicians.

Borrowing from a legal statement, *res ipsa loquitur,* the facts speak for themselves, it becomes increasingly clear why it is vitally necessary to develop and complement an adequate advising system.

---

[11] Curtis, J. L.: *Blacks, Medical Schools and Society.* Ann Arbor: The University of Michigan Press, 1971.

[10] *Medical School Admission Requirements 1978-79, United States and Canada.* Washington, D.C.: Association of American Medical Colleges.

CHAPTER 6

Special Undergraduate Programs
for
Minority Medical Aspirants

Richard P. McGinnis

INTRODUCTION

Where are they? The twelve percent minority students who were
supposed to be enrolled in U.S. medical schools by . . . was it really
1975?

Who wants to know the answers? Certainly medical and dental
schools have displayed some interest. Various mixtures of genuine
commitment, faddism, and cold financial reality have assisted those
most conservative of educational institutions, the guardians of the
sacred caduceus, U.S. medical schools, to involve themselves in one
of the most significant social movements of our time. For the first
time since Flexner, the doors would be opened wide and medical
schools would become concerned about the health, not just the
diseases, of all the population, and were training people with
special sensitivity toward the poor. . . .

But there were problems. You see, it's not just *what* you learn, but
how you learn it that counts. You see, it says here in the book that in

Richard P. McGinnis, Ph.D., is Professor of Chemistry and Premedical Advisor,
Tougaloo College, Tougaloo, Mississippi.

order to be crowned you have to do all the hard stuff in two years . . .
after that you can forget it all—basic sciences have had their
chance at you. And the only way you can show what you know is by
marking the proper pattern on the little circles on the answer sheet.
Understand, it's not that we aren't *very* concerned about what kind
of a practitioner you'll be, but we just haven't figured out how to
put that onto the answer sheet. Besides, I've got much too much
happening in my lab to waste my time with this stuff. . . .

Yes, professional schools *are* interested in minority students, but
they are scarcely a high priority where research funding or
averages on the National Boards might be at stake. And it will
continue that way as long as we allow medical schools to gorge
themselves at the federal trough, ostensibly to promote better
health care for Americans.

If society has not helped medical schools to redefine their roles, it
certainly has left them with a real mess of problems in trying to
train "non-traditional" students. Reading deficiencies, inadequate
test-taking skills, and poor study habits, on top of the almost
unavoidable social and cultural isolation of the minority student,
cause grave difficulties for students and for the professional
schools who are committed to educating them. For those reasons,
as well as the small and static minority applicant pool, there are a
number of programs designed to bring minority students into
medical careers.

Medical and dental schools sponsor the majority of special
programs for minority medical aspirants. A few, including the
three programs discussed in this chapter, are sponsored by undergraduate schools.

These programs—the Harvard Health Careers Summer Program, the United Negro College Fund Pre-Medical Summer Institute at Fisk University, and the Tougaloo College Pre-Health
Program—are all trying to deal with the many problems which face
the talented but underprepared minority student.

These programs all share a common objective, increasing the
pool of minority students who enter and successfully complete
health professional school. They address real problems: the lack of
knowledge about health careers in many high schools and colleges,
inadequate preparation in mathematics and communication skills,
low standardized test scores both entering and leaving college, and

lack of information and counseling about curriculum requirements and application procedures for health professional schools.

There are some common threads in these programs. Recruitment, for example, is a far more seriously considered task for these programs than for some others. These programs must not only identify those already planning a medical career but also try to stimulate those with no prior interest.

All these programs, particularly those centered at Black colleges, lay great stress on reading, mathematics, and problem solving. Yet these skills are so difficult even to define, and their measurement so crude, that it is not surprising that none of these programs has been able to erase poor test scores.

The success of these programs is due to many factors, but central to them all is the high self-expectation which successful participants carry away with them. These programs identify for their students what must be learned for success. Once the student is convinced of the necessity of that learning, smoother sailing is ahead.

HARVARD HEALTH CAREERS SUMMER PROGRAM

General

Begun in the summer of 1969, the Harvard Health Careers Summer Program (HCSP) was the first large scale, nationally recognized summer pre-medical program for undergraduate minority students. It represented a cooperative effort on the part of Harvard Medical School and Harvard Summer School to increase the pool of minority applicants to U.S. medical schools. The Harvard-Yale-Columbia Intensive Summer Studies Program, targeting on graduate schools in the arts and sciences, was in many respects its predecessor during 1966-69.

The Harvard HCSP is designed to identify talented minority students to medical and other health professional schools. Because many of these students may be underprepared, or may be attending schools of which the medical schools may have little knowledge or whose pre-professional curricula may be suspect, Harvard gives these students the opportunity to perform in a setting which is more familiar to those schools, and also gives the students a chance to take courses which may not have been taken at their home institutions. In addition the program provides the opportunity for students to be introduced in depth to the medical school setting and to learn about the applications and admissions process.

Recruitment and Selection

Students are recruited from a national pool. Publicized by posters sent around the country, the program now attracts some one to three thousand applications per year for its 120 to 160 places. The program seeks to identify "disadvantaged" students whose chances for entry to a health professional school would be substantially enhanced by program participation. A special effort is made to find representatives of all groups underrepresented in the health professions. These typically include, in descending order of participation, Blacks, Hispanics, native Americans, Asian Americans, and disadvantaged Whites. Successful applicants to the program must not only demonstrate financial disadvantage and inadequate secondary school preparation, but also must be felt likely to benefit from the Harvard program, especially if the nature or quality of the pre-professional education they are receiving might be questioned. The majority of students selected in recent years have been college post-sophomores and post-juniors.

Program Organization

HCSP lasts eight weeks of the summer, its starting and ending dates coinciding exactly with those of Harvard Summer School. The program consists of five major components: regular courses in the summer school, academic tutorial (or seminar) courses, clinical tutorials, meetings with medical and other health professional school representatives, and a variety of other seminars and workshops. Each student takes one regular summer school course, one academic tutorial, and one clinical tutorial. All transportation, living, and educational expenses are provided to the students, along with a living allowance.

Summer school courses are chosen to meet individual student

needs compatible with the student's prior preparation, although courses taken during the first summer usually seem to be those necessary for pre-professional course requirements. In these courses students are taught along with other summer school students and are not graded any differently from others. Summer program students enroll in Introductory Zoology or Botany, Genetics, Cell Biology (the most popular course), mathematics (Elementary Mathematics, College Algebra, or Calculus I), or Nutrition, each of these courses counting four semester hours. A few students enroll in eight-hour courses: General Chemistry, Organic Chemistry, or Physics. In most of these courses HCSP students make up only a small portion of the course enrollment, and in none do they represent the total enrollment.

The academic tutorial is a small group course with about five students, taught by a graduate or medical student. They typically meet six to nine hours per week and consist of a variegated mixture of lectures, discussions, written and laboratory work. The topics cover a very wide range. In the summer of 1978, for example, tutorials were offered in genetics, pre-organic chemistry, immunology, physiology, neurophysiology, biochemistry with clinical relationships, calculus, the circulatory system, general microbiology, and human neuroanatomy. Many of these courses had clinical or laboratory components. The tutors also act as advisors and counselors and facilitate student adjustment to the summer environment.

Clinical tutorials are a very strong component of this program. Run in conjunction with the teaching hospitals, laboratories, and clinics of the Harvard Medical, Dental, and Public Health Schools, they take place at least two half days per week at various sites within the Boston area. Usually they are arranged to meet student interests—psychiatry, surgery, dentistry, or obstetrics, for example. The small group (two to four students) allows the student to see operations, autopsies, and childbirths, to visit emergency rooms, research laboratories, etc. Altogether this activity promotes student involvement with medical activities which is usually intense and very satisfying for the students.

Noteworthy among the other activities are the visits of representatives of professional schools. Often medical or dental schools conduct official interviews with post-junior applicants during these visits, saving the students the expense of interview trips later on. A number of other seminars are held throughout the summer on medically related subjects.

Workshops are held throughout the summer for review for the Medical College Admission Test and the Dental Aptitude Test, utilizing the review manual which Harvard developed and is continually updating. The manual is an important addition to the "literature" of test review; one cannot help but speculate what would occur if only a small portion of the effort which goes into analysis of why minority students do poorly on tests were instead placed into helping students to do better on them. This manual is an excellent example of what can be done.

Accomplishments

Perhaps most important, Harvard's HCSP has not only helped to identify top-notch minority students but also has suggested to other institutions means of improving the preparation of minority students and identifying them to health professional schools. The "spin-off" of Harvard's program has been very significant in terms of inspiring many other programs, most of which are very different in means but have the same ultimate objective.

The program has had a really enviable record of success in the placement of its participants in health professional schools. In a survey of the program's 789 participants from 1969 to 1977, 91% of the 614 students reporting the completion of pre-professional requirements had been accepted to medical or dental schools, including such schools as Harvard, USC, Meharry, New York Medical College, and the University of Iowa. About five percent of participants are now working in other medically related fields.

It is possible to ascribe the success of this program to its selectivity and to the Harvard name, but credit is certainly more than due to two people who have been largely responsible for that success. William Wallace, former project director of the program, is a skilled, dedicated, and warm individual whose influence on many students has been very beneficial. The vision and commitment of Thomas Crooks, the former summer school director who helped shape the program and continued to guide it through the years, has had a significant impact on U.S. medical education.

UNITED NEGRO COLLEGE FUND PRE-MEDICAL SUMMER INSTITUTE AT FISK UNIVERSITY

General

The UNCF Pre-Medical Summer Institute is unique among special programs in that it is sponsored by an organization which represents some forty-one private colleges and universities (thirty-nine have undergraduate programs), all of which have predominantly Black enrollments. Thus the program acquires special significance because it draws from those colleges which traditionally have provided the greatest proportion of Black science graduates and health professionals, and which certainly are going to continue to be a major source of such students in the future.

The program aims to increase the numbers of qualified minority students who gain access to medical schools. It does this by (1) maintaining and stimulating the interest and motivation of able students toward the health professions, (2) improving their abilities to be successful in pre-professional course work, thereby augmenting their chances for admission to and success in health professional schools, and (3) arousing interest in the allied health professions. Its students are all at the post-freshman and post-sophomore levels in college, critical years during which most of the attrition in pre-medical curricula takes place.

The program began in 1971 and is located at Fisk University in Nashville, Tennessee. A member of UNCF, Fisk is located directly across the street from Meharry Medical College, giving it direct access to one of the highest concentrations of Black medical students, health professionals, and biomedical faculty and researchers in the United States.

Recruitment and Selection

The program is interested in enlarging the pool of minority applicants and in stimulating interest in the health professions among those who might not formerly have even considered the possibility seriously. As a result the method of selection is quite unusual. The president of each UNCF school designates a liaison person to head a group of faculty representing the natural and social sciences and the humanities. The faculty act as recruiters within the school, collect applications, and then rank the applicants. After applications are submitted to the program director, students are accepted in the order recommended by the committee until the slots available have been filled. While an effort is made to equalize the number of participants from each college, in practice the number of students from each institution can vary from one to nine, depending on the number of applications submitted and the availability of the applicants once the offer is made. There are usually about 150 participants in the program annually.

The method has several advantages. Especially for freshmen and sophomores, there is precious little available on paper which can tell of a student's potential, ability, or interest. The multidisciplinary faculty group helps to ensure that students from many different backgrounds will be selected, without the traditional bias in favor of science students.

Program Organization

The Pre-Medical Summer Institute lasts eight weeks during the summer. Transportation, living expenses, and educational expenses are provided to all participants, and in addition each student receives scholarship funds to be used the following year at the home institution. The program has academic, skills, and motivational components. Grades and credit hours are assigned by Fisk and are usually transferred by the student's own school.

The academic portion of the Fisk program is designed to complement rather than duplicate curricular offerings at the colleges. Courses are designed to stress the relationships between those standard pre-professional courses and medicine. Thus first year students choose from among Medical Cell Biology (3 semester hours), Organo-Biochemistry (3), or Selected Topics in General Chemistry (3), while second year students have options among Organo-Biochemistry, Psycho-Biology (3), Physical Biochemistry (with computer lab) (3), or Human Biology (3). Special Projects (1 or 2) and Reading (1) are also offered. Students usually take a load totalling eight or nine credit hours.

The faculty is both multidisciplinary and multi-institutional. In addition to those from Fisk, Meharry, Vanderbilt, and UT Nashville, several faculty fellows from UNCF schools also participate in the instructional program. All courses are team taught, usually pairing a "basic scientist" (a chemist, for example) with someone who can draw in clinical and medical correlations. The Institute's director teaches in the progam.

Curriculum

Courses designed for this program warrant some description.

Medical Cell Biology discusses a variety of topics which emphasize biological and biochemical concepts necessary to the understanding of life processes and the diseases of man. A special stress is laid on quantitative thinking and methods as applied to cellular processes and cell disorders.

Selected Topics in General Chemistry is designed for students who have had no prior chemistry. The course again stresses quantitative thinking and mathematics as applied to chemistry. Problem solving, graphing, and statistical data treatment are covered.

Organo-Biochemistry is open to students with some college chemistry and mathematics training, as determined by a special test. Students learn sufficient organic chemistry to appreciate its biological relevance. After a discussion of organic bonding, structure, and stereochemistry, the functional groups are presented. The second half of the course then deals with the biochemical functions of those groups and their role in metabolic processes.

The Physical Biochemistry course is laboratory centered. The course introduces students to the instrumentation commonly used in biomedical research. Projects were designed which involve the writing of simple FORTRAN computer programs for data analysis. This is the only laboratory course in the program.

Human Biology is an interdisciplinary systems approach to the systems of the human body and to their malfunctions.

Psycho-Biology, staffed by two anatomists and a pharmacologist, treats the anatomy and physiology of the nervous system. The staff has the opportunity to discuss with students, from a medical perspective, the dangers and effects of illicit drug experimentation.

Special Projects gives students exposure to problems within the health care system, at the same time developing the students' library research and communication skills. Each small group (four students) is assigned a topic, and each group then subdivides that into individual assignments for each group member. The student presents his paper to the group. The group then makes a presentation, in some form, to the entire assembly of participants.

Reading is a most important component of the program. Using only scientific materials, students are trained in acquisition of vocabulary and speed reading. They are trained in note- and test-taking techniques. The center is open throughout the day and even at night for students to practice. The course is required of all students.

Other Activities

Seminars are of two types, "professional" and "research." Professional seminars include speakers on such topics as admissions, financial aid, retention, curriculum, and social/psychological aspects of medical school. Research seminars, a very popular addition, deal with biomedical topics of current interest.

Clinical experiences are provided by both Vanderbilt and Meharry. Students visit the Matthew Walker Community Health Center, a tumor clinic, a cardiac conference, a nuclear medicine laboratory, and surgery, to name a few. The small special project groups are utilized for this purpose.

Field trips go to Mound Bayou Comprehensive Health Center in Mississippi annually, a model of comprehensive health care. At various times the group has travelled to Atlanta and Washington, D.C., visiting medical centers and research facilities. Such trips can be enormously stimulating to students.

Faculty Fellows

The faculty fellows program has been recently added to the institute. Five faculty, each from a different UNCF school, assist in the teaching of some of the courses. They are also able to work in curricular matters of interest to all the institutions. One summer faculty worked out a detailed syllabus for an interdisciplinary science course for the non-major which they plan to use at their home schools.

Accomplishments

The UNCF Pre-Medical Summer Institute is one of the most important programs operating. Its close relationships with Black schools, the nature of its supplemental activities, and the really powerful motivation it imparts to its participants are unsurpassed.

Since the program's start in 1971 until 1976 more than 650 students have been served by the program. Of the 310 who participated in the program in 1973 or before, 143, or 46%, are *known* to be in graduate or professional school, and the whereabouts of 54 of the 310 is not known. Of the 310, 92 (30%) are in medical school, 15 (5%) are in dental school, and 36 (12%) are in other graduate programs. Another eighteen (6%) are in a science-related career. Altogether it is a most impressive record for a program with its objectives and selection methods.

Finally the close linkages between the home institutions and the program are very significant. Evaluations and grades, provided to the liaison officer for each participant, assist each college to assess its curriculum. And the faculty fellows program helps to prevent the colleges from becoming isolated from each other, and instead assists them to work together to solve common academic and institutional problems.

This program is very indebted to the energy, enthusiasm, and organizational ability which its former director, Prince Rivers, has brought it. Formerly on the faculty at Fisk, Dr. Rivers is now at the National Institutes of Health. His care, ability, and concern are evident throughout.

TOUGALOO COLLEGE PRE-HEALTH PROGRAM

General

Tougaloo College is a small (800 enrollment) predominantly Black college located on the outskirts of Jackson, Mississippi. The

Pre-Health Program grows out of the college's long-term commitment to providing health professionals for the Mississippi area, and capitalizes on its good placement record with medical schools, especially during the period 1969-71. It attempts to improve the number and the quality of students from the college who enter health professional schools. Since the college typically draws 90 percent of its students from the state of Mississippi, the program maintains a regional focus. Likewise, in accord with the college's quite active role in the Mississippi civil rights movement and more recently in community organizing, there is a strong social action orientation to the program, emphasizing rural and community health. Started in 1971 with the encouragement of the Josiah Macy, Jr. Foundation, the program has grown over the years from a simple health professions advising and counseling program to include a summer academic program and preceptorships, achieving its more or less current form by 1973.

The primary objective of the program is to alleviate the shortage of Black and other minority health professionals in the state. Specifically the program tries to place twenty minority students per year into medical, dental, and other health professional schools. The need is serious: in 1973, when the program was started, there were only 43 Black physicians in the state to serve a Black population of over 800,000, a physician to patient ratio of 1 to 20,000. The average age of these physicians was over 60 years, and in a state which already had the fewest physicians per capita of any in the nation.

The program includes activities for recruitment, motivation, retention, skills building, orientation, advising, and counseling. It is presumed that a program of this type can help to unearth talent which otherwise might not be directed toward health professions. This is especially true in the Mississippi high schools where scarcely a handful provide adequate education in English or the sciences.

Program Description

The program consists of several components: recruitment and identification, academic reinforcement both for pre-freshmen and for pre-professional college students, advising and counseling, a pre-health club, and preceptorships. The program is envisioned as a four year continuum starting prior to matriculation at Tougaloo

College, when the student participates in a summer reinforcement program. During the academic year students participate in tutorials, and attend pre-health club talks and activities. During the summer students can acquire knowledge of health care delivery through preceptorships in the community; others attend summer programs at other institutions; a few serve as tutors in the summer pre-college academic reinforcement program. During the second semester of the junior year students begin to receive extensive advising and counseling about application procedures to medical, dental, and other health professional schools, and in-depth reviews for standardized exams are held. Students may enter the program at any point, and may participate in only some of the activities if they desire.

Recruiting and Identification

Initial recruiting in high schools is carried out by student teams who work in cooperation with the college recruitment office. The students talk about the summer program, talk about the college's placement record with health professional schools, and answer general questions about college life. The student recruiters generally seem to be able to communicate very well with high school students, and this seems to be a most effective means of recruitment. Efforts are made also to talk to the science teachers and guidance counselors, often the bottlenecks in the identification process. When time is available Therman Evans' film "Code Blue" has been very effective, though the musical background and the message are both showing signs of age.

Recently the program has put out a newsletter, in newspaper format, which describes the experiences in the previous summer program. A national testing program distributes these by mail to students who indicate interest in science-related areas and who live in the nearby geographical region.

Summer Academic Reinforcement

All but a few Mississippi high schools do a superb job of denying Black students access to a high school education. The purpose of the summer program is to try to overcome that damage, and to introduce talented entering college freshmen to the possibilities and opportunities in the health professions. The program is called Health Sciences Summer Program, and lasts for six weeks during the mid-summer. It gives the students an intensive introduction to course work they are likely to encounter in courses in biology, chemistry, mathematics, communication skills, and problem solving. Students are also provided with an introduction to college life, and they become aware of the opportunities in the various health-related professions.

Courses are not offered for credit, and are staffed by faculty of the college and by recent college graduates. A number of undergraduate tutors are available to assist students with course work. Mathematics is taught at three levels: basic algebra, advanced algebra/trigonometry, and calculus. In biology a review of organismal biology is presented, followed by a discussion of molecular cell processes at an elementary level. The relationships between biology, chemistry, and mathematics are stressed. The chemistry course is really a course in problem solving with chemical applications, and encourages students to make commonsense connections between chemical concepts and the real world. Writing and speech are stressed in the communication skills course, along with readings from elementary scientific literature at the *Scientific American* level.

The problem-solving course warrants special discussion. Using materials developed by Arthur Whimby (author of *Intelligence Can Be Taught*), students work in pairs to solve a variety of problems. One student works as "problem solver" and the other as "listener." The "problem solver" explains the detailed logical processes which he is using to solve the problem step by step, and the "listener" is only supposed to indicate when he doesn't follow his partner. Roles are reversed for the next problem. The method is designed to improve student capacity to reason carefully. Whimby argues that thinking is a process which can be taught like any other, and by exposing it to the detailed scrutiny of another, one learns that even difficult problems can be solved with careful, systematic reasoning.

Other summer program activities include forums on health care delivery, a health careers fair with local professionals and educators, and student debates. An annual trip goes to Meharry Medical College in Nashville. Students are counseled about the pre-medical programs which they will be following in their college years, the admissions process, and financial aid.

Of the approximately fifty participants each summer, approximately forty return to the college in the fall. Most of those who do (80 to 90%) decide to stay in health career or science curricula.

Academic Year Activities

During the academic year there are a number of academic support and informational activities. Tutoring is offered for basic pre-professional courses (General Chemistry, Organic Chemistry, and Introduction to Biology). An audio-tutorial biology course has likewise been set up in the Introduction to Biology course.

The Pre-Health Club serves both as information center and as a conduit for student energy. Students hear recruiters, discuss health professions with alumni who are either in or out of school, and listen to discussions about difficulties and advantages to setting up practice in Mississippi.

For some years the program has offered a test review program for the MCAT and DAT. This is customarily offered to juniors. The publication, in whatever limited quantities, of the Harvard review manual has been quite helpful in these sessions. Reviews proceed throughout the spring semester.

Students in the pre-health program are strongly encouraged to take part in other sponsored programs in related areas. For example, the NIH Minority Biomedical Support program gives students the opportunity to be paid for assisting in research, for which they also gain credit. Other students do research in the NIH-sponsored Student Research Training Grant program which targets them toward biomedical research in graduate school. These programs are a most important complement to the regular pre-health program, although administratively these are separate entities.

Preceptorships

The preceptorship program, open to post-freshmen and above, offers students hands-on involvement in health care delivery in their home setting. Most of the preceptorships are during the summer (usually twelve to fifteen). County hospitals, local physicians and dentists, and county health departments have all assisted in placing students in their home towns. Students do lab tests, position patients for X-rays, act as receptionists, and occasionally even take trips with their supervisor. Evaluation from both students and supervisors has been overwhelmingly positive.

The preceptorship program, because it is done at home, makes participants aware of the needs and the opportunity for their participation in that system, and hopefully for its improvement.

Advising and Counseling

A faculty committee oversees all program activities and advises the director. The committee also is kept informed of pre-professional curricula so that course advising is coordinated. A major function of the committee is to compile and write pre-medical and pre-dental letters of recommendation. It is perhaps important that, since Tougaloo is such a small college and the degree of involvement so intense, faculty *always* know students, even those they have never taught. As a result the letters always reflect real knowledge of the student, and faculty provide often insightful and knowing comments about their students.

Other Programs

An important part of the pre-health program is that it encourages its participants to take part in others. Tougaloo students are kept apprised of summer programs everywhere, and few are the competent science students who do not have a summer placement somewhere. Tougaloo students are regular participants in the other two programs mentioned in this chapter, MEdREP at Tulane and the Meharry Biomedical Science Programs. In addition to pre-medical summer programs, students find industrial positions or research positions. In this way students get a chance to explore many options instead of being channeled into only one career area which may not suit everyone equally well.

Some interinstitutional arrangements have been made as a part of this program. The Pre-Health Program has established a cooperative medical technology program with Meharry Medical

College. Brown University's Program in Medicine selects Tougaloo participants for their Early Identification Program. In this program two sophomores are selected annually to enter Brown's Medical School upon graduation, with admission all but guaranteed provided the students do acceptable work in their subsequent years.

Accomplishments

The Tougaloo College Pre-Health Program is an example of what one small college has done to encourage students to enter health careers. It has accomplished several tasks. First it was able to set up a *comprehensive* pre-medical program which tracks its students from their first day in the summer program to the day they enter medical school. That, coupled with the flexibility of working with an entire college, allows programs which can be individually tailored to student needs. Second, it has created in the process a definite awareness among Tougaloo students, and among high school students, of the opportunities in medical careers, especially medicine and dentistry. Most Tougaloo students now know, well in advance, about curriculum requirements, test dates, and application procedures for health professional schools. Awareness has risen to the point where now nearly half of the college's 250 freshmen plan on entering a health career. While the proportion drops to 25 percent by the sophomore year, there has been an approximately threefold increase in the enrollment in the pre-professional courses, largely as a result of this program.

Perhaps most significant for the college, the program seems to have begun to establish a track record equal to or surpassing what it achieved in the 1969-71 period, when times were very different. Since 1973, approximately 75 to 80 percent of Tougaloo's medical and dental school applicants have matriculated in professional school. Thirty-six students have entered medical schools (1973-1978), including one M.D./Ph.D. student, thirteen have entered dental school, five have entered medical technology, and six others have entered other allied health professions, and the program is now reaching its objective of placing 20 students annually in health professional schools. While the program can take little credit for it, the number of Black physicians in Mississippi has nearly doubled since 1973 (to 80), the majority Tougaloo graduates returning from their medical training out of state.

The program has very serious deficiencies, too. MCAT and DAT scores, most importantly, are still not significantly higher than when the program began. The program has yet to deal effectively with apathetic attitudes characteristic of many students in the late seventies.

The Tougaloo program, like others, owes much of its success to the support from the institution and from the community, especially President George Owens and the campus physician, Dr. Robert Smith, whose dedication to improving health care delivery inspired a faculty member to design this program.

CONCLUSIONS

All the programs here represent rather special efforts by schools which do not have to be in the minority pre-medical business but are anyway, and it is pretty clear that it is because of the strong commitment of their sponsoring institutions, or at least parts of them, that they operate and are effective. There are other notable undergraduate programs but it is no accident that almost all of these are at minority institutions.

All the programs have as their goal increasing the pool of minority health professionals. Less explicitly stated, but clearly underlying each of these programs, is a common analysis of "the problem." It is simple. Most minority science students are not attending college where most medical schools want to find them. They are, in fact, in schools about whose curriculum a large portion of most medical faculties have doubts.

In this chapter we have presented three undergraduate college sponsored pre-medical programs. All, in one way or another, are engaged in making students visible who otherwise would not be, assisting students who otherwise might be passed over to acquire proper credentials. Primarily, too, all three programs address the minority colleges, understanding that it is these colleges whose students will have the greatest gap between ability and visibility.

These programs have a remarkable degree of success in stimulating interest and in identifying students who are likely to be successful in gaining entrance to health professional schools. The specific academic problems they are dealing with are not easy to solve, but they are making serious and often successful attempts to deal with them. Now that successful models of recruitment, motivation, and skills building have been developed, it is especially unfortunate that medical school and societal interest should be declining.

Programs like these will certainly be necessary in the future if minorities are to continue to hold places in medical schools. Ten years after the institution of the Harvard program, most medical schools are scarcely more knowledgeable of the Black colleges and other minority schools than when it began. Every effort will have to be expended to continue to make minority students well prepared and *visible,* in order to keep the attention of those who might prefer to look in more familiar places for their minority students. Only in this way can we maintain the remembrance of a commitment.

CHAPTER 7

Summer Programs for Undergraduates in a Professional Medical Education Environment

Joseph C. Pisano
and
Anna Cherrie Epps

Recognition of the scarcity of minority health professionals, and the overall uneven distribution of health personnel throughout the United States, prompted the development of reinforcement and enrichment summer programs which were implemented initially in minority health professional training institutions and ultimately adopted and incorporated in proposals submitted to the federal government. These Health Career Opportunity Programs were made possible by the concerns of Congress as reflected in the

Joseph C. Pisano, Ph.D., is associate Professor of Physiology and Associate Director, Medical Education Reinforcement and Enrichment Program, Tulane University Medical Center, New Orleans, Louisiana.

Anna Cherrie Epps, Ph.D., is Professor of Medicine and Director, Medical Education Reinforcement and Enrichment Program, Tulane University Medical Center, New Orleans, Louisiana, and Vice Chairperson (1978-1979) and Chairperson-Elect (1979-1980), Minority Affairs Section, Group on Student Affairs, Association of American Medical Colleges, Washington, D.C.

Health Manpower Education Initiative Awards in the Comprehensive Health Manpower Training Act of 1971.

However, it must be pointed out that such organizations as the National Fund for Medical Education, the Josiah Macy, Jr. Foundation, the National Urban Coalition, and a few other private philanthropic organizations, were among those to recognize early in the 1960's that there were health manpower problems and significant barriers associated with the education of the underrepresented minority in the health professions. These organizations realized that the alleviation of these health manpower problems depended on innovative educational efforts, such as summer reinforcement and enrichment programs that are presently in operation throughout our country's medical centers, where there is commitment to eradication of inequality of opportunity in education for underrepresented groups, such as minorities and the socioeconomically disadvantaged, in the field of medicine. These reinforcement and enrichment programs generally have operated throughout the summer months in most institutions. However, there are a few which continue their program activities throughout the academic year. These programs are designed to identify, inform, recruit, retain, and ultimately graduate an increased number of minority and socioeconomically disadvantaged youths in the fields of heath care throughout our nation.

Today, many examples of these types of health career opportunity projects are found within the environments of our institutions of higher education, particularly medical centers. Exclusive of our own, which is known as the Medical Education Reinforcement and Enrichment Program (MEdREP) of Tulane Medical Center, we would like to turn your attention to a few we consider similar in format. They include the following: the MEDPREP Program of the University of Southern Illinois at Carbondale; the Harvard University Health Careers Summer Program at Cambridge, Massachusetts; the University of Texas Medical Branch Health Careers Opportunity Program, at Galveston, Texas; the PREP Program of Barnard College in New York City, New York; the Baylor University School of Medicine Health Careers Opportunity Program at Houston, Texas; the University of New Mexico Prematriculation Program at Albuquerque, New Mexico; the Temple University RAR Program at Philadelphia, Pennsylvania; the Summer Program of the College of Medicine and Dentistry of New Jersey at

Newark, New Jersey; the Cornell University Medical College Summer Program at Ithaca, New York; the Howard University Colleges of Medicine and Dentistry Reinforcement and Enrichment Programs at Washington, D.C., and others. (See table for further listings.)

These summer program activities serve to identify and recruit into the health professions and other related fields, the socioeconomically, culturally, and educationally disadvantaged students, especially from among minority groups whose background and interests make it reasonably certain that they will engage in the delivery of health care in severe shortage areas. In addition, the summer programs serve to inform and introduce undergraduate disadvantaged students to the practical and simulated experiences associated with the pursuit of a health professions career, thus providing these students with a more realistic approach to the requirements for entrance into the health professional fields. These summer programs are aimed at salvaging and making inclusive these segments of our population in the educational processes, leading to a professional career in the field of medicine and related fields of health.

Having become aware of the potential of the disadvantaged youth of our nation, there has developed over the past decade a growing desire to face the problems related to increasing the underrepresented in the fields of medicine and science. There is overwhelming evidence which demonstrates the need to continue the development of health manpower, especially physicians, from among the underrepresented minorities and economically disadvantaged. These physicians can respond to the unmet demands of medical care and health maintenance among the nation's minority populations. These demands are evidenced especially in the inner city and rural areas where the impoverished and poorly educated live.

Health career summer programs address these problems. They are directed to the development of the academic prerequisites and personal qualities which are essential characteristics of those in pursuit of a health profession. Through these programs there is a reinforcement of interest in the health professions, enhancement of motivation, and assurance of academic performance expectations for those students participating in summer program activities. These objectives are achieved through the introduction and utilization of education skills, academic reinforcement and enrichment activities, exposure and experiences in the medical school environment, as well as introduction to the health care delivery system and teams, thus expanding the horizons for those aspiring to serve others in need of health care.

The above is a general description of innovative and revolutionary approaches to providing educational opportunities through summer program experiences, which are in themselves exciting and rewarding educational experiences for all involved. Thus, it is obvious that these programs have the potential capability of creating a pool of applicants whose enriched experiences will allow them a better chance at succeeding in the health professional career of their choice. This goal can be accomplished by creating a more comprehensive premedical and prematriculation medical education opportunity and experience which will assist in assuring future success and ultimate participation of a greater number of minority and disadvantaged in higher education pursuits and the system of health care delivery. Summer programs such as Tulane's MEdREP, and others similar in format, best operate when located in medical education institutions, where the student has immediate access to educational opportunities and experiences that portray the real environment and characteristics of health professional training, as well as provide the opportunity to observe the development of the health professionals in the delivery of health care at close range. This unlimiting and constantly unfolding experience in such an atmosphere has the potential to stimulate as well as reassure participant motivation, enhance self-confidence, and ultimately produce a well-informed, highly educated, and competent health professional for the future from among the underrepresented minorities and disadvantaged youth of our nation.

A rather extensive search of the existing literature has revealed that each of the summer programs described has similar goals and objectives, and the results to date, as reported, are usually of a positive nature. The literature surveyed also revealed that the formats of such program activities are quite similar, with minor modifications in one or more of the program components. In order to describe these types of summer programs which are provided for undergraduate pre-professional and science majors, usually located within the medical school environment, one must consider the across-the-board program objectives in their relationship to the programs as conducted. In discussing these summer program components, the reader must be cognizant of and cautious about accepting these program components as strictly distinct entities.

When categorizing the major components of summer program activities for the medically motivated and aspiring youth of our nation, one must recognize that the variety of programmatic objectives encompassed in these programs generally traverse all categorical areas and are indeed dependent upon each other for efficacy. The components may be categorized as follows: identification, information, dissemination, motivation, recruitment, and retention; all of which are designed and conducted for the socioeconomically, culturally, and educationally disadvantaged individuals interested in pursuing one of the major health professions, namely medicine, dentistry, osteopathy, podiatry, optometry, veterinary medicine, pharmacy, and others in the public health and allied health fields.

Most preadmissions and prematriculation summer program activities emphasize motivational, didactic, and socialization experiences to improve the chances for admissions to health professions training and to further the assurance of retention for those participating.

Summer program components must provide a challenging educational environment, which will rise to the level of the student with superior intellect and produce both the opportunity and adroitness of approach, which will enhance performance at both the premedical and medical levels. Participation in summer programs throughout our country is essentially dependent upon early identification, dissemination of information, and recruitment of potential participants. This is generally accomplished by most project directors through out-reach activities, with presentations given before student audiences, early in each academic year. The out-reach activities involve on-site visits with dissemination of detailed information to key persons, such as presidents, deans, pre-professional advisors, and counselors. These visits are most effective in those institutions of higher learning where minority and disadvantaged student populations are highest. The most crucial step in recruitment is the presentation of accurate and up-to-date information to the students and advisors, and the provision of in-depth advice and counseling about both health careers and summer program activities. As a follow-up, recruitment representatives usually meet with preprofessional advisors at the undergraduate institutions visited, all of which ultimately leads to assistance in early identification, recommendation of potential applicants for participation in summer program activities, and eventual admission to medical school.

Most summer program activities, particularly those located within medical centers, select their participants from among those demonstrating potential and capability for the pursuit of a health professions education, as well as those newly admitted medical students requiring strengthening of their basic science backgrounds to insure their ability to complete a health professions education.

Health career summer program activities are probably the most underestimated and yet profound of the recruitment tools, which most assuredly lead to actual increases in enrollment levels of those individuals who have the ability to complete a health professions education. These programs also assist in reducing or eliminating many of the major barriers encountered in the course of the admissions process, and eventual admissions to health professions training.

Motivational aspects of these summer programs utilize the services of role models and extensive exposure to the health professions through the presentations of films, lectures, and seminars. In addition, preceptorship experiences with health professionals and introduction to health care delivery, in-depth counseling and guidance directed toward immediate and subsequent matriculation in a health professions training program, as well as academic and personalized support services, are provided. The introduction to medical school life in the basic sciences, enhancement of communication skills, study skills and test-taking techniques, and exposure to the research environment contained within the health professional environment, also help to make up the experiences of summer program participants. The functions of these experiences and exposures are to convey accurate and up-to-date information and to provide some insight into performance expectations, as well as reawaken, reinforce, and ultimately maintain the participant's interest in pursuing a health professions career.

The didactic component of summer programs provides the means for strengthening a student's prerequisite knowledge, comprehension, and application of scientific information to the study of the health profession of his or her choice. This component also serves to reassure the student participant's acceptability of self and of the academic setting from which he has received preprofessional training, which should ultimately assist the participant in successfully competing for admission to and completion of a health professions training program.

The socialization aspect of summer program activities helps student participants gain a broader view of the variety of cultural differences which exist in our populations, and helps develop a deeper concern for and consideration of their fellow man, as well as a heightened sense of competence in their educational training and backgrounds. Thus, the socialization activities of summer programs provide a firm foundation for the development of future personal attitudes as these participants continue their educational pursuits in preprofessional and professional training.

It should be re-emphasized, and it is well illustrated, that no one summer program component can fit into any one category to the exclusion of the others. There is no absolute substitute for the achievement of academic preparedness, the development of skills to insure competitiveness and equality of opportunity for admissions to health professional training, and the reawakening of a subdued desire to enter into these pathways. The recognition of the surfacing of a student's aspiration and reaffirmation of the commitment to pursue a career choice plays a rather significant and determining role in most pre-professional and professional students' lives. These characteristic results, generally achieved by summer programs, profoundly illustrate the complexities and rewards of these special educational opportunity activities, which are especially designed to meet the needs of the socioeconomically disadvantaged and the academically deprived of our nation. It is essential that all parts of a summer program experience mesh and reinforce the other components to achieve the desired transformation observed in many summer program student participants. The necessity of reinforcement of one component by another makes it obvious that there is no single most important element of a summer program; only the entire program experience will accomplish the ultimate objectives and achieve the goals desired.

In the discussion to follow, we shall place much emphasis upon the Medical Education Reinforcement and Enrichment Program (MEdREP) at Tulane. We feel that the MEdREP Summer Program encompasses all of the components previously described, and meets the demands of most student participants by impacting the academic, emotional, and personal needs of the participants. Thus, it is the opinion of the authors that such programs provide each student participant with a better chance at success in the pursuit of a health professional career, as well as an enhanced ability for the completion of health professional training and eventual practice in the professional field chosen. The emphasis on the MEdREP system of summer program activity is not only because the authors are most familiar with it, but we also admit to an attitudinal prejudice in terms of its success.

It has been observed by those associated with MEdREP that to recruit and retain individuals, both at the preprofessional and professional levels, and to create a pool of professional applicants whose enriched experiences and exposures will allow them a better chance at succeeding in admission to professional training and the ability to complete a health professions education, a summer program experience is the best approach to achieving that goal.

The MEdREP Summer Program staff includes directors, a summer program staff coordinator, medical student assistants, an academic and personal counselor, and a financial aid advisor. In addition, research faculty advisors and a consortium of local college and university undergraduate faculty assist in offering the academic means for strengthening the student's prerequisite knowledge, comprehension and application of information, as well as more personalized educational opportunities, for eventual competition in pursuit of the health professions. The summer program experience affords the student participant meaningful and personal interaction with the administration, faculty, and students within the medical center environment, exposure to research, lectures and the clinical aspects of that environment, and accurate and up-to-date information as it concerns medical school life, the curriculum, and the application process. There is also extensive information provided on financial assistance, communicative skills, basic learning skills, and study and test-taking skills, in addition to the reinforcement of interest in the health professions and determination of personal motivation.

Program methodology involves early recruitment of participants by health professions institution representatives during the academic year with the assistance of advisors, counselors, and students, as well as repeated dissemination of information to target institutions and interested organizations and individuals within the United States, utilizing posters, brochures, application materials, and personal contacts.

Eligibility and selection of student participants is determined by a committee composed of the directors, medical student assistants, staff coordinators and a counselor, with the advisory assistance of administration and faculty of the nominating institutions. Health professions oriented and motivated students are carefully selected through the assessment of application information, demonstrated commitment to a health professional career, utilization of faculty appraisals, and demonstrated potential and ability to pursue a health professions education.

Notification of summer program application status is made early in the spring of each academic year, and students selected for participation (usually rising junior or senior undergraduates) are requested to confirm acceptance in writing. Immediately following receipt of confirmation, the participants are advised of housing accommodations, provided a list of possible research exposures, the amount of per diem provided and travel information, as well as details concerning the summer experience.

The MEdREP summer experience lasts for ten weeks, beginning early in June and ending in mid-August of each calendar year. The program is organized to include basic science and clinical science research, prerequisite course review sessions, clinical exposures, and preceptorship experiences, films, lectures and seminars, role model activities, interviews, and in-depth academic, personal, and financial aid counseling. Students who have been selected for participation in the summer program are involved in an established research program designed to foster their interest in the study of the health professions, particularly medicine, or alternate health careers. Each student participant is assigned, at the beginning of the summer experience, to a faculty advisor conducting research in his or her field of interest. Using academic transcripts, as well as the student interest preference list, submitted by each participant after hearing brief faculty presentations, each individual is assigned to a specific research laboratory. Students are generally placed in a research laboratory which best suits their individual interests and academic backgrounds. For the duration of the program, the students spend a large percentage of their time in their individual laboratory environments. This intense research laboratory exposure enables student participants to become acquainted with at least one or more fields of research interest, in-depth information in terms of technique, and exposure to the scientific method. In order to monitor each student's research progress, the student is required to make an oral and written presentation at the conclusion of the program. These presentations are considered to be a valuable part of the summer program experience because they allow the student to exercise his ability to communicate ideas to a group, with appropriate sophistication and poise, despite some degree of pressure. In addition, these presentations also enable the students participating to learn about valuable techniques and on-going research in laboratories other than their own. All presentations are made before an audience of student participants, staff, student coordinators, visiting research faculty, and other interested persons.

Written reports, which are required at the conclusion of the program, are read critically by each student's research advisor and returned with written criticism to the student at the end of the summer experience.

The prerequisite review sessions allow the student an even greater opportunity to strengthen prerequisite knowledge and prepare for the standardized admissions tests required for competition for admission to the health profession training program of his or her choice. These sessions are designed not only to review the basic principles in the disciplines covered on the admissions examinations, but also to furnish the skills that will enable students to improve their performance in competing for admission to health professional training and their future academic and professional competence. In addition, these sessions assist in the early identification of students' deficiencies or inadequacies and allow sufficient time to provide individualized academic reinforcement when necessary.

Clinical exposures and preceptorship experiences are a part of the total motivational program. As part of the clinical exposure phase, each student participating in the summer program is given an opportunity to spend an evening in the emergency room of a large community hospital under the supervision of participating medical students. This activity is primarily designed to allow the student a better chance to observe what goes on in a large health care delivery facility, and how the health professional and other supporting staff interrelate in the emergency room environment. The one-to-one ratio of medical student to summer program participant allows for active exposure and information exchange as it concerns the clinical experience. The summer program also offers several clinically-oriented tours and field trips.

The preceptorship experience, which is offered to each student participating in the summer program, provides an opportunity for a student to spend an entire day with a practicing physician within the local community. Physician volunteers allow one or two students to join them in their daily routine. This phase of the program provides the student with an understanding of the daily activities of the practicing physician, particularly in primary health care. Additional clinical experience involves an eight-hour program devoted to a surgically operable disease state, such as the resection of the small bowel in the dog. This experience includes informal lectures given by medical school faculty on the anatomy and physiology of the organ system involved in the case to be studied. This is followed by a discussion of clinical aspects and illustrated relationships to the human. These demonstrations are further enhanced by videotapes of the operable procedure to follow. The summer students participate under the supervision of senior medical students and help in the operative procedure, which takes place in the vivarium operating rooms of the medical center. All students have the opportunity to assist the medical student surgeon throughout the procedure. The final clinical exposure involves the experience of weekly grand rounds at one of our large medical institutions within the immediate environs.

Films, lectures, and seminars are all a part of the weekly experience of each of the participants in the summer program. These are held every Friday afternoon over the ten-week period. The films, lectures, and seminars expose the students to the medical environment, which includes medical students, basic and clinical science faculty, local practicing physicians, and other health professionals. It is a time which is designed to give the students an accurate perception of the requirements and the preparation necessary for entrance into health professional training.

Information is provided regarding the application process, admissions policies and procedures, medical school curricula, financial aid available, the interview process, and an opportunity to meet

TABLE 1. A PARTIAL LISTING OF SUMMER PROGRAMS FOR UNDERGRADUATES IN A PROFESSIONAL MEDICAL EDUCATION ENVIRONMENT

COLLEGE OR UNIVERSITY	RECRUITMENT/ GEOGRAPHICAL CONCENTRATION	TARGET POPULATION GROUPS	PROGRAM COMPONENTS						STUDENT SUPPORT SERVICES	
			FORMAL COURSE WORK	REVIEW SESSIONS	LEARNING SKILLS DEVELOPMENT	RESEARCH EXPERIENCE	CLINICAL EXPOSURE	COUNSELING	PRE-MATRICULATION	MEDICAL MATRICULATION
U. of Arizona Tucson, AZ	ARIZONA	NA, MA 1, 2, 3	X		X		X	X	Summer Program	
U. of So. Calif. School of Medicine Los Angeles, CA		B, Ch 1, 2, 3	X		X		X	X	Tutorial Services Summer Workshop Guest Speakers	
U. of California San Diego. CA		All 5, 6								Summer Program
Metropolitan State College Denver, CO	COLORADO	B, NA, MA 1, 2, 3			X				Student remains until career program has begun	
Georgetown U. School of Medicine Washington. DC	WASHINGTON. DC	All 2, 3, 5		X				X	Summer Program	Tutorial Services
Medical College of Georgia Augusta. GA		B 1, 2, 3	X		X	X	X		Pre-Med Tutorial Summer Program	Supports the minority affairs program for enrolled students
U. of Hawaii School of Medicine Honolulu. HI	HAWAII (SOUTH PACIFIC)	All 2, 3	X	X				X	Tutorial Services Summer Program	Works especially with Micronesians and Polynesians
Southern Illinois U. Carbondale. IL	In-House	All 1, 2	X		X			X	Tutorial Services	Focus on undergraduate/ medical student interaction
Indiana U. Bloomington. IN		All 2, 3					X		Summer Program	
U. of Kansas School of Medicine Kansas City. KS	KANSAS	B, All 4, 5			X			X	Tutorial Services Summer Program	Emphasis on support to minority medical students
Tulane U. School of Medicine New Orleans. LA	NATIONAL	All 2, 3, 4		X	X	X	X	X	Tutorial Services Summer Program	Tutorial Services Academic Year Reviews

Institution	Groups / Levels					Program	Services
Boston U School of Medicine, Boston, MA	All 1, 3, 6						Summer Program
Tufts U, Boston, MA — MASSACHUSETTS	All 2, 3, 4	X	X	X		Summer Program	Tutorial Services
Harvard U, Cambridge, MA — NATIONAL	All 2, 3, 4	X	X	X		Tutorial Services / Summer Program	
Wayne State U School of Medicine, Detroit, MI — MICHIGAN	B 1, 2, 3, 4	X	X	X		Tutorial Services	Tutorial and Support Services
U of Minnesota School of Medicine, Duluth, MN	NA 1, 2, 3, 4	X				Tutorial Services / Summer Program / Free tuition to NA	Tutorial and Support Services / Works closely with enrolled NA students
U of Mississippi School of Medicine, Jackson, MS	All 2, 3					Summer Program	
U of Nebraska Medical Center, Omaha, NE — NEBRASKA	All 1, 2, 3	X				Tutorial Services / Summer Program	Tutorial and Support Services / Emphasis on motivational activities
U of Nevada Div of Health Sci, Reno, NV — NEVADA	NA, All / All	X	X	X			Works with agencies in NV health care areas. Accents motivational & retention activities
U of North Carolina School of Medicine, Chapel Hill, NC	All 2, 3, 5, 6						Summer Program
U of North Dakota School of Medicine, Grand Forks, ND	AI, All 1, 2, 3	X				Summer Program	

LEGENDS

AI: American Indian
B: Black
Ch: Chicano
F: Female

H: Hispanic
MA: Mexican American
NA: Native American

1. High School
2. Junior College (freshman, sophomore)
3. Senior College (junior, senior)

4. Post-Baccalaureate
5. Pre-Matriculation
6. Other

TABLE 1. (continued)

COLLEGE OR UNIVERSITY	RECRUITMENT/ GEOGRAPHICAL CONCENTRATION	TARGET POPULATION GROUPS	PROGRAM COMPONENTS						STUDENT SUPPORT SERVICES	
			FORMAL COURSE WORK	REVIEW SESSIONS	LEARNING SKILLS DEVELOPMENT	RESEARCH EXPERIENCE	CLINICAL EXPOSURE	COUN-SELING	PRE-MATRICULATION	MEDICAL MATRICULATION
College of Medicine & Dentistry of NJ Newark, NJ		All 3, 4	X		X			X	Tutorial Services Summer Program	Work-Study Program
U. of New Mexico School of Medicine Albuquerque, NM	NEW MEXICO	All 5	X					X	Tutorial Services Summer Program Pre-Entrance Prog.	
Cornell U. Medical College New York, NY	NEW YORK	B, H 2, 3				X		X	Tutorial Services Summer Program	
New York Medical College New York, NY	NEW YORK	All 3, 5	X		X	X	X	X	Tutorial Services Summer Program	Works with post-baccalaureate students not accepted into medical school
Ohio State U. Research Foundation Columbus, OH	In-House	All	X				X	X	Tutorial Services	
Okla. State Regents for Higher Educ. Oklahoma City, OK	OKLAHOMA	All 1, 2, 3, 4		X	X			X	Summer Program	
U. of Oklahoma Health Sci. Center Oklahoma City, OK	OKLAHOMA	All 1, 2, 3	X			X		X	Tutorial Services Summer Program w/ academic credit	
Medical College of Pennsylvania Philadelphia, PA	PENNSYLVANIA	F 2				X	X		Tutorial Services Summer Program	
Temple University School of Medicine Philadelphia, PA	GREATER DELAWARE VALLEY	All 5	X	X	X			X	Pre-Matriculation Program Summer Program	Tutorial and Support Services
Brown U. Providence, RI		All 1, 2, 3								Summer Program

Institution	Region	Minority Groups	Level						Program	Program
Medical U. of South Carolina, Charleston, SC		All	2, 3, 5, 6				x	x	Summer Program	Summer Program
Meharry Medical College, Nashville, TN	NATIONAL	B, NA, MA, H	2, 3				x	x	Tutorial Services Summer Program (three summers)	
Baylor College of Medicine, Houston, TX		All	2, 3, 6		x	x	x		Summer Program	Summer Program
U. of Texas Medical Branch, Galveston, TX		B, MA	2, 3		x				Summer Program	
U. of Utah College of Medicine, Salt Lake City, UT	UTAH	All	1, 2, 3, 4		x	x		x	Tutorial Services Summer Program	Students are reinforced in medical school basic science courses
Eastern Virginia Medical School, Norfolk, VA	VIRGINIA	All	3		x	x	x	x	Tutorial Services Summer Program	
Howard University, Washington, D.C.		B, All	1		x	x		x		
U. of Washington, Seattle, WA	NATIONAL	All	5		x	x		x	Interaction with med. students and medical faculty	Emphasizes interaction between medical students and medical school faculty
Medical College of Wisconsin, Milwaukee, WI	WISCONSIN	All	5		x			x	Tutorial Services Summer Program	
U. of Wisconsin School of Medicine, Madison, WI	WISCONSIN	All	All		x				Summer Program Pre-Matriculation Programs	Tutorial and Support Services

LEGENDS

AI: American Indian
B: Black
Ch: Chicano
F: Female

H: Hispanic
MA: Mexican American
NA: Native American

1. High School
2. Junior College (freshman, sophomore)
3. Senior College (junior, senior)

4. Post-Baccalaureate
5. Pre-Matriculation
6. Other

with role models and recruiters from other health professional institutions and fields. An invaluable feature of the summer program is the exposure of the student participants to a variety of role models found within the medical center environment, as well as in the local community. This exposure affords the student an opportunity to see administrators, students, faculty, practicing physicians, and facilities which form the environment in which he or she will train, if he continues his interest and academic pursuits. Furthermore, participants are required to live within the medical student residence of the medical center, allowing them a better chance to exchange information and work with medical student assistants who are available on a 24-hour basis, to assist with any problems that might arise.

In addition to the day-to-day exposure of the program participants to the medical school environment, motivational speakers, especially those representing minority groups in the various health professions, are invited to provide helpful insights into the professions they represent through the utilization of panel presentations.

The summer program not only exposes students to the medical environment, but also provides the opportunity to participate in and observe mock interviews, which are followed by scheduled interviews with the Dean of Admissions and two other faculty members within the medical center. During the mock interview sessions, students are given a briefing on the medical school interview process, so that they are made aware of the proper interview behavior and attire, as well as the kinds of questions that will confront them, thus assisting students in preparing to cope with the interview situation without unnecessary anxiety. Interviews may be made official for all students interested in applying in the following academic year.

During the summer program, the counselor, financial aid advisor, as well as the director of the program, are available for academic career and personalized counseling on a formal basis. These sessions are scheduled for each summer participant, one at the beginning of the summer, and one at the conclusion of the program. An additional counseling session is scheduled with the director of the program to review academic records, to discuss future course selections, resources, and the personal comments section written by each participant in a simulated application process. Counseling provided throughout the summer covers a wide range of areas, including information on careers in the health care field, financial aid resources, medical school admissions and application procedures, and discussion of personal barriers, if any.

In summary, summer programs which are broad in scope offer students a well-rounded educational environment and a comprehensive view of health professional school life. Students who have participated in summer program experiences gain a realistic understanding of what it means to pursue a health professional education and career. This greater insight is often accompanied by a personal reaffirmation of interest and maintenance of motivation to pursue a health career. Moreover, it enables the student to make an intelligent decision about his career interests and abilities. Finally, adjustment to a health professions institutional environment should be easier as the result of the student's increased self-confidence and enhancement of self-image, particularly as he crosses the threshold of health professional training. In essence, the summer program experience reinforces a student's potential for success in completing health professional training and as a health professional in health care delivery.

BIBLIOGRAPHY

Summer Programs

Aranda, T. and Henry, J.L. "Academic Reinforcement Program." Journal of Dental Education 39(1975):782-785.

Ballard, D.P. et al. "The University of Kentucky SAMA Summer Program in Health Careers." Kentucky Medical Association 72(1974):215-217.

Birch, J.S. and Wolfe, S. "An Enrichment Program for Minority Students." Journal of Medical Education 50(1975):1059-1060.

Bryans, A.M. "The Summer School of Frontier Medicine, CAMSI Exchange—Inuvik 1967." Canadian Medical Association Journal 100(1969):512-515.

Bruhn, J.G. et al. "Follow-Up of Minority Pre-Medical Students Attending Summer Enrichment Programs in a Medical Setting." Texas Medicine 72(1976):87-90.

Davidson, C. and Creson, D.L. "A Summer Program for Minority Students in a Medical Setting—A Progress Report." Texas Reports on Biology and Medicine 29(1971):443-450.

Epps, A.C. "The Howard-Tulane Challenge: A Medical Education Reinforcement and Enrichment Program." Journal of the National Medical Association 67(1975):55-60.

Feldman, L.A. and Burnett, F.F. "Students for Medicine: A Program for the Preparation of Disadvantaged Students." Journal of Medical Education 48(1973):945-947.

Gaines, V.P. "Minority Recruitment and Retention." Journal of Medical Education 50(1975):416-417.

Jackson, R.E. "The Effectiveness of a Special Program for Minority Group Students." Journal of Medical Education 47(1972):620-624.

Lea, J. and Farias, H. "A Summer Health Sciences Experience for Minority Group Students." Journal of Medical Education 47(1972):903-904.

Levine, H.G. et al. "Six Years of Experience with a Summer Program for Minority Students." Journal of Medical Education 51(1976)735-742.

Ortiz, G. and Kendler, K.S. "The New York Medical College Summer Program: Remedial Education for Medical School Admission," Journal of Medical Education 49(1974):694-695.

Perry, R. et al. "A Follow-Up Evaluation of a Summer Health Career Program for Minority Students." Journal of Medical Education 51(1976):178-180.

Philips, B.U. et al. "A Formative and Summative Evaluation Model for Special Education Programs." Journal of Medical Education 51(1976):836-843.

Read, J.H. and Strick, F.L. "Medical Education and the Native Canadian: An Example of Mutual Symbiosis." Canadian Medical Association Journal 100(1969):515-520.

Roberts, D. and Plunkett, R.A. "Selected Keys to Open the Door to Minority Student Participation in Health Careers." Journal of Allied Health Winter 1974: 40-49.

Walker, T.J. "Pilot Summer Program in Medical and Life Science for Black Students." Journal of Medical Education 46(1971):537-539.

Waymouth, R.J. and Wergin, J. "Pilot Programs for Minority Students: One School's Experience." Journal of Medical Education 51 (1976):668-670.

Special Programs

Diekema, A.J. "The Medical Opportunities Program Revisited: An Assessment of Admission, Enrollment and Retention of Minority Students in Health Professional Schools." Association of Collegiate Registrars and Admissions Officers 50(1974):60-75.

Evans, T.E. "Training Black Physicians: The Current Status." Hospital Practice Sept. 1976:13.

Gardner, K.D. et al. "Minority Student Education at the University of Hawaii School of Medicine." Journal of Medical Education 47(1972):467-472.

Geertsma, R.H. "A Special Tutorial for Minority Medical Students: An Account of a Year's Experience." Journal of Medical Education 52(1977):396-403.

Heller, L.E. et al. "Academic Achievement of Baylor Work-Study Students." Texas Medicine 71(1975):92-94.

Jarecky, R.K. "Medical School Efforts to Increase Minority Representation in Medicine." Journal of Medical Education 44(1969):912-918.

Johnson, C.W. "Meharry's Special Medical and Research Programs," Journal of the National Medical Association 65(1973):307-308.

Kimball, C.P. "Yale's Program in Intracultural Medicine." Journal of Medical Education 45(1970):1032-1040.

Klapper, M.S. "The Alabama Experience in Minority Recruitment." Journal of the National Medical Association 65(1973):322-326.

Marshall, C.L. "Minority Students for Medicine and the Hazards of High School." Journal of Medical Education 48(1973):134-140.

Plagge, J.C. et al. "Increasing the Number of Minority Enrollees and Graduates: A Medical Opportunities Program." Journal of Medical Education 49(1974):735-745.

Quinones, M.A. and Harmon, W.H. "Training Minorities for Health Careers: The Newark Experience." Journal of Allied Health Fall 1975:19-24.

Richard, A.J. "Recruitment and Retention Programming for Minority Students Pursuing Allied Health Careers." Journal of Allied Health Fall 1975:36-38.

Robinson, J.D. "Meharry's Health Care Administration and Planning Program." Journal of the National Medical Association 65(1973):306.

Standeven, M. and Keck, K. "Developing Social Sensitivity through an Experiential Approach in Professional Education." Journal of Medical Education 48(1973):951-953.

General References through 1974

Adams, J.K. "Physician's Assistant: New Medical Profession." Opportunity August 1972:17-19.

Applewhite, H. "A New Design for Recruitment of Blacks into Health Careers" American Journal of Public Health 61(1971):1965-1971.

Blewett, W.E. "Minority Students' Special Needs and Recruitments." Journal of Allied Health 31(1974):22-25.

Bowers, John Z. "Negroes for Medicine: Report of a Conference." Journal of the American Medical Association 202(1967):141-142.

Diekema, A.J. and Hilton, W.J. "The Medical Opportunities Program: An Approach Toward Increasing Minority Enrollments in Health Professional Schools." College and University Spring 1972:201-211.

Early, J.L. "The Minority Experience." Journal of the American Pharmaceutical Association NS13(1973):87-88.

Evans, T.E. "Black Health Manpower: A Critical Concern." Black Collegian September 1973:22-26.

Golin, S. "Project Self-Esteem: Reactions of Middle- and Lower-Class Black Parents to an Elementary School Black Studies Program." Community Mental Health Journal 7(1971):331-338.

Grant, L. and Bennett, H. "The Buck Hill Falls Conference on Medical Education and the College-Medical School Interface." Journal of Medical Education 43(1968):1258-1267.

Green, R.A. "Solutions Needed for Medical School Admissions Problems." Journal of Medical Education 47(1972):974-976.

Haynes, M.A. and Dates, V.H. "Educational Opportunities in the Health Professions for Negroes in the State of Maryland." Journal of Medical Education 43(1968):1075-1082.

Hutchins, E.B. et al. "Minorities, Manpower and Medicine." Journal of Medical Education 42(1967):809-821.

Johnson, D. (National Committee for Careers in the Medical Laboratory) "Up the Career Ladder: How To Get the People Where They Want To Go." Modern Hospital 117(1971):75-89.

Johnson, D.G. "Conference in Preparation for Medical Education in Traditionally Negro Colleges." Journal of Medical Education 43(1968):933-935.

Lee, P.R. "Equal Opportunity—A Reality for Minority Students in the Health Professions?" Journal of the National Medical Association 61(1969):461-465.

Murphy, B. "Minorities in Medicine." Opportunity August 1972:4-16.

Nelson, B.W. et al. "Expanding Educational Opportunities in Medicine for Blacks and Other Minority Students." Journal of Medical Education 45(1970):731-736.

Nelson, B.W. et al. "Educational Pathway Analysis for the Study of Minority Representation in Medical School." Journal of Medical Education 46(1971):745-749.

Plaut, R.L. "Closing the Educational Gap." Journal of the National Medical Association 57(1965):447-451.

Ramsay, F.J. "Minority Recruitment to Medicine: The Maryland Experience." Journal of the National Medical Association 65(1973):497-500.

Richardson, E.L. "Meeting the Nation's Health Power Needs." Journal of Medical Education 47(1972):2-9.

Scott, K.R. and Rogers, A.L. "Recruitment and Retention of Black Students." Journal of the American Pharmaceutical Association NS13(1973):83-86.

Stepto, R.C. "Recruitment for Medicine by National Medical Fellowships, Inc." Journal of the National Medical Association 57(1965):444-446.

Swanson, A.G. "Black Student Recruitment at the University of Washington." Journal of the American Medical Association 209(1969):1077.

Thomas, A.L. "Project 75: A Program to Increase the Number of Minority Medical Students in U.S. Medical Schools." Journal of the American Medical Association 219(1971):1816-1818.

Thompson, T. "Curbing the Black Physician Manpower Shortage." Journal of Medical Education 49(1974):944-950.

United States Department of Health, Education and Welfare, Bureau of Health Manpower Education, Division of Physician and Health Professions Education. "Minority Groups in Medicine: Selected Biography." June 1972.

General References: 1975 through Present

Bingham, R.S. "Equity of Access." Civil Rights Digest 10(1978):772-775.

Bleich, M. "Funding of Minority Programs from the Private Sector, 1966-1976." Paper presented at the Annual Meeting of the AAAS, February 1976.

Bruhn, J.G. and Hrachovy, R.A. "Black College Students' Attitudes Toward Opportunities in the Health Professions." Journal of Medical Education 52(1977):847-849.

Burke, Y.B. "Minority Admissions to Medical Schools: Problems and Opportunities." Journal of Medical Education 52(1977):731-738.

Culp, R.W. "The Genesis of Black Pharmacists in America to 1900." Transactions and Studies of the College of Physicians of Philadelphia 42(1975):401-411.

"Dental School Enrollment." Bulletin of the Philadelphia City Dental Society December 1975:14-17.

Dresden, J.H. et al. "Cognitive and Non-Cognitive Characteristics of Minority Medical School Applicants." Journal of the National Medical Association 67(1975):321-323.

Dube, W.F. and Johnson, D.G. "Study of U.S. Medical School Applicants, 1974-1975." Journal of Medical Education 51(1976):877-896.

Evans, D.A. et al. "Traditional Criteria as Predictors of Minority Student Success in Medical School." Journal of Medical Education 50(1975):934-939.

Evans, D.A. et al. "Deans of Minority Students Affairs in Medical Schools." Journal of Medical Education 51(1976):197-199.

Feldbaum, E.G. et al. "Recruitment Strategies in the Health Professions." Program of Health Services Delivery, Bureau of Governmental Research: 209-214; 287-292; 376-383.

Johnson, D.G. "Recruitment and Progress of Minority Medical School Entrants, 1970-1972. A Cooperative Study by the SNMA and the AAMC." Journal of Medical Education 50(1975):713-755.

Johnson, D.G. and Sedlacek, W.E. "Retention by Sex and Race of 1968-1972 U.S. Medical School Entrants." Journal of Medical Education 50(1975):925-933.

Melnick, Vijaya L. and Hamilton, Franklin D. *Minorities in Science: The Challenge for Change in Biomedicine.* Plenum Press, New York, 1977.

Scott, H.W. "A Banner With A Strange Device, Excelsior!" Annals of Surgery 12(1977):772-775.

Sullivan, L.W. "The Morehouse Medical Education Program." Journal of the Medical Association of Georgia 64(1975):386-387.

Sullivan, L.W. "Testimony Before the Subcommittee on Health, Committee on Labor and Public Welfare, United States Senate." Journal of the National Medical Association 68(1976):250-251.

Sullivan, L.W. "The Education of Black Health Professionals." PHYLON 38(1977):181-193.

Weissmann, G. "Are We Reverting to the Pre-Flexner Era?" Hospital Practice 11(1976):35,43,46.

CHAPTER 8

Improving Your Study/Learning Skills

Laia Hanau

INTRODUCTION

There are three things with which I would like to open this chapter. One is that students are always complaining that their teachers only want them to regurgitate facts and don't allow them to think; and teachers are always complaining that students only regurgitate facts and don't know how to think. The teachers are right but the students are not at fault. All their lives teachers and parents say, "THINK!" and never, or rarely, tell them how to do it.

The second thing is that you must realize that it is no use to tell yourself that now you're going to really get down to studying and organizing your school work if you don't know *how* to study or organize material. You have to remember that motivation, counseling, affection, guidance, and sympathy are no substitutes for having the tools of learning.

The third thing is that a professional attitude toward studying/learning is something we all need to develop. We don't expect, in later life, at work or at home to have one excuse or another for not

Laia Hanau, M.A. (in Ed.), is Study Skills and Writing Consultant, and author of *The Study Game: How To Play and Win*, Lexington, Kentucky.

doing the job for which we are being paid. It is assumed that the teacher, whether the cellar has flooded or the pet dog has disappeared, will come into class and teach without whining or wailing about the problems of home or life. It isn't a bad idea to train ourselves to set aside our own whines and wails and do the work we have to do whether we like it or not. A student must be able to learn from any kind of teacher, loved or hated; learn any kind of material, interesting or mind dulling; organize any kind of information no matter how it is presented, ordered or chaotic. If we can't do this, then we've got problems, because no one else is able to do it for us.

THE STUDYING/LEARNING PROCESS

> Studying/learning is a process in which you
> (1) take in endless pieces of information
> (2) compact this information
> (3) establish routes for retrieving this information
> and (4) prepare yourself to reproduce this information.

It is a process which can easily be learned, like music, tennis, dancing, and basketball—but it takes time to perfect, as any activity of the body or mind takes time to perfect.

For the unskilled student the chill of Academic Shock, the first "D," hits sooner or later. For the best of students as for the worst of students, it usually hits at college in the early years. Since the best students tend to gravitate to the more difficult, competitive schools, their experience of Academic Shock is often greater than that of the less brilliant student's experience in a less competitive school.

The material in this chapter is therefore both for the less brilliant unskilled student and for the more brilliant unskilled student. If you are unskilled, whichever category you fall into, it is first useful to find out what the symptoms are that indicate you are unskilled, that you have study problems.

SYMPTOMS OF STUDY PROBLEMS

The symptoms of study problems are easily recognizable since they show up in various common situations. The basic problems are those of Organization, of Memorization, and of Time. They occur equally often: in the lecture-lab situation, the test-taking situation, the reading or talking (writing) situation, and the note-taking situation.

The Lecture-Lab Study Problem Symptoms

If you complain that the Instructor is disorganized, or throws in irrelevant material, or doesn't explain the stuff well enough, you may be saying that you have problems organizing information.

If you complain that the Instructor just wants you to regurgitate facts, or gives you too much unnecessary detail, you may be saying that you don't know how to memorize or retrieve information.

If you complain that the Instructor goes too fast or gives you too much work, you may be saying you are overwhelmed by the whole process of studying: you neither know how to organize or memorize material, and therefore Time becomes a study problem. But, give yourself this consolation . . . the sense of being over-whelmed means you have intelligence, although it is intelligence without adequate study skills.

The Test-Taking Study Problem Symptoms

If you complain that the test questions are ambiguous or that the test is not a fair one, you may be saying that you have problems organizing, memorizing, and retrieving information.

If you find yourself complaining about too many questions on insignificant details, it generally means that you don't know the significance of those details—which, in turn, means you don't know how to organize *details* of information (though you might do well on the organizing of *topics* of information).

If you find that tests are too long, it probably means the whole process of retrieving, organizing, and reproducing information quickly is something you don't know how to do.

If you "freeze" in an exam, if you "don't take tests well," if you are "test-shy," these are all nice words for saying you are an unskilled student. The reason why skilled students don't freeze in exams is because they have a sharp, clear command of their information, and know they can recall it through their test-taking skills. The intelligent but unskilled student freezes or panics because he/she does not have *conscious* techniques for retrieving information, and is panic-stricken about whether or not recall will come.

The Reading-Talking-Writing Study Problem Symptoms

Most people exhibit some symptoms in this general reading-talking-writing situation, whether in school or out. Some of us can't concentrate when we need to. Some of us can read rapidly, but write slowly. Others write rapidly but read slowly. Some of us answer a question with too much detail, others with too little detail. Most of us can understand what we read or hear, but can't tell anyone else with any kind of precision what was said. Others "feel" there's something wrong in what they're reading, but can't pinpoint the error without re-reading the article several times. Very few people know how to check out whether they actually know what they've been studying. (And many people study by constant repetition, going over notes, re-reading material . . . when, to study efficiently, you should never do the same thing twice with the same material.) If you hear any of these complaints from someone, you are hearing the symptoms of someone with a major study problem.

THE NOTE-TAKING STUDY PROBLEM SYMPTOMS

Most students take notes in a combination of outlining and getting down the key words. Unfortunately, very few lectures, discussions, or books stay rigorously with the standard school form of outlining. In the attempt to force the material into the standard outline form, you come up with a confused and misleading set of notes. Unfortunately, too, almost no students can tell you what a Key Word is, nor how to recognize it. In their attempt to eliminate all but the Key Words, they leave out the critical, essential words that would make their note information correct and easily retrievable to the mind.

For example, these are notes taken by a college freshman in an ancient history course. They are the work of an unskilled student—a combination of outlining and Key Word note-taking:

Only former authority for knowledge of ancient world—
Herodotus and Bible
  Scientific Method
    1. Ancient stone—key
Discovery of Rosetta stone, giving key to hierogylphic and
demotic language opens up antique history—19th century,
knowledge of antiquity *now* gained by actual research.

Egypt discovered solar year in 4241 BC, July 19
    1. Life in Thebes and Memphis
        Knowledge gained from remains, pictures, etc.,
      houses high, grain sorted by being thrown in air,
        Trinkets used for money
      Age of Unification had 3 causes: Nile—natural
      roadway, shut in from outsiders, fertile country

        In Assyria—case is opposite. Euphrates open
        to ingress

    History of Euphrates Valley began after Egypt's
      civilization

These notes give us a series of facts. These notes also tell us that the student uses sentences sometimes and sometimes not—but doesn't know why he does either. He hears facts, but doesn't know how they tie together. To "go over" his notes he will have to (1) re-read them verbatim, (2) read a text to figure out why each fact was given when it was (e.g., there are three causes of unification given: Assyria is stated as opposite to Egypt—but in how many ways? Only one opposite is given), and (3) he will end up talking to other students to find out what was missing in his own notes. He will then pray that it has all somehow gotten into his head by osmosis. And he still won't know, from his key-word-and-outline notes, the three essential things a skilled student knows within fifteen minutes of looking at his notes: what he knows, what he doesn't know, and what is fuzz in his head.

A skilled student would have taken his notes in class like this, with the words in parentheses added soon after class when he looks over his notes:

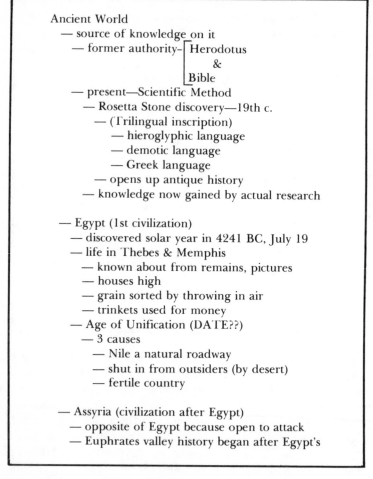

```
Ancient World
    — source of knowledge on it
        — former authority-⌈ Herodotus
                          |        &
                          ⌊ Bible
        — present—Scientific Method
        — Rosetta Stone discovery—19th c.
            — (Trilingual inscription)
                — hieroglyphic language
                — demotic language
                — Greek language
            — opens up antique history
            — knowledge now gained by actual research

    — Egypt (1st civilization)
        — discovered solar year in 4241 BC, July 19
        — life in Thebes & Memphis
            — known about from remains, pictures
            — houses high
            — grain sorted by throwing in air
            — trinkets used for money
        — Age of Unification (DATE??)
            — 3 causes
                — Nile a natural roadway
                — shut in from outsiders (by desert)
                — fertile country

    — Assyria (civilization after Egypt)
        — opposite of Egypt because open to attack
        — Euphrates valley history began after Egypt's
```

These notes, which incidentally have exactly the same number of words as the first set, are the notes of a student who knows how to listen, how to find/recognize the key words, how to use a skillful variation of outline form, and how to cut his study time in half. But the first set of notes indicates that that student should improve all his study skills so that he can at least take efficient notes.

AREAS IN WHICH STUDY PROBLEMS
SHOW UP

There are six areas in which students need the skilled techniques of studying/learning:

BEFORE EXAM TIME
— *Lectures* require an ability to deal with
— Definitions
— Note-taking
— Organization of content

— *Reading* requires an ability to deal with
— Definitions
— Note-taking
— Comprehension
— Speed

— *Laboratory* (x-rays, graphs, diagrams, charts . . . visual information)
         requires an ability to deal with
— Directions
— Memorizing (and recall)

AT EXAM TIME
— *Exam preparation* requires an ability for
— Organizing on a larger scale
— Checking out what has already been memorized
— Memorizing (and recall)

— *Exam taking* requires an ability for
— Question analysis
— Recall (and memorizing)
— Writing for essay-type answers

FOR COMMUNICATING YOUR INFORMATION
— *Writing-talking* requires an ability to deal with
— Definitions
— Note-MAKING
— Organization of content

To check out your level of study skills, compare your own study time with that of a skilled student, below. When a student is really in command of an efficient, conscious system for organizing and memorizing material, the time required to complete his studying and get above B grades is as follows:

. . *each lecture* will need about 10-15 minutes for after class organization of material, and no further review of the lecture will be necessary until a topic (from several lectures) is completed.

When a topic is completed, about 30 minutes is required to do the larger scale organization as preparation for an exam on that topic.

. . *textbook reading* on supplementary material covering the *same* information as that in the properly organized lecture notes can be read at the rate of 30-50 pages an hour.

. . *lab material* (visual information) including specimens, graphs, etc., of average difficulty can be learned in about one minute, and the student will have about 70% recall at exam time without review. With review the recall will exceed 85%.

. . *exam preparation* will take 3 to 6 hours for an hour-exam. If it takes longer than this amount, the student does not know how to consciously prepare his material from lecture, lab, and text.

. . *exam taking* will have a specific procedure for the student to follow for both essay-type and multiple-choice type questions. Peace should exist, not panic, in the exam taking situation; the student will know how to start the retrieval of information, and the organization of it for answers.

. . *writing* is an orderly process that can be carried out at broken intervals. It is not necessary to clear a space in time such as a full evening, or a weekend in order to organize and write a paper. All changes and revisions are done in the note-making stage, and all outlining is checked out constantly as it is revised. (We are talking here about writing-to-convey-information, not writing with or for literary style.)

If you can't complete your studying within the time frame given above, and get B or better grades, then you don't know how to study properly and efficiently.

THE BASIS OF THE STUDY PROBLEMS in these six areas (above) is always the same: a lack of efficient, *conscious* techniques for organizing or memorizing information. In the laboratory area, in the exam preparation area, and in the exam-taking area, memorizing and recall are two sides of the same coin: in the process of memorizing material you should be setting up the patterns for recalling or retrieving it. In every other item that must be dealt with—definitions, note-taking, checking, reading directions, etc.— the problem is one of "conscious organization."

> (In the most basic sense, all study problems come down to not knowing how to compact information into error-free, organized, hierarchic patterns, because efficient memorization and information retrieval will only occur from the development of such patterns.)

If you do not have conscious techniques for organizing or memorizing material that comes at you in lecture and lab; that has to be dug out in reading and in exam preparation; or that must be created in writing and talking, you are relying on your subconscious mind to do the work for you. If your method of studying is to read and re-read, underline and re-read the same material over and over, this is a strong indication that you do not consciously know how to learn.

The problem becomes more acute as you move from elementary school, through high school, college, career training, professional school, and on-the-job training in whatever area of the working world you find yourself. The problem can at any stage become acute and devastating to both your performance and your self-image because as you move along, the content you get is greater, the repetition is less, and you have less time (in school or in jobs) to read, re-read, and re-read. Therefore, your subconscious mind has less time in which to do the work of organizing the material for you. And you can never count on the stuff somehow getting itself organized in your head in time for the exam. This, in turn, puts many students into a state of anxiety which, in its turn, causes the "freeze" at exam time.

CAUSES OF THIS BASIC STUDY PROBLEM

Technical Causes

The first of the technical causes is this reliance on our subconscious minds to absorb and organize the material to be learned, and therefore our failure to develop conscious techniques for learning.

Most of us have had the experience of reaching the end of a course and having a sudden insight into what it was all about and how to study for it—too late to do it, but suddenly realizing how it could have been done easily. This is about what happens when we rely on our subconscious minds to finish their work, and hand up the organization for us to use. You somehow feel like an idiot for not figuring out how to study the course earlier. But, as long as the work of organizing information is being done by your subconscious mind, you have no control over the time schedule. When you have efficient and conscious techniques for learning, you can control your own time schedule, and you don't need time "to absorb the material." The courses do not go too fast.

We have come to this reliance on the subconscious by subtle pathways. (1) While we were young we came to think that that was the way organizing got done—through the subconscious mind. All through school years, our parents, teachers, and other students have spoken with awe and respect of the student who didn't crack a book, or of someone who looked over the material once, and topped the class. There was an aura about the student, about people with an intuitive, innate ability to learn. (2) Our subconscious reactions, instead of our self-directed mental processes, were and are constantly being brought into play by our environment which is constantly asking "What do you think about it?," and "Think about that chapter," and "Tell me what you think."

Since you have no idea what you're supposed to do "to think," you wait for something to formulate in your mind, i.e., you wait for your subconscious mind to do something and flip up something for you to say. In all this constant questioning and telling you to think throughout your school years, your reactions are being called into play, not your self-directed, conscious capacity for organizing and then analyzing what you have organized—which is the process of thinking. The questions that should have been asked were "Precisely what was *said*? How do you know that is what was said? Are there any flaws in what was said? How do you know that is a flaw?" These questions, at least, would require the development (and teaching) of conscious methods of learning.

The second of the technical causes for the basic study problem is the reliance on repetition of a process as a study technique. At some point repetition will collapse as a study technique. When you read and underline, then read and highlight, then read and review, then read and memorize, time eventually becomes your enemy. If there were all the time in the world, the subconscious mind could deal with large amounts of material, but there is never enough time. Repetition of a process dulls the mind. You could double the amount of time and repetition you put into your studying and still not do much better on an exam. With few exceptions, the students who use repetition as a study technique overwork and under-achieve.

The third of the technical causes is the lack of knowledge on how to take notes and fix them up. The techniques of skilled, hierarchic note-taking are not generally known. (Taking notes in the hierarchic format* places the various items of information on comparable levels of classifications.) The standard school outline format cannot be counted on to deal with the variety of lectures and texts with their endless variations of "outlines." It is essential that a student face the reality that neither people nor books can be counted upon to write and talk in an outline form that suits the student's knowledge. Therefore, fortunately or unfortunately, it becomes the business of the student to learn how to take notes from any kind of speaker and book.

Assuming, however, that you are a student who gets down fairly complete and accurate information from a lecture or text, the question of skill in fixing up those notes then comes in. Most students don't know how to fix up their notes so that only a glance at them is needed to recall and review the material (hierarchic format*). Most students "fix-up" their notes by underlining what they feel is important or to be emphasized. As a rule they have no conscious criteria for why they feel this or that is important, should be indented, should be underlined, should be memorized, etc.

---

* For those who want to learn more about the techniques I recommend for improving study skills, I refer them to my book: Hanau, L., *The Study Game, How To Play and Win,* Harper & Row, Publishers, Inc., 1978, New York, N.Y.

A fourth of the technical causes is the lack of conscious test-taking techniques. This subject is discussed elsewhere in this book.

Psychological Causes

The belief or feeling that the material you have to learn should be made interesting to you may be, psychologically, one of the most damaging ideas that has ever evolved in the head of any student: it becomes a persistent excuse for not studying something that doesn't interest you.

In the early grades a great deal of effort is expended to interest the children in what they are doing and what they have to learn. This may be correct for children in the very early grades, but after Sesame Street time is passed, you should not expect your instructors or your books to interest you in the material you have to learn. Unfortunately, many of us don't get past the Sesame Street stage of expectation . . . we feel we have a "right" to have material made interesting to us. Why should stuff be made interesting to us? We're the ones who need the knowledge, not the teacher. The facts remain: to pass your courses, in school or in on-the-job training, you are often going to have to learn from teachers you find uninteresting, and books you find enormously dull. Poor teachers and dull textbooks are things a skilled student learns to deal with as efficiently and as rapidly as possible. For example, never cut the class of a subject you're not interested in. If you go to class, take proper notes, and spend fifteen minutes fixing them up,* you will save yourself four or five hours of reading in the subject you're not interested in.

One of the most profound psychological causes for not developing conscious study techniques is that we like the Aura of Potential which we, and others, have draped about us. "He has potential," and "She really has tremendous potential," and "He isn't working up to his potential," and "Very quick," "Very bright" . . . all these phrases settle very quickly over masses of young children because the environment—parents, teachers, friends—in an honest effort to give us a good self-image, encourage and praise us. And we take out of that praise and encouragement the idea that in some way we

---

* Hanau, *ibid.*

are special, gifted, have high potential. Then, very naturally, we come to enjoy the aura of "special" that envelopes us. It is a shock when we come up against the stiffer competition of high school and college where we are no longer able to maintain high grades.

You know you studied for the tests—you studied secretly, but you studied—and the grades you made weren't A's, sometimes not even B's. You also know you're not going to run around shouting at the world, "I'm not as smart as you told me I was!" So what is left is a choice between two opposites: You can work like the devil, get good but not brilliant grades, and have people murmur that you don't have potential after all. Or you can quit working, let the grades come out poor to failing, and have people murmur, "Tsk . . . such a waste . . . not challenged . . . such potential . . . psychological block."

If you decide to quit working, there are lots of phrases left around by those who preceded you on the not-working path, such as: "This stuff isn't relevant." "I could get the grades but I don't feel like putting in the work—I've got more important things to do." "I'm going to quit school and see what life is all about." It is hard to give up the aura of potential.

We would all live up to our potential if we knew how. As far as school is concerned, there is no accurate way to gauge your potential, what you have the capacity to achieve, unless you have first tackled the school work with a set of skilled, conscious techniques for studying and learning.

A third psychological cause of study problems is the poor self-image, the feeling of ineffectualness. It is as incapacitating as the I-have-potential problem, but it is far more easily solved. A poor self-image in relation to the school-world comes essentially from a lack of good study techniques. It is not, at first, an image picked up from other people's concept of our capacities. It usually grows as a result of being in school and having no voice in the right-or-wrong decision making process. For example, in school, at whatever level of note-taking, outlining, or interpretation, the *teacher* is the one who says whether you are right or wrong in what you've done. You have *no method of checking* your own work, no method of fighting the teacher's decision. Other students get it right, but the reasons are never crystal clear to you why his outline is right and her outline isn't as right. You begin to think that everyone also knows something you don't because you're never able to tell whether your notes, or your outline, or your interpretation is correct until the teacher tells you one way or another.

Choosing the main idea, finding the key words add to our sense of ineffectualness. The teacher or the book says what the main idea is and what the key words are. If you differ, you are wrong. Why you're wrong, you don't know. So the feeling grows in you that you just aren't much good at school stuff because trying doesn't get you anywhere. Pretty soon you give up trying.

Then you get yelled at to "THINK!" and "CONCENTRATE!" Since you don't know how to do either, and no one tells you how to do either, you figure you're just deficient not only about rights-and-wrongs, main ideas and key words, but also about thinking and concentrating.

Actually the only deficiency you have is that you never found a set of good, skillful study techniques that would show you how to check out the rights-and-wrongs, the main ideas and key words and interpretations. And show you how to think and concentrate. Almost without exception, not-thinking and not-concentrating both come from not knowing the sequence of processes through which the mind learns academic material.* It is perfectly natural for most of us to find our minds wandering during the second and third times we re-read our textbooks and notes. Why shouldn't it wander? We haven't told it what else to do, where to go, how to proceed, what new task to complete with the new re-reading of the material. Of course the mind wanders. And it takes a great deal of will power to make it keep coming back to the page.

The trick about concentrating, and the trick about thinking, is the same as the trick about efficient studying: *Never do the same thing with the same material twice.**

WHAT TO LOOK FOR IN STUDY SKILLS MATERIALS ON THE MARKET

Of first importance is to recognize that our study problems can be solved. The basis of these problems is our reliance on unconscious techniques and on repetition for organizing and memorizing material. If we know how to study and learn, *consciously* know what

---

* Hanau, *ibid.*

procedures to follow and in what order, then the technical causes of study problems can be consciously dealt with. Once they are taken care of, the psychological problems can be looked at realistically because we will at last find out what our actual learning potential is, and realistically deal with the praise or the condemnation that our environment feeds into us.

A study system that works for us must be a clearly stated, self-checking, and conscious system that we can depend upon to be there in times of crisis (tests, papers, reports, deadlines, etc.) There are many study systems presented in and out of the schools. The national evidence of poor scholastic achievement suggests that the systems most in use are not working well, and the overwhelming numbers of students suffering academic shock their first years in college will vouch for the fact that the study systems they were taught in high school were not adequate for college and career level work.

Examining a study system to see if you want to use it means looking at whether it will teach you how to handle very large amounts of material, whether it is self-checking, and whether it establishes routes for retrieving information. *The Study Game*, already referred to,* deals with these problems in a simple enough manner so that a student can learn the system on his own or with an instructor. It breaks information into two elements, then uses these two elements to organize, analyze, write, deal with essay-type and multiple-choice questions, recognize and write definitions, and using these elements tries to show the reasons for different grades that students get in the same course. Most importantly it is a self-checking system that gives the techniques of compacting information (hierarchic system) in such a way that it is easily retrievable. The Hanau system essentially identifies the sequence of processes through which the mind of a good student moves to learn material today. All knowledge exists in a hierarchy which is constantly shifting—a series of units of information encompassed in larger and ever larger units. The direction of *The Study Game* is to teach the student how to compact knowledge for the Information Age in which we now exist—to compact information in an ordered hierarchical system that makes the information easily retrievable to the mind.

---

* Hanau, *ibid.*

Outline Series books are excellent study aids, and should be looked at and if possible used in all your courses. These books condense and outline the factual knowledge, extracting the essentials of the course materials. Many skilled students use them all the time as reference guides, being careful to adapt the outline series book to the requirements and information of their course.

These outline materials, like the outlines and charts that you borrow from other students, are similar to having a tutor for the course. They will help you through the course but will not teach you how to learn a course on your own. And some courses, and most job-training courses, do not have Outline Series books for their material.

Reading Development courses are designed to improve your capacity to deal with written and spoken material by increasing both your vocabulary and your comprehension skills. They are not designed to teach you how to compact large bodies of information into easily retrievable material. But, it is self-evident that you must be able to read well enough to understand the course work before you can apply any study system to it. The Hanau book will help speed up comprehension, but not teach the basics of the comprehension skills.

CONCLUSION

We are not all born scholars or intellectuals, and the great highways of the mind cannot be traveled by all of us. Most of us don't want to travel those great highways; we want to know how to handle the ordinary work of the world, in school and out. And all of us can, if we know how to learn.

CHAPTER 9

Preparing Students for Examinations

Barbara M. Jarecky

INTRODUCTION

Taking examinations is a fact of life for all students. As early as grammar school and certainly by high school, students have been tested and retested in order to evaluate their performance in a variety of subjects and skills. Many students experience difficulty in performing well on examinations. For these students test taking is a highly anxiety producing and ego shattering experience. Minority and other culturally and educationally disadvantaged students, as a group, consistently have achieved somewhat lower scores on nationally administered multiple-choice examinations than have their more advantaged majority counterparts.

In an effort to overcome this differential between groups, a variety of ameliorative measures have been tried, including the development of an entirely new examination for medical school admissions: the "New" Medical College Admission Test. Persons who are involved in programs of recruitment and retention of minority and disadvantaged students have developed various

Barbara M. Jarecky is Coordinator for Academic Support Services, Health Career Opportunity Office, University of Kentucky, Lexington, Kentucky.

methods to help these students perform well on examinations. On the path to becoming a practicing physician, there are two national examination hurdles which must be crossed: the Medical College Admission Test (MCAT) for admissions and the Medical National Boards or the Federation Licensing Examination (FLEX) for licensure. In addition, medical students are faced with the on-going challenge of course examinations while they are in medical school.

As a result of the move during the early 1970s by the majority of medical schools to admit more disadvantaged and minority students, it has become increasingly important that these students do well first on the MCAT to be competitive for a place in a medical school class and then, once admitted, to do well enough in course examinations that they will be graduated and then licensed to practice.

Schools which are particularly interested in establishing admissions and retention programs for the disadvantaged include in their programs opportunities to teach test-taking skills. The purpose of this chapter is to describe how students may be prepared to take examinations. Observations of students encountering problems with test-taking show that they are deficient in either or both of two areas, information needed to answer the questions and skills related to taking multiple-choice examinations. The most common problem students have with exams is a lack of sufficient information to answer the questions. It may be that the information was never acquired or it was learned and then forgotten, or the student knows the information but fails to recognize when it is appropriate to use it to answer a particular question.

In order to overcome the information problem, any examination preparation program should include diagnostic procedures which will allow a counselor or tutor to pinpoint those topics which a student never learned, forgot, or did not organize sufficiently to answer the questions. If this diagnostic procedure is successful, then the student on his or her own or with the help of a tutor can fill in the information gaps.

There is also a significant number of students who have learned and remembered enough information to do well on an exam but are so distracted by the way in which a question is asked or by the format of the item that they perform poorly in spite of their knowledge. It is for these students that examination-taking skills are taught. These skills should include strategies for interpreting directions, selecting the "best" answer from among the possible choices, managing time in order to answer all the questions, and making use of "guessing" techniques when the correct answer is not immediately obvious.

In addition, even skillful, knowledgeable test-takers can have a sufficiently high level of anxiety concerning the examination-taking experience that it interferes with their performance. A number of examination-preparation programs teach students physical relaxation techniques and/or desensitization procedures so that the students can lower their anxiety levels. Physical relaxation techniques usually involve methods by which students are trained to relax specific muscle groups. Part of the training involves heightening student awareness of those muscles that are contracted when they are tense and anxious. Students learn that when this happens, the tension building behavior can be interrupted by relaxing the whole body or the tense muscles only. Test anxiety desensitization procedures are usually very specific. The general procedures, however, could be applied to any anxiety-producing situation once the student has become skillful in the technique. The techniques themselves involve forming pleasant associations and pleasing mental images of real or imagined experiences. The students are directed to focus their thoughts on such images as soon as they feel anxiety related to a testing situation. In this way pleasant rather than anxiety-producing thoughts come to mind. However, some anxiety is often helpful to keep students working carefully through the test. Students refer to this as being "up" for an examination, that is, alert and ready to select their best answer for every item.

Preparing students for examinations can be done on a one-to-one basis with a counselor or tutor, or it can be done in large or small group meetings. The selection of the mode of preparation will depend upon student needs and, of course, upon the resources available. For an overview of the information and skills needed for a particular examination, a group setting is sufficient. For an individual student who needs to improve a past performance, the one-to-one situation is indicated in order to gear the sessions to help solve individual problems.

If an institution wishes to offer only group sessions for an overview, it can hire outside consultants to give one or two-day workshops. However, if several students need to improve their test performance, a person should be employed by the school preferably full-time. The person so employed will most likely be the one who has responsibility for the general learning skills program of which examination preparation is a part. The financial burden to an institution will depend on the salary or consulting fee for the instructor plus whatever materials are needed to conduct the group or individual work sessions.

TYPES OF EXAMINATION PREPARATION PROGRAMS

Pre-entrance Preparation Programs—MCAT

The first type of examination preparation program that either an undergraduate or medical school might initiate is a program for the Medical College Admission Test (MCAT). An undergraduate school may wish to develop such a program in order to enhance its students' opportunities for acceptance to medical school and its own reputation for having a sound premedical program. A medical school might provide instruction in test-taking as part of its recruitment of non-traditional students, either in a summer program or as a series of one-day workshops during the school year.

The MCAT assesses student knowledge and skills in four parts: science knowledge, science problems, reading skills, and quantitative skills.

Science Knowledge

Items in this subtest require "one best answer." The items include a stem, which may consist of a short paragraph, a diagram, a chart, or a formula. The stem is followed by three to five alternatives, one of which is the best or keyed answer. The student needs to recall factual information very rapidly to complete this test within the time allowed. The information should have been acquired in courses in biology, general and organic chemistry, and physics, and most of it will be at the first-course level.

Science Problems

The test items in this subtest also require "one best answer." Scientific information is presented mostly in paragraphs and formulas and followed by three test items pertaining to the information. They test the students' ability to apply factual information in solving problems in biology, general and organic chemistry, and physics.

Reading Skills

The items in this subtest require the student to (1) identify the "one best answer" or (2) determine whether a statement "supports, contradicts, or neither supports nor contradicts" information presented in a reading passage. Each passage is followed by several items. Students should apply only that information presented in the passage, not any prior information they may have, in selecting responses to these items. This section of the MCAT tests students' skills in comprehension, evaluation, and use of various types of information. The content of the reading passages may include subject matter from the natural and social sciences and medically related topics similar to what is found in medical textbooks.

Quantitative Skills

The items in this subtest also require the student to (1) identify the "one best answer" or (2) determine whether a statement "supports, contradicts, or neither supports nor contradicts" information presented mostly in charts, tables, or graphs. Students will need to apply only data presented in the test booklet for the necessary computations and interpretations. This part of the MCAT tests ability to carry out calculations on scientific data and to interpret and synthesize scientific findings.

Scoring of the MCAT

A student who has taken the MCAT receives six scaled scores, each of which may range anywhere from 1 to 15. A separate score is reported for biology, chemistry and physics, science problems, reading skills, and quantitative skills. There is a tendency for both a student and a school to average these six scores. Such an average is meaningless in assessing overall performance because items on the science problems subtest are counted twice, once to the total score for the science problems subtest and once again in the achievement scores in biology, chemistry, and physics. All the reported scaled scores reveal about an applicant is his or her performance in relationship to the other individuals who took the examination. An applicant's relative standing can also be compared for each of the six areas of assessment. The scaled scores are a conversion of the raw scores which have little or no meaning in assessing performance.

Reported percentile scores range from 0 to 99.9. This allows for comparison of all students sitting for a particular administration of the MCAT. Students can easily determine where they rank vis à vis all other candidates on each subtest.

Uses Made of the MCAT Scores by Admissions Committees and Students

Medical school admissions committees use MCAT scores to assess student potential for success mainly in the basic science portion of the medical school curriculum. The MCAT is the only totally external evaluation device that a school has to compare knowledge and skills as tested on a national examination that is identical for all students taking it at one specified time. In most cases, students who do well in college and have high GPAs should expect to perform acceptably on the MCAT. Admissions committees use the test to a certain extent to confirm college performance. A student who has a modest GPA can impress a committee with high scores on the MCAT. On the other hand, someone with a high GPA and low MCAT scores often makes committees uneasy about the soundness of the applicant's academic preparation.

Students can use their reported scores to assess their own performance and to make decisions about whether or not to retake the examination. If they decide to retake it, they can use the first scores to pinpoint those areas in which they need to improve their performance. Since scores are reported separately for biology, chemistry, and physics, students are able to determine which subject(s) they need to review.

Methods to Overcome Problems with the MCAT

The more familiar a student is with a particular type of examination, the more comfortable the experience of actually taking that examination becomes. The test-taking process is a process of applying information and skills that one has learned or developed prior to selecting answers to a series of any test items. During the item-answering process, the student does not acquire any more information than he or she already knows about a topic, nor does he or she learn any new skills but can only use to the best advantage knowledge and skills previously acquired. Therefore, in order to maximize the opportunity to do well, examination preparation programs are helpful. Basically they serve three purposes: first, to present sufficient information about the topics to be covered; second, to teach examination-taking techniques for answering different item types and formats; and third, to help the student feel comfortable with the examination-taking process so that feelings of anxiety do not interfere with performance. Examination preparation programs for the MCAT should address each of these three general purposes.

1. *Information*

The New MCAT Student Manual published by the Association of American Medical Colleges in Washington, D.C. contains the most accurate set of questions that can be used to analyze a student's level of information, particularly on the subtests of science knowledge and science problems. The questions are related to the science subtopics which appear on pages 6 through 11 in the Manual. Areas of weakness can be determined by how many items a student misses in each subtopic. For the reading and quantitative subtests, descriptions of the specific skills tested are given on pages 16 through 18. These descriptions can be used to analyze student performance by noting which skills were the weakest as determined by items missed. In order to help students fill in the gaps in their skills and knowledge, review sessions which teach content information can be held. In lieu of or in addition to the review sessions, there are commercially prepared review books on the general textbook market which give additional practice items. In many cases, these review books also include summary information about the science and mathematics topics. For those students who have previously performed poorly on the MCAT and who in addition have both time and money, there are review courses given by commercial concerns at centers throughout the United States. Students should not depend solely on an undergraduate or medical school to provide formal review sessions; a counselor or a tutor can provide direction för much of the content and skill preparation to be done by the students on their own.

2. *Skills*

There are two item formats used for the MCAT. The items are either "One Best Answer," that is, a stem followed by three to five possible alternative answers or completions, or a statement "Supports, Contradicts or Neither Supports nor Contradicts" information given. Workshops and practice sessions for these two types of items help students develop skills in the decision-making process needed to select a best answer or to make a determination about the quality of the information given. On the day of the examination, skills should be sufficiently automatic that all the students' energy can be used in applying information. In order to help students develop skills, MCAT items types can be included in regular undergraduate course examinations during the school year.

Examination-taking preparation for science knowledge and science problems subtests should include instruction for analyzing the stem, the intent of the question, and for turning each of the alternatives into a series of true-false statements in order to improve the students' decision-making process. Since on the MCAT there is no penalty for guessing, students should be directed to mark answers for all the questions, particularly if they are in danger of running out of time. Since speed is essential the techniques should include pacing and time-management skills in addition to strategies for guessing or applying incomplete information.

Examination-taking techniques for the reading and quantitative skills subtests should include instructions to students on how to make true-false decisions for each of the item alternatives offered and to become efficient in making these decisions. Students should be told to read the test items first and then the passage or problem to which the items relate. This will help students identify the information they need to select the correct response. In addition, students should underline pertinent words in the reading passage or problem and make margin notations to help them relocate the critical information.

3. *Anxiety*

Since the MCAT is 7½ hours in length, it is both intellectually and physically demanding. One of the ways to overcome anxiety associated with this experience is to offer a simulated testing situation which parallels the actual administration. In order to do this, practice tests in the Manual can be used. Other ways are to familiarize the students with the directions which accompany each subtest, the time limits associated with each part, and how many items must be answered in the allotted time. Students who have prepared for the MCAT by checking their level of information and are reasonably confident they know enough to answer most of the questions, who through practice are skillful decision-makers with each item type, and who maintain a low level of anxiety about the examination-taking process should be able to do well on the test. Since the MCAT examination is so lengthy students should be counseled to make plans to get sufficient sleep not only the night before the test, but the two previous nights as well in order to be rested, fresh, and relaxed. Test anxiety is more difficult to handle if the student has gone without sufficient rest for a relatively long period of time. If restful sleep is not possible for some students before an examination, then physical relaxation techniques can be taught to aid these students to secure proper rest.

COURSE EXAMINATIONS DURING
MEDICAL SCHOOL

Once students have been admitted to medical school and are taking first-year courses, they are faced with their second type of major examination-taking situation—medical school course examinations. These examinations are constructed by departmental faculties at the individual medical schools. Most of the examinations are multiple-choice and are usually patterned after the National Board Examinations. These item types include "One Best Answer," "Matching," "Matching Pairs," and "Multiple True-False."

One Best Answer items consist of a stem which is an open-ended statement or a direct question followed by four or five alternative answers, only one of which is the best or correct answer.

The Matching item is a list of four or five alternative answers followed by a series of items, each of which matches with only one of the alternatives.

Matching Pairs items consist of a leading list of two answers plus the statements "both" and "neither," followed by a series of questions which relate to one or both or neither of the two possible answers.

Multiple True-False items consist of a stem followed by four alternative answers, any number of which can be correct answers for the stem of the item.

In addition to the five most commonly used multiple-choice item formats, most medical schools make use of some student-generated response items. These include "Essay," "Short answer," and "Fill-in-the Blank." Essay questions require a student to organize general principles as they relate to planning a method, a process, a procedure, a theory, or an idea. Students are often called upon to contrast and compare methods and steps in this item type. In short answer and fill-in-the-blank items, students are more often called upon to recall only specific details about a structure, formula, or technique.

There are two basic methods of evaluating student performance. A school or individual department may choose either criterion or norm-referenced examinations. Criterion-referenced examinations generally have a predetermined pass level and the questions are all referenced to written behavioral objectives which are given to each student prior to the examination.

Norm-referenced examinations generally have no predetermined pass level and may or may not directly relate to previously stated objectives. In this case students are competing against each other for grades, and usually some percentage of a class will fail the examination because their information was considerably less than the majority of their fellow students. On the other hand, with criterion-referenced examinations it is possible for all students not only to pass but get 100 percent correct (although they rarely do so).

Medical school examinations are used to evaluate individual students' performance in each of their courses and to monitor their progress through a particular curriculum. Course examinations can be used to help a student to assess his or her own performance relative to other classmates and/or the learning objectives set forth by the course instructor. Besides reflecting course performance, medical school course grades are frequently used as an important element in selection for graduate medical education, such as residency and post-doctoral fellowship programs.

From time to time in medical school, students experience difficulty with course examinations. The question always asked is: "How is it possible that students could experience difficulty with course examinations when to be admitted to medical school in the first place they had to have demonstrated such superior ability in undergraduate school and on the MCAT?" The answer seems to be one of degree, not of kind. The medical school curriculum requires students to learn more information in a shorter period of time than was ever required before. In addition, they must have a greater understanding of relationships among details of information. For these reasons, examination preparation sessions are most successful as a part of a larger learning skills program such as is discussed in Chapter 8.

Methods to Overcome Student Problems with Course Examinations

If a medical school has someone available to help students overcome examination-taking problems, then when a student experiences such difficulty an appointment can be made to assess the problem and to begin remedial procedures. Unfortunately that is not always an easy thing for a student to do because of pride or embarrassment. In order to help the student overcome reluctance, if any, to work on a test-taking problem, a referral service is helpful. The student's advisor, course instructor, Dean of Students, or the school's Academic Performance Committee can be helpful in this regard. However, it is best to identify students with test-taking problems during freshman orientation when examination-taking techniques are presented by the same individual who will offer that support service during the school year. Such an individual can identify quickly students who need assistance and start them promptly in a correction program.

When students experience problems on course examinations and come to the learning skills counselor for help, the problem, from their point of view, is usually that they really know the information but the questions were so poorly written that they were not able to demonstrate their full range of knowledge. Rarely is this entirely true. Most often the problem lies with either a lack of information or of examination-taking skills.

Method 1. In order to determine specific problems, an analysis of the previous performance is necessary. These sessions must be done with an individual student on a one-to-one basis. A determination should be made for each question that was missed as to whether the student really did have sufficient information in order to answer it. If he/she had the information, was it lack of skill in determining what was being asked for or was it distraction by the item type which caused an incorrect answer?

Method 2. If the problem was a lack of information, a return to the course objective which covered that item should point up the deficits in the information. If there are no objectives, a return to the classroom lecture notes, syllabus, or textbooks would be necessary.

Method 3. In the case of the student who has sufficient information but doesn't seem to be able to apply it on the examination, then test-taking techniques should be taught. These sessions should include techniques for interpreting directions, analysis of item intent, and a technique for turning each multiple-choice item into a series of true-false statements. In the case of student-generated response items, the techniques should include methods for analyzing the items and organizing answers.

Method 4. From time to time we see students who are knowledgeable and skillful but find both the pressures experienced in medical school and anxiety over the test-taking situation so overwhelming that they interfere with their performance. For these students sessions in either test-taking desensitization or physical relaxation techniques are helpful.

Yet another way to reduce anxiety is, from the very beginning, to include as a part of the medical school orientation program, such features as general test-taking techniques and the matching of test items from previous years with course objectives or text and syllabus. An analysis of and some practice sessions on the use of the item formats a student is likely to encounter in first-year courses tends to reduce some of the anxiety caused by fear of the unknown and should reduce the number of problems encountered during the first series of examinations.

LICENSURE EXAMINATIONS

On the pathway to becoming a practicing physician, the final examinations are those for licensure. For students who have received the M.D. degree in United States medical schools there are two possible ways to become a licensed physician. One is to take National Medical Board Examinations Parts I, II, and III. The other is to take the Federation Licensing Examination (FLEX). Physicians are licensed by the individual states or territories. All states except two, Texas and Louisiana, accept for licensing an M.D. who passed Parts I, II, III of the National Boards. All states accept for licensure an M.D. who has passed FLEX.

Part I of the National Boards is a series of 800 to 1000 multiple-choice questions which cover anatomy, biochemistry, microbiology, pathology, pharmacology, physiology, and behavioral science. The students sit for the examination on two successive days for 6 hours each day.

Part II of the National Boards is a series of 800 to 1000 multiple-choice items which cover internal medicine, obstetrics and gynecology, pediatrics, preventive medicine and public health, psychiatry, and surgery. This series of questions is also given in a two-day period for 6½ hours each day. Both Parts I and II are administered twice a year, once in the spring and once in the fall.

Most students take Part I at the end of the second year of medical school and Part II near the end of their third year or during their senior year.

Part III of National Boards is a one-day examination whose objective is to evaluate a student's clinical competence. This examination is administered once a year and is usually taken in the spring of the first year of graduate medical education. Part III consists of a series of patient-management problems. The student is given information about a patient and then must make decisions about diagnosis and treatment for that patient. He or she chooses from a series of possible procedures those which the student feels are appropriate for the patient's well-being. In addition to the patient-management problems, Part III also includes two multiple-choice sections, one covering therapy and management, the other pictorial representations of lesions, ECGs, X-rays, charts, and graphs.

The FLEX examination is administered on three consecutive days and includes all of the features of Part I, II, and III of National Boards. The basic science disciplines are on the first day, the clinical topics on the second day, and the multiple-choice and patient-management problems on the third day. The examinations are scored by the National Board of Medical Examiners in Philadelphia, but it is left up to each state to determine its own pass level.

Even though there are two methods for licensure, most students, if given the opportunity, elect to take Parts I, II, and III of National Boards. If for any reason they experience failure in one or more parts, they have the opportunity to retake any part a maximum of three times. Should they still experience failure, the option is open to sit for the FLEX, which may be retaken differing numbers of times, depending on individual state requirements.

Examination-preparation programs designed to help students with the licensure examinations will depend to a large degree on the use individual schools make of the scores previous students have achieved. Medical schools confer the M.D. degree and states license physicians to practice within their borders; however, there are a number of different uses schools make of scores on National Boards. These range all the way from schools which require candidates for the M.D. degree to pass both parts I and II for both promotion and graduation to schools which have no requirement that the students sit for Boards or FLEX.

Medical schools which require passing Part I for promotion to the clinical years are those institutions most likely to have extensive National Board Examination preparation programs. Part I of the Boards has the highest failure rate, usually about 10 percent of the candidates who sit at any given administration. This is in contrast to a 2 percent failure rate on Parts II and III.

For students preparing for licensure examinations, there are two common programs in use at this time. One is a series of large-group workshops given before the candidates sit for the examinations. These workshops, to be effective, must include enough practice items categorized by topic so that students can identify gaps or weak areas in their information. In order to do this, there are available in bookstores and from national corporations large pools of National Board-type items. By paying particular attention to the topic outlines supplied by the National Board of Medical Examiners, formal review sessions can be scheduled where information is either taught or reviewed by faculty or upper classmen.

In addition to content identification and review sessions, workshops should include examination-taking techniques for each of the standard multiple-choice item formats which appear on Boards—"One Best Answer," "Matching," "Matching Pairs," and "Multiple True-False." If these item formats have been in general use in course examinations, students will feel more comfortable with the decision-making process for each item type.

Because National Boards and FLEX are such long examinations, two and three days respectively, many students find it a highly anxiety-producing experience. In order to reduce anxiety, the workshop leaders should include familiarization with the actual examination format. Although subscores are reported for each of the separate disciplines in the basic and clinical sciences, the examinations are written in an interdisciplinary format. Some suggestions for time management will also help reduce anxiety. In order to progress in a proper manner through the examination, it is necessary to answer about 75 to 80 items an hour. Timed practice sessions should be set up so the students get used to thinking and marking answers at that pace. For students with more severe anxiety, physical relaxation techniques can be taught.

For those students who experience failure on National Boards or FLEX, individual sessions for diagnosis of the adequacy of information and skills should be set up and the individual problems remedied before the student attempts a retake. Retaking the examination without additional preparation will improve the score very little if at all. If the problem is diagnosed as a lack of information and if the student has the time and the money, there are commercial review courses which can be taken at centers around the country. However, they are expensive and very time-consuming. Unfortunately, the expense places them out of reach for many minority and disadvantaged students.

CONCLUSION

Although many of the examination-preparation programs were initiated to help minority and disadvantaged students in their efforts to be admitted and retained in medical school, many other students have benefited from having such programs available. In schools which offer workshops or counseling in test-taking techniques, it is not unusual to have these services available to any student who wishes to participate in such a program.

All students find it helpful to be able to pinpoint information which they need to learn or review before an examination as well as to have an opportunity to learn or practice the test-taking skills they will need to enhance their decision-making ability for selecting answers on an examination. Lowering students' anxiety concerning the evaluation of their performance creates an atmosphere within a school which is more conducive to learning. Students who are anxious about forthcoming examinations tend to learn and re-member their current course work less well than students who are confident they have sufficient information and skills necessary to do well on impending examinations.

Since the cost of educating a student in medical school has escalated dramatically in the past few years, it is more important now than ever before to make sure that there is a reasonable expectation that students admitted to medical schools will in fact become licensed physicians. Proper and adequate preparation for examinations can help to retain in medical school and eventually help to license as many of those admitted as possible.

Schools which wish to initiate a program to help students prepare for examinations should first assess the students' needs. If almost all students are performing well on examinations, then a program which deals with problems on a one-to-one basis might be sufficient. For a school where a significant number of students are not performing as well as expected, group workshops in test-taking techniques and item analysis should be given regularly before each examination period. At a school where students perform well on examinations but run such a high level of anxiety that the atmosphere at the school is affected, then desensitization or physical relaxation sessions should be offered. Each of these programs should be conducted by individuals trained in examination-preparation methods to ensure the success of the program.

The focus of all learning-skills programs, of which examination-preparation is only one part, is to enable each student to achieve his or her maximum potential for success and to do it as easily and efficiently as possible. The extent to which examination-preparation programs contribute to the students' success is the final measure of their success.

REFERENCES

1. *The New Student MCAT Student Manual: New Medical College Admission Test,* Association of American Medical Colleges, Washington, D.C., 1977.
2. John P. Hubbard: *Measuring Medical Education: The Tests and the Experience of the National Board of Medical Examiners,* 2nd ed. Philadelphia: Lea and Febiger, 1978.

Admissions and Financial Aid

CHAPTER 10

The Medical College Admission Test

Paul R. Elliott

The control of power and of resources in western societies has for centuries been passed down through the powerful, the affluent, and the "well-born" via carefully controlled access to education. Eton and Cambridge begot Groton and Yale; the Athenaeum became Harvard Yard. And though no longer passed from father to son on the playing fields of Eton, access to the traditional benefits of our society is still achieved primarily through education.

In contrast, much of the evolution of American society stems from the Jeffersonian view of democracy as being dependent upon the education of all its citizens—a singularly non-elitist philosophy from a singularly well-born intellect.

So it was not at all surprising in 1954 that a new thrust of civil rights activity in this country was aimed directly at opening this "pathway to power"—the traditional educational system—to racial minority students. In the last twenty-five years in this country we have gone from Brown to Bakke and from Birmingham to South Boston, and our educational systems (fortunately) will never be the same.

Paul R. Elliott, Ph.D., is Professor of Biological Science and Assistant Vice President for Academic Affairs, Florida State University, Tallahassee, Florida.

COGNITIVE EXAMINATIONS

The democratization of higher education in this country, however, ably augmented by the development of subsidized public education in the form of our state universities, has been a painfully slow process for ethnic and racial minority groups—Catholics, Jews, Native Americans, Blacks, and the Spanish speaking. One of the most direct controls of access to higher education (and one of the most insidious) was the development of the cognitive examination as an entrance requirement.

Cognitive examinations are basically exclusionary devices which appear to be unchallengeable because they purport to measure intelligence in some form (aptitude, achievement, reasoning). In fact, they do measure such attributes, but they do so in a cultural and sociological context from which they derive their exclusionary character.

Stated in another way, such measures generally are designed by traditional persons to measure traditional languages, skills, and knowledge for traditional students in a traditional educational pathway. If one will substitute "White, male, upper middle class" for the word traditional, much of the history of cognitive measures for admissions, and much of the inherent bias of such measures when applied to other groups become apparent.

In this chapter we will review some of the history of the Medical College Admission Test (MCAT) and its offspring the New MCAT as it relates to medical admissions over the last thirty years, and to admission of racial minority students over the last ten years.

THE MCAT AND MEDICAL EDUCATION

With the exception of those colleges and universities of significant reputation, the admission of a student to undergraduate college is a relatively straight-forward process in which successful completion of a degree program (retention) is the foremost goal, and in which cognitive measures such as test scores are given some predetermined weight along with the student's prior academic record.

Admission to medical school, however, carries an additional implied goal of critical relevance—the training of a "good physician." Even the subgoal of retention carries added weight in medical education because of the high cost associated with the educational process, and the cost to society of an unfilled position. It was this latter problem of retention coupled with (and related to) a decreasing applicant pool which resulted in the development of the Medical College Admission Test (MCAT) in the late 1940's. The test was designed to assess the academic aptitude (Verbal and Quantitative) and the academic achievement (Sciences and General Information) of each applicant for medical school. It was scored in 60 intervals of 10 points each from 205 to 795 with an adjusted mean (initially) of near 500.

Although the limitations of the MCAT were carefully delineated by its developers almost from its inception, the test was criticized for its lack of predictive validity as correlated with (1) academic achievement in medical school, (2) performance in postgraduate education, and (3) performance in medical practice.[1] In fact, the original purpose of the MCAT was simply that of reducing attrition in the basic sciences, of making gross discriminations between those who would and would not survive this earlier part of the medical curriculum.[2]

In an earlier paper, I attempted to identify some of the valid and invalid uses of the MCAT.[3] Among the valid uses were: the assessment of ability and knowledge in certain areas of study to help determine the probability of completion of the academic requirements of medical school; to compare the students of a given undergraduate school if there existed a sufficient population of MCAT examinees from that school; and to validate the grades of applicants who attended institutions unfamiliar to the medical admissions committee.

Some of the things the test cannot do are: to measure motivation, character, or other noncognitive characteristics; to separate individual applicants with small score differences;* and to measure

---

[1] Gough, H. G., Hall, W. B., and Harris, R. E.: Admissions Procedures as Forecasters of Performance in Medical Training. *J. Med. Ed.*, 38:983, 1963.

[2] Cuca, J. M., Sakakeeny, L. A., and Johnson, D. G.: The Medical School Admissions Process: A Review of Literature, 1955-1976. Special Report, Association of American Medical Colleges, Washington, D.C., 1976.

[3] Elliott, P. R.: The Use and Abuse of Quantitative Criteria for the Selection of Medical Students. *Surgery,* July, 1969.

* The AAMC began publishing standard error bands with the MCAT score results in 1970.

clinical judgement or expected professional competence except in the very broadest sense that intellectual factors along with personal and social factors contribute to clinical competence.

In the late 1960's, the MCAT came under increasing criticism from a number of directions. The verbal and general information sections of the test were considered to have marked potential for cultural, ethnic, and socioeconomic bias. Further, the test was criticized for its emphasis on factual information rather than the concepts upon which the facts were based, and was criticized for the absence of problem-solving approaches.

In a broader view, the early 1970's found most admissions criteria (including the MCAT) subjected to increasing criticism for:

— failure to predict physician performance,
— failure to select students with a propensity for primary care specialties,
— failure to aid in the solution of geographic maldistribution of physicians,
— failure to predict the performance of non-traditional students, particularly ethnic and racial minorities,
— failure to take into account the socialization (demographic and socioeconomic) factors affecting student performance.

While there is some truth in each of those criticisms, it is also clear that apart from admissions criteria, medical education itself favors the training of highly specialized, hospital-based, acute care physicians destined to practice in urban and suburban settings. The use of the MCAT simply was in keeping with those objectives.

With the criticisms of admissions criteria at a high level, with applicants sitting on the doorstep in record numbers, and with external pressures to increase the heterogeneity of medical classes (more minority students, rural, inner-urban, low socioeconomic, and students interested in primary care) the Association of American Medical Colleges (AAMC) in 1972 announced a major effort to assess the entire medical admissions process.

A Task Force was established by the AAMC to furnish recommendations for this Medical College Admissions Assessment Program (MCAAP). Among its recommendations were the development of noncognitive assessment measures, training programs for interviewers from admissions committees, review of the area of biographical data useful in the admissions process, and the development of new tests for cognitive assessment to replace the MCAT. Unfortunately, but predictably only the last of these recommendations has been implemented.

The Task Force further recommended[4] that any new tests developed for cognitive assessment should be validated prior to use (minimally adhered to); should be offered to medical admissions committees on an optional basis (the New MCAT is required of all applicants); should provide fair treatment to all applicants; should be secondary to the influence engendered by the noncognitive characteristics of the applicant.

Following extensive discussions among the affected groups regarding the broad outline and philosophy of the proposed New MCAT, the AAMC contracted in 1974 with the American Institutes for Research of Palo Alto, California, for the development of these cognitive measures which were to replace the original MCAT in 1977.

THE NEW MCAT

Before describing some of its characteristics, it is appropriate to describe briefly the specifics of the New MCAT.

The test is a full day examination utilizing four test components:

1. Science Knowledge, with three consecutive subtests in Biology, Chemistry, and Physics.
2. Science Problems, with intermingled questions across Biology, Chemistry, and Physics.
3. Skills Analysis: Reading.
4. Skills Analysis: Quantitative.

Test 1 is 135 minutes in length, tests 2, 3, and 4 are each of 85 minutes duration. With lunch break and rest periods, the total time involved is 470 minutes, ten minutes short of eight hours.

The Science Knowledge and Science Problems tests attempt to assess the understanding of scientific concepts and principles identified as being important to medical education and medical

---

[4] Final Report of the AAMC National Task Force with Recommendations for the Medical College Admissions Assessment Program Study. AAMC, Washington, D.C., 1973.

practice. Separate scores indicate performance in Biology, Chemistry, Physics, and Science Problems; the scores in Biology, Chemistry, and Physics being derived by combining the Science Knowledge questions for each discipline with the Science Problem questions for that same discipline. (Thus, problem solving is doubly weighted in the scoring.)

The Skills Analysis tests attempt to measure the applicant's ability to comprehend, evaluate, and use information that is presented in a narrative or quantitative format. They do not test reading speed or general knowledge.

The narrative format uses selected readings from the sciences, social sciences, and medical sciences; the quantitative format requires mathematical knowledge of high school algebra II, trigonometry, and descriptive concepts of statistics. Calculus is not required.

Each of the Skills Analysis tests is presented as one score, making a total of six scores, each ranging from one (lowest) to 15 (highest).

Changes in the New MCAT

As the New MCAT progressed through the developmental stages, a number of significant differences emerged in comparison to other cognitive examinations and in particular to the original MCAT. Among these differences are the following construed to be positive.

Test Development:

1. The test content for each section was uniquely determined by a broadly representative evaluation panel including medical students, residents, practicing physicians, undergraduate faculty, basic science faculty, and clinical faculty.
2. The test (and subtests) are designed as "power" tests rather than "speed" tests. This necessitates a longer examination period, but eliminates some potential rate-dependent biases more likely to occur in students with weaker educational backgrounds.
3. The old MCAT had the limited objective of attempting to predict success for the examinee in the basic medical sciences. The New MCAT is constructed around specific

skills and knowledge important to clinical training and, hence, presumably to the practice of medicine as well.

Test Content:

4. The test content (outlines and specifications) was developed around specific criteria (criterion referenced): relevance to performance in the medical curriculum and relevance to performance in the practice of medicine. If the criterion referencing is successful, the New MCAT may have improved predictive value.

5. The tests incorporate the measurement of skills important to being a medical student and a physician as well as the measurement of knowledge (content). These skills include the recognition of relevance, consistency, accuracy, objectivity, relationships, trends, and corroboration of the information presented. In particular, the emphasis on reading skills rather than work knowledge should furnish a valuable measure.

6. Science problem solving is a major element of the three science subtests and is reported as a separate score.

7. The readings and information presented in the subtests are taken from the sciences, social sciences, and medically related topics—roughly evenly distributed. Among students of varying cultural backgrounds, such readings are more likely to represent common experiences.

Score Reporting:

8. The scoring system has less potential for abuse, with 15 intervals rather than 60. This means that students with equivalent abilities and knowledge are more likely to achieve the same scaled score, and therefore that comparison of individuals is a more defensible procedure and less likely to be abused than on the original MCAT.

9. The reporting of separate scores for the three science subtests allows the identification of the examinees' strengths and weaknesses among the tested areas, and should result in improved advising and self-evaluation as well as specific academic reinforcement. Also of value, if a student has not yet taken a course (for example, Physics) the reason for a low score in that subject is easily detected. In the past, ignorance

of a subject simply lowered the score for the entire science section, a perilous position for an applicant.

Preparation for the Exam:

10. The complete content outlines for the science subtests are published, and a New MCAT practice test (80 percent of a complete testing) is furnished in *The New MCAT*^{SM} *Student Manual*.[5] This should offset the disadvantage of low socioeconomic group students who cannot afford a prep course for the New MCAT. Unfortunately, the AAMC has elected to charge for the Student Manual which restores part of that disadvantage.

Cultural Bias

One of the positive aspects of the development of the New MCAT was (and continues to be) the involvement of non-traditional groups at all levels of test development and validation. In all committees advising the project and in the development of content outlines, specifications, et al., approximately 20 percent of those involved were racial minorities. Further, the writing and the testing of questions for the New MCAT had extensive input from minority group students, faculty, and physicians.

This is the first major cognitive assessment test in which an effort was made to include minority input in every stage of the developmental process and in the continuing validation studies. Let us turn now to the evaluation of the New MCAT results for 1977 and 1978.

Validation and Evaluation

Contrary to the recommendations of the MCAAP Task Force, the New MCAT was placed in use in 1977 with only minimal validation studies having been carried out. As indicated in the New MCAT Interpretive Manual,[6] a research form of the New MCAT

---

[5] *The New MCAT*^{SM} *Student Manual:* Association of American Medical Colleges, Washington, D.C., 1977.

[6] *New Medical College Admission Test: Interpretive Manual;* Association of American Medical Colleges, Washington, D.C., 1977.

was administered in the fall of 1976 on a voluntary basis to students enrolled at a number of U.S. Medical Schools.

Within the rather marked limitations of that research study (which the authors indicate "certainly does not constitute an adequate validity study in the best sense of the word"[6]), positive relationships between New MCAT scores and other measures of medical school performance were observed. Given the immense effort that is necessary to develop an entirely new standardized measure such as the New MCAT, especially one which is criterion referenced, one would certainly hope that predictive validity for medical school performance would be detected.

However, with or without sufficient validation, the test instrument was first offered in 1977. Predictive validation studies at the national level will continue as students who have taken the New MCAT move through medical school into postgraduate education and then to medical practice.

It is worth noting that the most important validation studies occur at the local medical school level, since the predictive utility of any testing instrument is essentially a local matter. As individual medical schools ascertain the value of all or portions of the New MCAT scores in predicting performance in various aspects of their own medical education and training program, it will become a more useful instrument to each school. This will be particularly true if these results are passed on to potential students via their preprofessional advisors.

In the report of the AAMC Task Force on Minority Student Opportunities in Medicine,[7] an important recommendation is: "Admissions Committees should use the New MCAT Test results with judicious caution prior to completion of validation studies by the AAMC and by individual medical schools." That is a gentle statement, since caution should be used any time cognitive test scores are involved in an admissions process; the point is that particular caution need be used prior to completion of appropriate validation studies.

Evaluation and Interpretation

If we cannot yet speak with confidence about the predictive validity of the New MCAT, we can at least look at some of the

[7] Elliott, P. R.: Report of the AAMC Task Force on Minority Student Opportunities in Medicine, AAMC, Washington, D.C., 1978.

results of the first offerings of the test in terms of national reference groups. With the appropriate evaluations, one could then compare an individual's score with the total group of examinees taking the New MCAT or with various national subpopulations.

Evaluations have been carried out by the AAMC and reported for national subgroups by racial self-description, undergraduate major, sex, and college class level.

In general, there are predicatably few surprises in reviewing scores for national subpopulations by major and college class. For example: Humanities majors do better on the "Skills Analysis: Reading" than do other majors. Physics and Mathematics majors do better in "Skills Analysis: Quantitative." Likewise, third year undergraduate students who are nearest in time to those courses which relate to the science section do better than students who are graduated from college.

New MCAT Scores by Racial/Ethnic Background

Table 1 presents the scaled score means and standard deviations for each of the subtests by racial/ethnic subpopulations on the two 1978 testings of the New MCAT.

It is apparent that racial minority groups (other than Asian/ Pacific Islanders) perform on the average at a lower level than do white majority students; in fact the magnitude of the difference (in standard deviations units) between minority and majority populations parallels the magnitude of differences observed in the original MCAT, and parallels the observed differences of grade point average for the same groups.

Before discussing further these results, it is important to point out some special cautions. The racial/ethnic descriptions utilized in Table 1 are from the examinees' self-descriptions which may lead to some error, particularly for American Indian and for the various Hispanic subpopulations. Further, since test scores provide insight into only one dimension of an applicant's characteristics, generalizations drawn from the aggregate performance of any racial/ ethnic subpopulation could lead to an erroneous assessment of the qualifications of any single applicant as well as an incorrect assess-

Table 1. Mean Scale Scores and Standard Deviations for the New MCAT by Racial/Ethnic Subpopulations; Spring and Fall, 1978 Testings

	BLACK	AM. INDIAN ALASKAN NATIVE	WHITE	ASIAN/ PACIFIC ISLANDER	HISPANIC— MEXICAN AMERICAN	HISPANIC— PUERTO RICAN MAINLAND	HISPANIC— PUERTO RICAN COMMON- WEALTH	HISPANIC— OTHER
	N=3787 7.5%	N=210 0.4%	N=41,698 82%	N=2637 5.2%	N=702 1.4%	N=269 0.53%	N=678 1.3%	N=865 1.7%
Biology	5.36* (2.16)	7.25 (2.42)	8.25 (2.23)	7.71 (2.34)	6.80 (2.20)	5.67 (2.34)	4.98 (2.24)	7.24 (2.45)
Chemistry	5.29 (2.02)	6.77 (2.32)	8.04 (2.41)	8.35 (2.53)	6.47 (2.27)	5.82 (2.15)	5.01 (1.96)	7.12 (2.54)
Physics	5.55 (1.78)	7.13 (2.19)	8.26 (2.31)	8.43 (2.45)	6.69 (2.13)	5.96 (1.87)	5.34 (1.62)	7.29 (2.35)
Science Problems	5.48 (1.85)	7.25 (2.21)	8.29 (2.23)	8.29 (2.36)	6.74 (2.15)	5.75 (1.94)	5.10 (1.78)	7.22 (2.32)
Skills Analysis: Reading	5.08 (2.71)	7.66 (2.47)	8.46 (2.13)	7.04 (2.74)	6.85 (2.48)	5.26 (3.05)	3.66 (2.57)	7.02 (2.73)
Skills Analysis: Quantitative	4.86 (2.08)	7.04 (2.44)	8.34 (2.30)	7.62 (2.53)	6.38 (2.28)	5.01 (2.32)	4.13 (1.92)	6.74 (2.53)

*Upper figure is the mean score; lower figure is the standard deviation.
Data obtained from Division of Educational Measurement and Research, Association of American Medical Colleges.

ment of the potential for the study of medicine for any given subpopulation.[6]

But to return to the question of cultural or racial bias in the New MCAT: in retrospect, to have hoped that the significant and positive inclusion of racial minority students, faculty, and practicing physicians in the development of the New MCAT would reduce or eliminate the differences in the mean test scores of majority and racial minority populations represents a remarkably naive view of the sources and complexity of racism in our country.

It is equivalent to an assumption that if we were to involve sufficient "Southerners" in the test development, the differences in average New MCAT scores between Southern and Northeastern populations would disappear (Table 2).

Among many contributing factors, the educational systems of the South are simply not as good as those in the Northeast. Better representation by Southerners in test design and development would not alter that significant difference. The analogy for racial minority groups is oversimplified, but none the less appropriate.

I believe the efforts made by the American Institutes for Research and by the AAMC to eliminate cultural and racial bias in the New MCAT were impressive and sincere. In the face of that effort, since there remain marked differences in the mean scores of racial minority students and majority students on the New MCAT, we should recognize that this difference may be a real measure of the crippling nature of racism, and of the distance we must yet travel in our efforts to eliminate the devastating effects of racism in our society. I would contend that these performance differences do not measure cultural bias, but in fact measure "social bias": the aggregate effect of a multiplex of socialization phenomena resulting in a real disadvantage for persons who for racial, cultural, and socio-economic reasons are deflected from the mainstream of traditional institutions in our society.

Ironically, by incorporating in the New MCAT the measurement of skills critical to the reasoning required in medical education and medical practice, we may have further compounded the problem. Most would contend that this new approach to testing is at the least an interesting experiment compared to the relatively simplistic "content" questions of the old MCAT. Yet these skills are the very ones which are most difficult to nurture and which may be most affected by socialization processes (the family, the school, the demographic region) in the developing child and young adult.

**Table 2.   Mean Scale Scores For The New MCAT By State Of Residence:
Combined 1977 Spring And Fall Testing Dates**

	STATE A	SOUTHERN STATES STATE B	STATE C	STATE D	NORTHEASTERN STATES STATE E	STATE F
Biology	6.9	6.1	7.0	8.2	8.2	8.6
Chemistry	6.8	5.9	6.6	8.2	8.2	8.5
Physics	7.2	6.7	7.2	8.1	8.2	8.7
Science Problems	7.0	6.2	7.0	8.1	8.3	8.7
Skills Analysis: Reading	7.5	7.0	7.8	8.4	8.4	8.9
Skills Analysis: Quantitative	7.2	6.7	7.6	8.2	8.4	9.4

Data obtained from Division of Educational Measurement and Research, Association of American Medical Colleges.

169

They are some of the very characteristics which are least likely to be reinforced in poor schools, in broken families, in groups debilitated by the unintentional as well as intentional racism of our society.

Once again, it is appropriate to express concern regarding the use of New MCAT scores prior to completion of appropriate validation studies.

Preparation for the New MCAT

The topic of preparation for the MCAT is covered more extensively in Chapter 9, but a brief review here of the types of preparation utilized by many majority applicants is appropriate.

As indicated earlier in this chapter, one of the positive changes in the New MCAT testing program is the publication of the student manual[5] which includes complete content outlines, an extensive discussion of the skills being measured, and most remarkably, 80 percent of an actual test form with instructions for self-testing in a manner simulating the actual testing procedure. This openness should contribute to "test-wiseness" and could reduce some of the advantage furnished to those examinees who can afford commercial preparation and review courses for the New MCAT.

Since test-wiseness is important, and since the scoring system and the test composition are designed to aid the student in self-evaluation of content strengths and weaknesses, taking the examination twice is not inappropriate. Careful counseling with a pre-professional advisor should allow the examinee to make maximum use of the intervening time between the two examinations. Taking the New MCAT twice within one year is not advisable, since the intervening time is of insufficient duration to allow for the work necessary to show score improvement.

Discussion

As with other cognitive examinations, the New MCAT carries with it many limitations, and is most likely to be misused by being overused. It is but one of many important components of the evaluation of preparedness and aptitude for the study and practice of medicine. It most assuredly is not the most important of those components when compared to noncognitive characteristics such as motivation, realistic self-appraisal, empathy, honesty, maturity, positive self concept, sensitivity, and positive interpersonal skills. Unfortunately these personal attributes are not easily measured in an eight-hour, multiple-choice examination.

Further, whatever is measured in traditional cognitive examinations appears to be most useful when applied to the evaluation of traditional students (white, male, upper middle class). For non-traditional students, particularly racial/cultural/ethnic minorities, the direct assessment of certain *noncognitive* attributes may be of equal or greater value in predicting success in medical school. Evidence for this contention is presented in the work of Sedlacek and Brooks[8] of the University of Maryland Cultural Study Center.

A model developed to reconcile this discontinuity in the predictive value of cognitive examinations for minority and majority students is based on the assumption that attributes in the noncognitive domain are the most predictive of success in any human endeavor, including education. For traditional students in our educational institutions, these noncognitive attributes are positively and continuously reinforced in ways that link the noncognitive domain to measurable behaviors in the cognitive domain such as grades and test scores.

For non-traditional students in our society, those behaviors may be non-reinforced or capriciously reinforced (unintentional racism) or deliberately and negatively reinforced (intentional racism). The resultant is a disconnection of the linkage between the noncognitive predictors and those cognitive measures so frequently used as admissions criteria.

In the Simulated Minority Admissions Exercise (SMAE),[9] developed under the auspices of the AAMC, the authors argue that to achieve fairness for racial minority students in the admissions process, one should take into account this interrupted linkage, and should attempt to evaluate and utilize those noncognitive predic-

---

[8] Sedlacek, W. E., and Brooks, G. C.: *Racism in American Education: A Model for Change.* Chicago: Nelson Hall, 1976.

[9] Prieto, D. (ed.): Simulated Minority Admissions Exercise. AAMC, Washington, D.C., 1978.

tors* as appropriate adjuncts to the traditional, cognitive measures used for all students.

THE ADMISSIONS SYNDROME

The final topic of this Chapter was entitled "Preparation for the New MCAT." In response to this topic, one would have hoped to be able to say that the best preparation for the New MCAT is an excellent education. Unfortunately, when separated from socio-economic and demographic background, the contribution of a quality education to cognitive test scores is still unclear. What is clear is that there are important contributions—negative contributions—to such test scores attributable to being poor, or Black, or brown, or red, or rural. At this time, the New MCAT, as other cognitive examinations, is quite unable to account for or make adjustments for those who suffer from the insidious effects of a society which is not yet open, and certainly not yet equal.

Yet, in the absence of methodologies for the predictive evaluation of noncognitive attributes, medical admissions committees will continue to use (and over-use) the cognitive tools with "real" numbers. Thus, the problem for racial minority students continues to be one of how to compete within the traditional system.

That means, in part, competing with students whose primary goal is to gain admission to medical school; students who will select their courses not to broaden their education, or to increase their understanding of humanity but simply to gain admission to medical school; students who will obtain a job in a hospital not to learn about the profession and their fitness for it, but to gain admission to medical school; students who will join clubs and organizations not to develop their skills in leadership or as members of a team,

---

*1. Positive self-concept or confidence
2. Realistic self-appraisal
3. Understands and deals with racism
4. Prefers long-range goals to short term or immediate needs
5. Availability of strong support person
6. Successful leadership experience
7. Demonstrated community service
8. Demonstrated medical interests
(Taken from SMAE; Reference 9).

but simply to improve their chances of admission to medical school. And of relevance here, students who will spend outlandish sums of money not to improve their education but simply to improve their scores on the New MCAT, and thus to enhance their probability of admission to medical school. These behaviors collectively describe a disease we should call the "admissions syndrome."

Of one thing I am certain, whether the students are majority or minority, we should not condemn them for those compulsive and barren behaviors ascribed to the "admissions syndrome." That disease is perpetuated by an admissions process, a medical education system, and a profession which elicits and rewards such behaviors by misapplication of criteria such as scores from the New MCAT.

CHAPTER 11

Student Recommendations and Evaluations

James D. Dexter

INTRODUCTION

During the past decade medical schools have found themselves in the paradoxical position of being required to increase their educational product, i.e., medical students and residents. This has included new training programs such as Family Medicine and increasing postgraduate programs in Continuing Medical Education. This demand for increased education production has occurred concomitant with the decrease in the necessary funding for clinical service and research, the other major functions of any medical school.

This has occurred during a period of time that has seen the professions such as law and medicine become much more attractive as career choices because of the image of financial reward and security. This increasing desirability has provided a pool of very highly qualified applicants from which medical schools can choose students. Medical school faculties have only this one guaranteed factor in their planning data, i.e., adequate numbers of qualified

James D. Dexter, M.D. is Associate Professor of Neurology, School of Medicine, University of Missouri, Columbia, Missouri.

students. This has led to an attitude of accepting the "best of the best" because they will provide the least stress to an already tense institutional environment.

In light of these factors, it can be seen that the problems of admissions processing and decisions frequently carry a very low priority for medical school and university administrators. This places the primary responsibility of medical school applicant advocacy on the premedical faculty and advisors.

THE STUDENT PACKAGE

While the task of choosing the best of the best may seem to be an easy task, it is not. This task is made difficult because of the diversity of the data supplied to the admissions committees. At a time when the concept of due process is mandatory under the law, committees are required to be prepared to justify their decisions and, consequently, make their decision on the basis of data that are common to all applicants. These common data are what I have termed the "student package."

The data which have been historically the most common are the American Medical College Application Service (AMCAS) application, transcripts of academic performance, and Medical College Admission Test (MCAT) scores. These are the most common data; not that this is all that is required, but it is what most medical schools require in a given format. Because these data are most common, they do serve as the base of the student package.

While it is generally accepted that the AMCAS application (which contains both academic transcripts and MCAT scores) is the base of the package, I know of no admissions committee which is willing to make a final decision based upon this material alone. Most admissions committees will, however, use this as the base for the first step decision. This is most frequently referred to as a "screening procedure," which is based on the question, "Will the applicant be a good student?," believing that a good physician must be first a good student.

With the first question answered affirmatively, the admission committee is faced with the task of choosing among the good students, and of making that always tenuous judgement of who will make the good physician. This decision utilizes nonacademic characteristics such as maturity, energy, communication skills, motivation, ability to establish a rapport with other people, and humaneness.

While at first glance these may be seen as very subjective, they are real characteristics which we can all recognize but cannot quantitate sufficiently to be considered objectively. The assessment of these characteristics is the justification for the letters of evaluation and personal evaluations which medical schools require as part of the admissions process.

This completed package may be quite small, only five or so pages (with four pages of the AMCAS application and the academic letter of evaluation and recommendation). It is for this reason that many schools require supplementary applications to expand these data, and the interview is used by most admissions committees to test the integrity of the student package.

THE EVALUATION

A great deal of time and effort over the past two decades has been spent with the problem of standardizing the evaluations from premedical advisors or premedical professors. This has largely been without result, primarily because medical schools have difficulty with people attempting to quantitate those human characteristics which require the concerted effort of honest feedback to the evaluators. This type of communication requires personnel stability which is rare on the part of both premedical advisors and admissions officers.

How do medical school admissions committees want the applicants evaluated by their colleges? If you were to ask every admissions committee member this question you would hear no two agree in detail; however, most committee members would agree that after they have read a letter of evaluation, they would like to know the applicant as a student, as a leader, as a peer, and as a person.

There are many evaluations received by medical schools each year which are composed entirely of the applicants' academic transcript transcribed into prose and even near poetry, and many letters that assume that the transcript speaks for itself and leaves nothing for commentary; of course, this is rarely the case. Many students at all levels are concerend with compiling an attractive transcript with very little true scholarly energy expended and, likewise, there are students who are promising scholars whose grades are not the yardsticks of accomplishment. Most students are somewhere in the middle of this spectrum. This variation requires a commentary on the applicant's academic performance.

The successful physician of tomorrow will need to be a scholar whose rewards for scholarship will be the practice of high quality medicine and the often quite limited praise which accompanies that. This physician must be able to motivate himself to study specific problems in depth as well as to maintain a broad base of updated information, both specific data and conceptual understanding. This is most optimally obtained by those students who have shown the ability to deal with both concepts and specific facts and who have shown some self-motivation to understand beyond the usual academic grade-motivated requirements.

The good physician of tomorrow will be as he has been in the past, a scholar in a community of physician scholars, and the integrity of his scholarship as well as his willingness to share his scholarship are critical to both his patients and the patients of his peers. The practice of medicine changes with such rapidity that a physician cannot maintain a constant review of medical information; however, the ongoing sharing of information among physicians has been a successful method of learning. The absence of integrity in this sharing process has been in the past lethal. Can the student who is in the competitive pre-medicine curriculum say "I don't know" and does he have the ability and energy to find the answer? These are the scholarly characteristics which go beyond the courses and grades of the transcript. And the premedical evaluator who does not speak to these characteristics does not only the student but society as well a disservice.

There are few transcripts that have any way of reflecting the student's leadership abilities; however, this is a major requirement for that applicant who desires to practice clinical medicine. The last three decades have seen the demise of the isolated physician who was able to practice in the absence of allied health professionals and has seen the emergence of the health care team which is a reality without signs of dissolution. This has required the physician to be a team leader; he may lead only a small office staff or a large staff of nurses, technicians, therapists, and secretaries. Can the applicant make individual decisions, participate well in group decisions, and is he sensitive to other peoples' need to participate in decisions? This goes beyond the usual campus political popularity contest and concerns itself with "Can he lead groups to accomplish a goal?"

It has been said in the past that there will always be room for the isolated genius in medicine; however, over the next several decades there will be a marked constriction of that space. Even those people who prefer the route of medicine to the chemistry or physiology laboratory will find that peer cooperation, peer sharing, and peer evaluation will become as important as it is to the clinical physician. Does the student turn criticism into creativity, can he be critical without being cruel to others or himself, can he show respect without withdrawal, is he sensitive without being overly condescending, is he interpersonally strong without a need to be overpowering? Most evaluators of medical school applicants hope we will always have room for the isolationists for they may be the great creators; however, it is a gamble that the taxpayer, personal contributor, and consumer of health care can little afford to take over the next several decades.

There is probably no more rigorous endeavor to undertake than the curriculum of medical school and the three to six years of postgraduate residency training. Among the saddest persons seen in medical education is that person with just enough intelligence to make him marginally competitive but enough strength to make him tenacious, or that person who has the intellecutal power to master medicine but with a personality which is dangerous to his patients and peers. Acceptance of such applicants is the most common error made by medical school admissions committees and is most often the responsibility of those persons who wrote the premedical evaluation or those committees who have not taken heed of an insightful premedical evaluation. This oversight has resulted in a large number of unhappy physicians who are providing inadequate service to their patients and are rogues of the profession.

Most people have never taken the time to realize that the practice of medicine, like the practice of law, consists of serving people who, while needing help, do not really want to be there and that the practicioner's professional life is spent with anxious and often hostile clients or patients. There is no way of judging who can fit this role; however, often a rule that might be of some help is to visualize the applicant in the role of a physician who is expected to be caring for the crying, hospitable to the hostile, serving to the suffering while maintaining a clinical if not a scientific objectivity in response to the patient's problem.

Only rare people have this personality when they apply to medical school. Part of medical education is to optimize these characteristics. However, when it is obvious that an applicant is overly egocentric, hostile, or self-suffering this usually negates the ability to develop into a good physician. Does the applicant have a realistic image of himself and does this image fit into caring for people?

THE RECOMMENDATION

There are very few words in our language which compare with the power of the word "integrity" and there is no more important characteristic needed in the process of choosing those to enter medical school. By integrity I mean a consistency and unity of behavior. Many medical school admissions committees have relatively simplistic, but pragmatically useful methods of testing this and it is called the "track record" for want of a better term. This track record has three important aspects: the record of the applicant, the record of the recommending institution, and the record of the individual recommender.

It is not infrequent to see an applicant's file that shows little chance that he could withstand the rigors of the medical curriculum, and yet the premedical recommendation judges the applicant as an excellent candidate. And frequently the reverse is the case, that students who may have performed very well may not be judged as competitive as some others. Both of these situations are quite ominous signs in the admissions process. This is not to say that only those persons with sparkling transcripts can be judged as competitive; however, when there is an inconsistency of either extreme is when the letter of recommendation is most important to explain these inconsistencies and to explain the rationale of the recommendation. This is the most frequent error when addressing the application of the educationally underserved.

When we evaluate a student's record, we must describe the environment in which his premedical scholarship was performed, and this should include at least his high school background.

Medical schools have far too long looked at only the numerical aspects of the academic performance and have paid little attention to the pre-college education. This must be evaluated on the basis of both (1) academic quality of instruction and (2) the basis of the expectation of the pre-college curriculum.

Many very capable adolescents find themselves in an educational situation whose goal is preparation of the student for a non-academic career. As a result, these students are categorized prematurely by establishing inappropriately low expectations of performance which result in inadequate preparation for the high expectations of most college curricula. Those students who have come from such educational systems should, I think, be classified as educationally underserved, recognized as such, and evaluated using this as the basis. There have been all too many good race horses discarded because people looked at only their times without evaluating their quality of training to run. Unless a medical school restricts its admissions to a very constricted geographic region, it has no basis of judging the quality of precollege education and can only obtain that understanding from the premedical letter of evaluation.

Just as there is a broad variation in precollege training in students within a college, there are also subgroups of students who are being evaluated by common criteria but who are receiving a different education within the same curriculum. Education is a different experience for that student with adequate outside support who lives on campus than it is for that student who must travel two hours per day and works four hours per day for his own support. Just as there is a difference between that student who has chosen to excel in a non-science area while fulfilling his premed requirements from that single goal-seeking premed "scientist," these non-academic forces are essential to understand and make up the environment of performance.

A letter of recommendation should consider these environments of performance and make an estimate of the applicant's ability to perform in medical school, postgraduate medical training, and the practice of medicine, i.e., has the applicant been running on the fast or slow portion of the track and what will his performance be if he is allowed to run on a fast track?

In an academic system which uses a common system as a measure of the level of performance, the prime evaluator is the grade point average. And perfection is most commonly defined as 4.00. This is an inadequate definition when we realize that it is dependent on a collection of diverse human opinions of what is excellence and what is adequacy. Considering the origin of this number which is based upon individual value systems, we then can understand that this is not as objective as we would like to believe. Admissions committees must evaluate an applicant's college as well as the applicant.

This evaluation of colleges is the most difficult task facing these people in the admissions process and if done adequately is impossibly time consuming. This results in an often unfair advantage given to the colleges which are well known to the admissions committee. This leaves many schools which have large numbers of educationally disadvantaged students at a disadvantage until they can establish a good "track record" of educating students who will do well in medical school.

Most admissions committees seek to solve this college evaluation by, first, the use of the MCAT performance of the college and by the evaluation of the college's record of producing successful medical students.

Both the MCAT and this "reputation" have much difficulty. It is well known that the MCAT performance of a college must be interpreted in light of the regional variation on the MCAT and upon the known social and economic variation of such tests. Those students from suburban schools do much better than the rural or inner city public high schools. The major limitation of the MCAT is that it is designed only to predict performance in basic medical sciences and in standardized National Board of Medical Examiners Examination and is not predictive of the student's performance in the clinical sciences. With the recognition of these limitations, many premedical students and many colleges accept their performance on this examination as fate, which is a disservice to themselves and their students. The performance on this examination can be improved by training in reading, reading comprehension, and test-taking skills. The successful applicant will be faced with this type of examination the rest of his life and these skills should be part of his armamentaria. Every medical school applicant should have training in those skills necessary to allow him to prove the adequacy of his information base and cognitive skills by this type of examination. Those people who say the MCAT is only a game, not an adequate examination, certainly owe it to their students to teach them to play the game the best they can. It does very little good to train a person who cannot pass a board examination due to lack of test-taking skills.

The other way admissions committees evaluate the college is by the number of successful medical students they have produced. It is quite obvious that those schools who graduate one premedical student per year will have a much harder time developing a reputation and good track record than a major university which is graduating 100 premedical students per year. This is not as difficult as it looks when it takes only one good medical student to start this reputation at one medical school. The converse is also true; it takes only one inadequate student who has come highly recommended to damage the college's reputation.

There is another track record that admissions committees usually consider and that is the individual evaluator. Many colleges are fortunate enough to have that rare faculty member who is willing to make a prolonged commitment to writing letters of evaluation and recommendation and who serves as the focus of communications with medical schools. Much of a major premedical school's success is due to the success of this person. This allows a school to have a constant evaluator who can measure a student against not only his peers but also against previous students who have been successful in medical school. While many individual professors within colleges become known to admissions committees, most committees learn to rely on that single person who compiles the total evaluation. A person in this position who has established himself with students, established communication with medical schools, and has a good track record with his recommendations is the singularly most important person in the admissions process except the applicant himself.

The last component of the letter of evaluation and recommendation is its ability to serve as a basis of the interview and needs to be consistent with the finding and impression of the interview. When there is an inconsistency between these two major components of the evaluation, this again serves as a disadvantage to the student's application. If a student has some characteristics that may appear in the interview that could detract, the interviewer should have the advantage of this knowledge prior to the interview. Remember, at best it is difficult for the applicant to interview well if the image in the evaluation and recommendation letter sets the wrong stage. If it is inconsistent the favorable interview is nearly impossible.

CONCLUSION

Those faculty members who are responsible for evaluating the medical school applicant have a responsibility to make the student as competitive as his basic academic talents, motivation, and personal commitment will allow. This is best done by not only solid education and high expectations but also by good evaluations and realistic recommendations. Those who write on behalf of students should be sensitive to those admissions committee members who must review sometimes several thousand of these applications. They should be consistent, honest, and present the admissions committee with a package which is complete so that they can know the applicant as a student, a peer, a leader, and a person.

CHAPTER 12

Admissions Interviews

Judith W. Krupka

Medical school admissions interviews are a mixed blessing for minority applicants. At present, the interview provides one of the few opportunities for applicants to be evaluated on some basis other than simply the undergraduate grade point average and the Medical College Admissions Test scores, the two most extensively used admissions criteria and the two criteria most likely to be damaging to the minority applicant. Seduced by the ease with which the data on these two criteria can be compiled and lured by the myth of "objectivity" which surrounds these two criteria, we who are involved in medical school admissions tend to forget that while it is true that they can predict reasonably well performance in the first two years of medical school, it is also true that they underpredict the performance of minority medical students. Furthermore, it has been repeatedly demonstrated that GPA and MCAT scores have little predictive validity in the third and fourth years of medical school or in other important areas such as choice of specialty, location of practice or quality of physician performance. Fairly administered interviews, focusing on relevant qualities can offer some balance to the cognitive criteria, and thus provide schools with

Judith Krupka, Ph.D., is Associate Professor and Associate Dean for Student Affairs, College of Human Medicine, Michigan State University, East Lansing, Michigan.

a means by which they can evaluate minority applicants on a more suitable basis. It should not be forgotten that interviews are not a one-way street. Rather, they also allow the applicant to ask questions about the medical school which will be pertinent to the decision of whether or not this is an appropriate place for that person to study medicine. In addition to the direct information obtained through questioning the interviewer, the applicant will be forming impressions about the kind of environment the medical school will be providing the student body, impressions based on the treatment the applicant receives by the various representatives of the medical school.

Unfortunately, interviews as currently conducted at many medical schools fail in two important aspects. They do not assess appropriate qualities and the treatment of applicants reveals a lack of concern for prospective students which is appalling. Often they have very real potential for introducing negative biases and can even result in the rejection of the very persons for whom we profess to be searching. Harrison Gough, who has conducted a number of important studies of the measurement of non-cognitive criteria in medical students, studied the decision-making processes of one medical school admissions committee which stated that the committee was most interested in selecting creative, independent-thinking, other-oriented students. The outcome data from this study suggested that, instead, the students selected tended to be conforming, compliant students who were not other-oriented. If a school has a commitment to the identification and selection of minority students, and wishes to apply uniform criteria to the overall applicant pool, it will be necessary for that school to review critically the entire admissions process in terms of its merit and the consistency with which stated objectives are achieved. It will further be necessary to understand that reliance on traditional cognitive measures alone will almost certainly exclude a good many promising minority applicants from consideration.

I am a proponent of the continued use of the interview in medical school admissions, not because I am not aware of its many fallibilities, but because at the present time, there are no adequate alternative measures. The cynics who indict the interview for its lack of reliability and validity, for the lack of expertise on the part of the interviewers, and for the potential for misuse are ignoring some very simple facts. They are ignoring the fact that there are no psychometric tests which can measure with any accuracy such qualities as empathy, motivation, or maturity, qualities which interviews under some conditions have been shown to identify. There are no psychometric tests which differentiate those applicants who are most likely to drop out before the completion of medical school from those applicants who are most likely to successfully complete medical school. There simply are no acceptable substitute instruments available to the admissions committee which permit the incorporation of alternative criteria or which permit the assessment of non-traditional applicants. These same critics also overlook the facts that there are ways to increase the reliability and validity of the interview and that it is possible to train interviewers. They fail to acknowledge the fact that the steps required of a medical school to institute a more racially fair, valid interview process are simple and inexpensive to implement. Needed changes should focus on two areas—the actual format of the interviews and interviewer training. By means of a few changes, it becomes possible for the school to construct interviews which are useful to the committee in making selection decisions and which are also perceived by applicants as meaningful.

DESIGNING AND CONSTRUCTING
ADMISSIONS INTERVIEWS

Regrettably, the interview is not the place for free-wheeling creativity, an approach currently favored by many interviewers. Selection interviews have two basic purposes which should be kept in mind at all times. They should be used to assess qualities which cannot be assessed by any other means, and they should assess qualities which have some bearing on the applicant's potential as a student and a physician. In developing the interview, the committee should attempt to meet to the fullest extent possible the following objectives:

1. *The Interview Should Be Structured.* By structuring the interview so that each interviewer is asking questions concerning similar topics, the committee has much greater uniformity of information at its disposal and there is a greater likelihood that the information obtained will be accurate. Another advantage of structuring the interview is that it encourages interviewers to adhere to appropriate

topics and questions and reduces the collection of nonrelevant data. Structure can be as minimal as establishing which topic areas should be covered or as rigid as actually requiring interviewers to ask identical questions of each applicant. The more structured an interview, the greater will be the accuracy of the information obtained. Agreement between interviewers judging the same applicants will also be increased, thus increasing the confidence of the interviewers in their ability to make sound judgments and increasing the confidence of the committee upon the recommendations of the interviewers. Sharply divided opinions of interviewers of the same applicant are more likely to signal a need for more careful review of the applicant than is the case when no control is exercised over the content of the interview. Beginning interviewers are able to function at a much higher level than would be the case if they were to have less guidance. In most cases, the committee will need to strike a balance between the need to acquire uniform and consistent data and the need to allow some latitude to the interviewer. I would assure the skeptical that structured interviews do not have to be dull or restricting.

2. *The Scope of the Interview Should Be Limited to Appropriate Criteria.* There is growing evidence that human beings can make sound judgments about other human beings, particularly if they restrict themselves to judgments concerning personal qualities. Although many of the studies supporting this have pertained to persons being selected for such programs as Officer Training School, or graduate students in clinical psychology, a recent study at the University of Missouri-Columbia medical school of their graduates demonstrated that admissions interviewers' ratings of applicants on the basis of maturity and motivation showed a significant correlation with outstanding evaluations of their overall medical school performance.

Although many will take issue with what I am about to say, I feel it is necessary to call attention to the considerable evidence which has been accumulated that numerical data such as GPA and MCAT scores cannot be evaluated consistently or accurately by human judges, and may even impair the ability of judges to make sound assessments of personal qualities. An excellent paper on this subject by Robin Dawes demonstrates this conclusively. In my own experience with an exercise in policy-capturing for use in medical school admissions interviewing workshops, this same phenomenon has been demonstrated repeatedly. I recognize the problem which exclusion of discussion of the GPA and MCAT scores may present to committees, but I would encourage committees to consider alternative means of using these data other than in the selection interviews. Schools which utilize routine administrative interviews as adjuncts to the selections interviews could very easily include discussion of the academic performance in the administrative interview.

3. *Criteria Should Have Direct Bearing on Medical School Performance.* In the case of minority applicants, this can be particularly critical. In their book, *Racism in American Education: A Model for Change,* Sedlacek and Brooks list seven variables not usually considered in selection which they feel to be essential in determining the likely success of minority students in an academic program. They conclude that because these factors are so universally present for non-minority students, we are unaware of their importance, and we also fail to realize that they are not automatically present for minority students. They are variables which can be assessed by means of the interview. The critical seven are: (1) Positive self-concept; (2) Realistic way of dealing with racism; (3) Realistic self-appraisal; (4) Prefers long-range goals; (5) Presence of a strong support person or group; (6) Successful leadership experience (the authors note that this is unlikely to be culled from a review of traditional campus leadership activities); (7) Demonstrated community service as a measure of identification or affiliation with a community.

4. *Criteria Used Should be Legal and Ethically Acceptable.* Persons tempted to use trick questions or exercises should consider very carefully the ethics of such maneuvers as well as the need for such ploys. The criteria should be applicable to the total pool of applicants and should be reviewed carefully to be sure that there is no possibility of unintentional bias for or against one group of applicants.

5. *Criteria Should be Defined.* It is extremely important that the criteria to be used are defined and that the committee has reached a consensus on the definitions. The definitions need not be elaborate, but attention should be given to possible confusion or overlap among criteria.

6. *Appropriate Questions Should be Generated.* The task of the interviewer will be simplified if a bank of questions has been developed which can be used by interviewers. There are at least two

advantages. This will help standardize the definition of the criteria and will enable the interviewer to have a reserve of suitable questions, relieving him or her of the pressure to continually improvise questions during the interview. The questions should meet the following standards:

A. The questions should assess on the basis of direct information or by means of observed behaviors rather than on assumptions.
B. The questions should be designed so as to minimize the effect of the attitudinal biases or opinions of the interviewer making the judgment.
C. The questions should be open-ended rather than requiring a "Yes" or "No" response.
D. The questions should not favor the kinds of experiences to which only one subgroup of applicants may have had access.
E. Questions should be specific, not global, and should deal with behaviors rather than opinions.
F. The questions should be legal.
G. The questions should not be offensive. Women and minority applicants are frequently offended by questions which imply assumptions of inferior academic abilities. Such insults are often unintentional, but they frequently reveal unconscious biases on the part of the interviewer.
H. The expected depth of responses should be realistic in terms of the age, education, and life experience of the applicant.

7. *Applicants Should Have Ample Time to Discuss Topics They View as Important.* The interview should include an opportunity for applicants to ask questions or to provide information which they feel would be important for the interviewer to know about them. Sometimes this will give the interviewer valuable insights about the applicant which might otherwise be overlooked. Even more important, however, it establishes a relationship between the interviewer and the applicant which recognizes the needs of the applicant as well as the needs of the committee. In short, it introduces the dimension of humanity to the treatment of the applicant.

8. *Evaluating the Responses.* Once the criteria have been selected and refined, and once suitable questions have been generated, the

committee must establish guidelines for rating the responses. The following five criteria have proved extremely useful:

A. Consistency of Response. Does the response of the applicant hold through various lines of questioning? How does the applicant respond when confronted with inconsistencies in his or her responses? Are the activities or behaviors which an applicant reports consistent with behavior throughout the interview or with the stated likes and dislikes of the applicant?

B. Depth of Understanding. Are the responses glib and shallow or do they demonstrate a real understanding of the issues or the problems being discussed?

C. Conviction. Are the responses wishy-washy or is the applicant able to hold to his or her convictions without being rigid?

D. Absence of Social Desirability. Does the applicant attempt to please the interviewer or is he or she able to respond in the absence of interviewer's cues or to maintain opinions which differ from those expressed by the interviewer?

E. Conceptualization of Questions. Is the applicant able to deal with concepts or does he or she require concrete examples? Does the applicant demonstrate an ability to extract from a range of facts some central meaning?

TRAINING INTERVIEWERS

Having developed an interview which uses desirable criteria and having established some ground rules for its use, the committee must now address the even more difficult half of their responsibility, that of insuring that the interviewers they will be using have the necessary skills, are relatively unbiased, and are able to judge their interview behavior accurately and honestly. I am firmly convinced that most persons have the capacity to become good interviewers. In order to actualize this capacity interviewers must be willing to acknowledge their shortcomings and understand in what ways these affect their ability to conduct fair and valid interviews. One of the most effective ways of helping an interviewer understand how interviewing style affects the outcome of an interview is to videotape several interviews with students and then, with the aid of a more experienced interviewer, observe the interviews. Most interviewers find much to their surprise that they are better than they thought they could be and most find the process enlightening and rewarding. It is important to remember that each individual will bring a different level and assortment of skills into the process. The goal is not to create identical interviewers but to enable each interviewer to achieve his or her own maximum level. Interviewers who consistently offend students or who are not consistent with the other interviewers should be informed of this and provided the opportunity to change, but interviewers who are unable or unwilling to change should not continue to be used. At least one medical school grades its interviewers on a series of criteria and continues to use only those interviewers with a consistently superior track record. Again, this type of monitoring is extremely critical in the case of those interviewers who are interviewing minority applicants. Such interviewers must be able to demonstrate the skills of good listening and the ability to understand and establish rapport with a broad range of individuals from widely differing backgrounds. They must be able to evaluate applicants in the context of their unique experiences, background, and previous opportunities or lack of opportunities and assess their accomplishments on a flexible rather than a rigid scale—not an easy job, but not impossible.

ADVICE TO APPLICANTS

Applicants who have been reading this chapter should note that I am not advocating trickery or deception on the part of interviewers, but rather the development of interviews which provide a systematic means of broadening the criteria used in evaluating applicants. Many of you will have heard all kinds of tales from other applicants, from friends, and even from advisors that may tend to make you feel very apprehensive about impending interviews. You will also have received well-meaning advice on what to expect and what you should do to impress an interviewer. For the most part, you will find it more helpful to forget the stories—they are often exaggerated or distorted—and to forget the advice. Remember, life has prepared you for the interviews. The more chances you have had to interact with authority figures on more or less equal terms, the more likely you are to be comfortable in an interview setting, even in an interview which is not going well. Maturity allows individuals to gain a more realistic perspective of the process and enables them to realize that a bad interview does not necessarily mean the end of their dreams. If you have this perspective, you are less likely to concentrate on the impression you are making and more able to concentrate on trying to respond to the questions, remembering that you want the interviewer to have as full and complete an understanding of you as possible.

The name of the game in this case is not to try to "psych out" the interviewer. It is to present yourself as honestly and completely as possible. I understand that the enormous range in format and the treatment you will receive at different medical schools can be very confusing and sometimes discouraging. At some schools each applicant who is interviewed will receive two one-hour interviews which are one-to-one. At other schools, you may be interviewed by a pair of interviewers or an even larger group. At other schools, there may be only one interviewer but as many as four applicants in the interview. The amount of time will vary from five minutes to well over an hour. The interview setting may be relaxed and informal or it may be designed to be more stressful. If at all possible, find out what the interviews will be like at each of the schools where you have interviews scheduled. You can do this by phoning or writing the admissions office. In order to get complete information, you may need to be persistent. You should find out what percentage of the pool of applicants is invited to interview and what percentage of interviewed applicants is accepted. You should get some indication of the length of time the interview will entail, as well as whether or not it is a group interview, a one-to-one, or some other variation. If the school is close by, you may want to visit the school a few days ahead of your interview date. This will give you an opportunity to become somewhat familiar with the setting, and perhaps even to talk to some students. Not only will this help you feel more comfortable on interview day, it will also give some time for you to think about what you would like to know about the school, its progams, and its curriculum. If the school is too far away to visit, be sure to have read the catalog or the prospectus before the interview. As you read try to anticipate what reservations you might have about what the school has to offer as well as what benefits there are. The interview is very likely to be the one chance you will have to get any questions you have responded to or clarified. As an applicant you have a right to be as completely informed about the school as possible, and you should exercise that right.

At the risk of making some of you feel unnecessarily anxious, I feel it is only fair to point out that difficult as admissions interviews are for all applicants, they may present a greater difficulty to minority applicants for a number of reasons. Although minority faculty and students do serve as interviewers at many schools, the interviewer may well be a non-minority person, and this increases the possibility that you may be confronted with someone with preconceived negative stereotypes which are difficult for you to counteract. The minority applicant may have to deal with remarks which are insensitive or insulting and so may have to contend with the resultant feelings of anger in a way which does not adversely affect the interview. The minority applicant is apt to have to take a more active stance in helping the interviewer understand the implications of past activities, and may have to translate these accomplishments into terms more understandable to the non-minority interviewer.

Earlier I stressed the importance of trying to be as complete and honest as possible in your responses during the interview. You are not expected to know the answer to every question, and the interviewer is more likely to be impressed with the answer, "I don't know" than with an answer which clearly shows that you did not know what you were talking about and did not have the sense to acknowledge that. That same advice should apply to your style of dress. It is not necessary to buy a new outfit. You should wear something you feel good in, something that is comfortable and that is neither excessively casual nor excessively formal. You will feel more relaxed and your behavior will reflect that good feeling. I would caution you that for the most part you will be interacting with a relatively conservative group of people who will not be impressed by flashiness or sloppiness in dress, and that should be taken into consideration when you are planning what to wear.

My final advice concerns what you should do if you feel you have been treated inappropriately or unfairly in the interview. If at all possible, you should make an effort to meet with the principal admissions officer before leaving the school. This might make it possible to schedule another interview immediately. If you are unable to do so, write to the admissions officer detailing your reasons for feeling the interview was unfair, and request another interview. You also have rights in the interview process and fundamental among those rights is the right to expect that the interviewer will treat you in a non-judgmental fashion and will offer you ample opportunity to discuss your views.

SUMMARY

In summary, despite their many shortcomings, interviews can be of value to those schools interested in broadening the range of individuals selected. They provide a useful means by which non-traditional applicants can be more fairly and adequately assessed. They permit the inclusion of the human dimension in a process which tends to dehumanize the applicant. The majority of medical schools currently using interviews have not made effective use of them even though the means to do so exist. Applicants can take heart in the fact that interviews are really not so mysterious or complicated after all. For the most part, they consist of meetings with persons who are trying to the best of their ability to select the best applicants possible. Although the job of communicating an accurate picture of the applicant to the interviewer may be more difficult for the minority applicant because of factors over which the applicant has no control, it is necessary that the applicant make the attempt. The results are well worth it.

CHAPTER 13

The Admissions Process

Norma E. Wagoner

Perhaps the greatest mystery to most students when applying to medical school is *what actually happens* to their applications as they work their way through a maze of procedures, where predictability of outcome often remains a mystery, or at the speculation level at best.

This chapter will address a variety of issues relating to the admissions process, including a definition of the "process;" what constitutes a "committee;" how it functions; and the roles and responsibilities of the "admissions director." Within the context of the discussion in each of these sections will be a question-and-answer format, since most of the interaction which students have with an admissions office comes in the way of questions posed to them. The objective of this chapter is in some way to help "demystify" the process and give students a more realistic framework within which to proceed.

Norma E. Wagoner, Ph.D., is Assistant Professor of Anatomy and Associate Dean, Student Services and Educational Resources, College of Medicine, University of Cincinnati, Ohio.

THE SETTING

Currently, there are 124 medical schools in this country with an all-time high enrollment in those three and four-year programs, with a total of 62,242 students. It is important to have a look at the composition nationally, because in many ways these percentages tend to get mirrored in the individual processes that schools operate. The total number of women enrolled in 1978 accounted for 24.3 percent, by comparison to 23.7 percent the previous year. There was little change in the racial/ethnic composition over the previous year; however, those minority groups targeted for increased representation amounted to 7.9 percent, as compared to 8.1 percent in 1977. The number of White students now enrolled in medical schools represents 86.4 percent of the total enrollment (53,746), with the number of Black students being 3,540 and the other nonwhites representing the remainder of the pool.*

THE PROCESS

The words "admissions process" can conjure up many meanings, and for some may encompass such things as the paper processing part of the application cycle, while for others it may connote an admissions office with its Dean and staff, or the interviews, or all of the components which lead up to the acceptance and entrance into medical school.

With this broad set of possibilities, let us look at the individual pieces by asking the following questions:

What is the best means for finding out about "the process"?

There are a variety of sources but two very reliable ones should be accessed by the students if possible. One contains general application information on each of the 124 medical schools and is known as the "Medical School Admission Requirements" book. An updated issue appears yearly. Most premedical advisors have a current copy in their offices, since school data on deadlines, percentage of nonresidents accepted, and tuition figures change yearly. Because of the importance of this book, a student may wish

---

* Davis G. Johnson: Memorandum—U.S. Medical School Enrollments as of October 15, 1978.

to purchase it directly (cost in the past has been around $5.00). The address to write to is:

Association of American Medical Colleges
Attention: Membership and Subscriptions
One Dupont Circle, N.W., Suite 200
Washington, D.C. 20036

The second publication of value is entitled "Minority Student Opportunities in United States Medical Schools." This, like the previous publication, can be purchased at the above address for around $3.00. It too is updated frequently and provides data on the number of minority student graduates for each of the 124 medical schools, as well as listings of opportunities for summer programs, financial aid, and the like at each school. The content of this publication is more fully detailed in the chapter in this book by Dario Prieto.

What kind of information is found in the "Medical School Admission Requirements" book?

This comprehensive manual has many sections in it, but can be divided into two major areas: (1) a general applicant information portion, and (2) a specific medical school informational profile section. The general material section includes suggestions on premedical planning; deciding on whether and where to apply to medical schools; the New MCAT and the AMCAS process; financial information; the nature of medical education; information for minority groups, as well as a discussion for those not admitted. All of this precedes the section in which the 124 medical schools each provide two pages of information on their school's program. It is here that the school will detail specific course requirements and sometimes the average grade point average of its enrolled students as well as their average MCAT scores are included, as well as application deadlines, tuition charges, and cost to the student for supplemental application fees. A student should know that deadlines vary from school to school, and that plans need to be made accordingly to meet these.

Where is the best place to obtain an application packet?

Ninety-one of the U.S. medical schools currently hold membership in the American Medical Colleges Application Service (AMCAS) in Washington, D.C. Packets can be obtained directly from them. Premedical advisor's offices will usually keep a supply on hand and pass them out to the students when they hold general orientation sessions for those about to submit applications, while medical schools will usually only keep a few on hand. The address for this service is: AMCAS, Suite 301, 1776 Massachusetts Avenue, Washington, D.C. 20036. As you review the "Medical School Admission Requirements" book and note which schools are members, you may also decide to apply to a nonmember AMCAS school. Since these schools are outside of the application service, it will be necessary to write directly to them for their materials. These school addresses are provided in the Admission Requirement book.

What is the length of time that applications are in process?

In order for most medical schools to select a class, the time involved may *exceed one year.* Medical school admissions are done in cycles of overlapping years. For instance, those students who entered in the fall of 1978 had the opportunity to submit their applications as early as June 15, 1977 if applying to an AMCAS school. Applications usually begin arriving at the medical schools in early July. The overall length of time for filing an application at any one school varies, but the closing dates begin as early as mid-October, with the latest being mid-December.

Is it worthwhile to apply early?

The answer to this is *most definitely!* This statement is made time and time again by admissions personnel, premedical advisors, etc. No doubt those who heed this suggestion will be more likely to achieve positive results. With so many schools participating in the uniform application service, this makes life considerably easier for the student. The student should be aware that the same statement can be made about early return of the school's supplemental forms. Most of the schools will not process the application until all materials are on file, and thus it pays *not to delay!*

What does it cost to apply?

Of the 37,000 students who applied to medical schools for the 1977-78 program, 90 percent applied to at least one of the 90 AMCAS schools, with eight as the average number being submitted. The AMCAS service charge is based on the number of participating schools to which a student applies, but the following scale obtains: $25 for the first school with $5 increments for each school up to five ($40), with an additional $10 fee for each school thereafter. For the average student applying to eight schools, the cost would be $70. AMCAS has not wished this to be a limiting factor for any student, and has developed a Fee Waiver Program for students from families who do not have the ability to pay. In order to apply for consideration of this program, the student should use the appropriate forms in the application packet.

Each of the schools has its own secondary screening fee which can range from no cost to $35, with the average being about $20. Thus, now adding the $160 onto the $70 figure, a total of approximately $230 will be needed for the paper processing portion of the application. Most of the medical schools, like AMCAS, do not wish to rule a student out because of limited funds to pay the secondary fee; thus if a student receives a fee waiver from AMCAS, schools will usually waive their supplemental fees as well. If a fee waiver is not granted, but the student has obtained considerable support in grants or loans from the undergraduate college, a visit to the Financial Aid officer to obtain documentation to send to the medical school may be sufficient to allow them to waive the secondary fee.

How many schools should a student apply to?

This is certainly one of the more critical aspects of the whole process, and not easy to discuss, since there are so many individual circumstances which are operational. While the burden of responsibility rests with the student to make the final selection of schools to which to apply, it is worthwhile to seek recommendations from your premedical advisor. Oftentimes the advisor has personal knowledge about a school's process as well as its strengths and weaknesses and can realistically guide you in your decision-making.

One of the major considerations in selecting schools to which to apply is the residence restrictions under which each school operates. State supported schools are usually allowed the least amount of latitude and are often required by state laws to take their own residents first. The restrictions on private schools vary, and again will depend upon the amount of state aid received. In states where there are no medical schools, both public and private schools in neighboring states may additionally give preference to students who reside in these states as well. Currently there are four such interstate agreements which provide special opportunities for residents of some states but only two will be discussed. For complete details of these programs, a student will need to write directly to each program. The names and addresses for these are found in the "Medical School Admission Requirements" book in the section on Whether and When To Apply.

WICHE - Students from Alaska, Arizona, Montana, and Washington who are accepted into accredited Western medical schools (with the exception of the University of Washington) who participate in the Western Interstate Commission for Higher Education can pay in-state tuition at public schools and a reduced tuition at private schools.

WAMI - Washington, Alaska, Montana, and Idaho have a cooperative program under the supervision of the University of Washington where students from these states take the preclinical phases of their course work in participating universities in their home state and clerkships in family medicine, internal medicine, pediatrics, obstetrics and gynecology, and psychiatry in rural communities in the four-state area.

Many schools, by virtue of their individual philosophy or types of students they seek, make it more likely for some students to be accepted at one school over another. Additionally, like many undergraduate schools, some medical schools are considered to be more highly competitive than others. Their reputations have been established over a long period of time, and thus they have a more commanding lead in the ability to attract the most competitive students. Traditionally, these will be students who have attended the most highly select undergraduate schools and who have the highest grades and MCATS. If at all possible, before a student applies to any school, the academic range of acceptable grades and MCATs should be determined so that students will be able to realistically assess how competitive they are for a position. Most advisors will suggest that students select a few in each range, with the major emphasis being placed on the schools in the student's state of residence. By ignoring these two major parameters of grades and residence and selecting inappropriately, a student could potentially face a year's delay.

What is the Early Decision Plan and should it be considered?

The Early Decision program is a contractual agreement by a

medical school and a student who wishes to participate in it. The student agrees to apply initially to one school only, and, if accepted, will attend that medical school. The acceptance date for this program is uniform and falls on October 1 of each year for all those who participate. There are obvious advantages to this program, not the least of which is the saving in time and money, as well as anxiety from not knowing about possible acceptance until a later time. Before selecting one school, it would be worthwhile visiting the various programs to determine if your notions of their offerings, the kinds of students attending, the facilities and costs are what you have perceived. It is additionally worthwhile to determine from each school what the academic credentials of students are who are being accepted during this program. Some schools make this known in their literature about the school, although others do not. If the latter is the case, it might be prudent to make an appointment with someone on the admissions staff to make sure that your candidacy is a realistic one. Since the schools stand to gain some commitments, they are usually happy to advise students about their own Early Decision program.

Is it important to let your undergraduate premedical advisor know you are applying to an Early Decision Program?

Some premedical advisors may require it, but by all means, you should use the resources of their office, since they may be able to provide you with some information that will allow you to direct your questions more appropriately to the admissions personnel when you make a visit. Secondly, the advisor can assist you in assuring that your letters are on file, so that once the medical school asks you for them, they can be obtained in an expedient manner. The next step is to discuss with the Registrar's office the importance of having your transcript sent to AMCAS (if your Early Decision School is an AMCAS school), since the processing will be held up if a *current* transcript is not available. This is true for all the undergraduate colleges in which some educational experience was obtained, so don't neglect asking for a transcript from the school(s) where one or two courses were taken.

What is the best time to send in an application for the EARLY DECISION Program?

There is a very short time period for applying during this program. As previously mentioned, AMCAS begins accepting applications about the middle of June, and all materials for the

Early Decision program must be in their hands by August 1. This gives the schools a very short time in which to ask the student to fill out supplemental materials and send letters of evaluation, along with being interviewed at that school. Most schools will try to complete all of this part of the process and reserve time for Committees to make decisions on the candidates during the last two weeks in September, so that final notification of how the students fared can be transmitted to them by October 1.

What happens if a student does not get accepted in the Early Decision Program; will there be opportunities at other schools?

The schools have three options in the Early Decision program—to accept a student, to defer the student to the regular applicant pool, or to reject that student, where he or she cannot continue in that school's application process for that year's cycle. On receiving either deferment or rejection, a student needs to submit immediately to AMCAS an alternate designation form, listing the other schools of interest. Since AMCAS has all the materials, processing additional applications to other medical schools will usually occur within two to three weeks. Unless a medical school begins its program in the early summer, students would not be likely to find themselves too late for consideration at these other schools.

There are a number of questions which are often asked by students about the application process that are of a more specific nature, but nonetheless get asked often enough to warrant short discussions.

If you have been told that a medical school only takes "certain types" of students, and that school is within your state of residence, is it worthwhile to apply if you don't believe you are "their type"?

By all means, a visit to the school is in order if you are at all in doubt about what they offer or what the prevailing philosophy is for their programs. Oftentimes rumors or misconceptions get perpetuated, and before a state school is ruled out, be sure to check the rumors. In many respects, this will greatly help when you are called to that school for an interview, since many schools will ask what you consider the strength of their program to be, or why you wish to come there for an education. If you have expended the effort to find out these things ahead of time, you will be in a better position to respond with accurate information. Before you visit any school, however, be sure to obtain the bulletins or handbooks published by that school, so that your questions will indicate a basic knowledge of the programs offered there.

How much should the school's cost of medical education or their ability to provide financial help influence whether an application is submitted?

The tuition figures are not too difficult to obtain, but the actual picture of how much assistance a school may be able to provide is very difficult to determine. Medical schools are faced with tremendous problems in finding dollars to assist students, and the whole picture is an extremely complicated one, so *don't* rule a school out on stated tuition costs alone. If the school accepts you, then explore the possibilities of financing, and if proposed aid is not acceptable to you at that point, then make a decision to discontinue consideration.

Should a student submit an application to an osteopathic school while applying to allopathic schools through the AMCAS process?

The answer to this one is somewhat difficult, although most osteopathic as well as allopathic schools appreciate that for students who truly wish to serve in a health professions setting, the number of places is still less than the number of qualified applicants. For the last two years, fewer students have applied to health professions schools, thus increasing the ratio of acceptance; however, there are still many more qualified students than places. If a student applies to an osteopathic school, clear differences in philosophy for these two branches of medicine should be determined. Osteopathic schools do not like to look upon themselves as second choice spots to allopathic medicine, should a student not be able to enter that one.

What about a second or third application to a medical school—is it realistic?

Medical schools differ in their philosophies about repeat applicants, particularly those in a year immediately after an unsuccessful attempt. From the student's perspective, it is certainly worthwhile to assess why acceptance was not granted on the first application. This is sometimes very difficult to do, particularly since there are many nuances used in the admissions process, and this information may or may not be shared with a student in a counseling session. It is certain, though, that medical schools will rarely turn down a student for a *single* factor. Analysis of the *whys* requires asking a series of questions, such as —was the selection of schools to which the student applied both sufficient and realistic? Were the grades in the sciences and nonsciences both of a sufficient level that there was a reasonably clear indication of success to the medical school? Were there any *withdraws, incompletes,* low grades, or an overall downward trend that might give some sign of inability to handle a medical school curriculum? Were the MCATs at the level of those students currently being accepted? Were there enough health-related or people-related activities to give indication of more than academic development alone at the undergraduate level? Studies show that the opportunity for a student to obtain an acceptance on the second try is about 31 percent. Some medical schools spend time counseling the nonaccepted applicant, and it may be worth a visit to the school prior to reapplying. Additionally, some premedical advisors' offices have an excellent publication entitled "The Rejected Medical School Applicant, Options and Alternatives" by Carlos Pestana, M.D. Overall, the general rule of thumb is that medical schools will most likely be interested in a second application if the student is able to show some substantial change over the first one.

Is it worthwhile to change state of residence for a second application if other states have better odds?

If a student is truly determined to seek entrance, and the residence variable was a major factor in the first round consideration, then it might be worth the effort. This is a route which has been successfully utilized by many students. There should be an understanding of how students obtain state residency at the medical schools, with the general recognition that public and private schools may have different guidelines, and that these are quite often different from those used for voting purposes, drivers license, state taxes, etc.

THE PAPER PROCESSING

Having spent considerable time talking about the ways in which applications can be generated by the student, it is now time to discuss what a school does when it receives the application. Some schools receive fewer than 1,000; there are some (largely private schools) where the number exceeds 8,000. Obviously the number received by that school has a lot to do with the way the application is processed. At this point it might be worthwhile to divide the discussion into two sections—that processing which is done by an admissions committee and the decisions they will make, and that handled by the admissions office.

THE ADMISSIONS COMMITTEE——WHO ARE THEY?

Students applying to medical school have somehow conjured up a great deal of power for this group, and have few notions of the checks and balances that occur to assure that the selection is representative of the wishes of the faculty of that college.

There are not many data in the literature to substantiate how medical schools actually constitute their committees. Most schools utilize one of two methods—that of having the Dean select the membership, or giving the responsibility to a standing committee which selects and sends the recommendations on to the Dean for approval. Usually the larger representation will come from the clinical departments with the smaller number from the basic sciences. Typically the committee would also include a Dean of Admissions or their administative officer as well as a psychiatrist or two, such that the total committee number may be as few as 10 to as many as 30. There is usually an attempt to "balance" a committee with an appropriate number of women, minorities, young faculty members, older faculty members, department chairpersons, community or health agency representatives, and students from the college of medicine. The belief is that these individuals will be able to provide insight into candidates whose backgrounds or experiences may be similar to their own.

Having talked about the Committee composition, what happens when the application arrives at the Admissions Office?

As mentioned previously, applications can be submitted as early as mid-June, and beginning around the first of July, medical schools will usually receive daily "batches" from AMCAS. These arrive with as few as one or two to as many as several hundred per day. The peak times in admissions offices occur in September through December. This is all the more reason for an applicant not to delay in submitting an application until this peak time. During these months, the process for an office is not only slower, but more likely for a letter or other piece of important information to go astray.

PRIMARY OR PRELIMINARY
SCREENING—STEP ONE

The first step is by necessity an office procedure, where each application is logged into the school's system, whether it be their own computer or a manual system. A file folder is then generated for each candidate, including the possibility of placing the bio-data card in a separate system for manual use and notation of activity. Some schools may elect to send out their own materials describing fee structure and processing schedule, as well as a request to complete supplemental materials and submit letters of evaluation.

Cognitive Screen

Whether a computer or manual screening process is employed, the scores (both grade point average and MCATs) can be an obstacle to any further consideration in the process, should these scores fall outside the range of the acceptable group. This type of screen, exclusive of other factors such as letters of recommendation, is most often used by highly selective schools and/or those who receive large numbers of applications. It serves as an effective means to "pare down" the applicant pool to a manageable size. Candidates with the desired state of residency are usually handled in a less rigorous manner and moved on into the secondary screening part of the process.

If the application appears competitive, the student will usually be asked to complete the school's secondary application form and submit letters of recommendation.

Once all of these materials have been returned, a complete evaluation of the application is done to determine who will be selected for interviews. However, this brings up the next logical question:

By whom and/or how does the decision get made as to which individuals will be interviewed?

SECONDARY SCREENING—STEP TWO

A look at the "who" part of the screening process first——this may be done by any one of the following individuals or combination thereof:

1. Director of Admissions and staff
2. Chairperson of Admissions Committee
3. Full Admissions Committee
4. Subcommittee of the Full Admissions Committee

There are many medical schools in which the Director or Dean of Admissions may also serve as chairperson of the Committee. If this is not the case, the Committee then tends to select one from among its membership to serve as chairperson, and the Dean or Director will serve in an ex-officio or advisory capacity. In some instances, one of the responsibilities of the Director or Dean will be to instruct the Committee on current admissions data and national guidelines, developing the school's own policies and procedures for committee work, and assist the committees in the screening process. Another but less common practice now is to set up subcommittees which are assigned the responsibility of assessing segments of the applicant pool. These constituted subcommittees tend to be asked to participate in these smaller work units because of particular expertise or understanding which they possess on a group or groups of candidates under consideration. Types of applicant grouping can occur through several means, which include using the designations on the AMCAS application, or by desire of candidates for certain kinds of programs that the schools might offer. Examples of some representative groups are as follows:

1. Candidates who are designated on AMCAS as coming from rural counties, or are interested in rural medicine.
2. Candidates who are designated on AMCAS as wishing to receive minority consideration.
3. Candidates who have an interest in a Ph.D./M.D. program at the medical school.
4. Candidates who have advanced degrees or are from other degree programs.
5. Candidates who are from other states.

The relationship of the subcommittee to the full committee is that subcommittees will usually serve in an advisory role when candidates are ultimately presented for vote. The implications of the subcommittee approach with the post-Bakke decision will be discussed in the last part of this chapter.

Regardless of the "who" part of the process when screening occurs, there is general cognizance about the relative importance of certain factors when selecting candidates for interview as well as a desire to select students with the greatest strengths in these areas. A listing of these follows, with a general discussion of a few of the more important ones.

ACADEMIC AND PERSONAL CHARACTERISTICS AFFECTING SELECTION FOR INTERVIEWS AND ENTRANCE

1. Selectivity index of college attended
2. Science grade point average total for all years
3. Science grades in required courses
4. Individual as well as composite MCAT scores
5. Nonscience grade point average over the four years
6. Difficulty in chosen program (honors, double major, etc.)
7. Number of hours carried per semester (quarter)
8. Honors or recognition in academics prior to entering college
9. Honors or recognition in academics during college
10. Upward trend in grades through all four years
11. Amount worked while taking full load of academic coursework
12. Extenuating circumstances which might have affected grades (illnesses)
13. Commitment to outside employment in the summer
14. Commitment to extracurricular activities
15. Honors or awards in extracurricular pursuits (varsity team, etc.)
16. Leadership roles in organizations or extracurriculars
17. Involvement in research while an undergraduate
18. Publishing a paper in a refereed journal
19. Pursuit of independent study programs in college
20. Writing an Honors thesis for a college program
21. Involvement in Community Affairs

22. Involvement in Health Care Activities
23. Involvement in Patient Care settings
24. Quality of personal comments on AMCAS (style, organization, content)
25. Quality of supplemental materials (including timeliness of return)
26. Letters of evaluation referencing:
    a. honesty or integrity of student
    b. motivation and willingness to learn
    c. perseverance and dedication to purpose
    d. team effort in classes as well as leadership skills
    e. style of learning
    f. ability at problem-solving
    g. ability to relate to others
    h. common sense, both personal and academic
    i. breadth and depth of character

This list is not intended to be inclusive, but certainly encompasses a large measure of personal and intellectual strengths sought in applicants. Several of these qualities will now be discussed in greater detail, as will the rationale behind their usage.

1. *Selectivity index of undergraduate school.* As a student might well appreciate, grades in and of themselves are not easily compared from one applicant to the other, because of the high degree of variability in schools, as well as professors teaching the courses. What an admissions director or committee members will have available to them is college reference guides, such as Cass and Birnbaum's *Comparative Guide to American Colleges* or Lovejoy's *College Guide* or any of several other references of this type which show the composite SAT or ACT scores of students attending that undergraduate school. Reference is usually made to the degree of difficulty in obtaining success at that campus. In addition, many of the premedical advisors provide the admissions committees with standards of reference about the courses, grades achieved in those programs for that year, number of students rated in the following categories, etc. These data are most helpful to committees in the screening process.

2. *Science courses and success in these* is a major consideration for most medical schools. Undergraduate schools know this as well, and thus, many of the courses that medical schools focus on are also

the most difficult to do well in academically. Since much weight is given to the outcome of these courses they should not be taken on the pass/fail basis. If possible, organic chemistry or physics should not be pursued during the summer at a local community or junior college, as medical schools will question the rationale for this since part of what a committee needs to know about students is whether they can handle difficult and demanding course work at their own college or university.

3. *If a student had to work while taking a full course load,* this should certainly be mentioned in the application. Many times students feel embarassed that they had to work their way through and may choose not to mention working. However, medical schools are realistic about the problems that this may pose for a student, particularly in reference to the science courses just mentioned. The same reference can be made to *extentuating circumstances* due to personal health or family problems. It is better to be open and honest about these situations, as this information will often be revealed in the interviews. The best advice is to share as much as possible of yourself and your academic and personal progress in the comments section of the application, which will provide your reviewers and interviewers with a better means to assess your coping skills.

4. Since the advent of the *New Medical College Admission Test* in 1977, there has not been a sufficient lapse of time to gather longitudinal data about which elements of the exam will be the best predictors of success. Even though predictive data are not available, medical schools will take these scores into consideration when selecting students, and they will be inclined to select those students whose scores fall within the range of candidates accepted in the previous year.

5. *Degree of difficulty of academic program* can be variously defined. Committees will carefully check those courses done at the honors level and evaluate these differently. When a student is elected to an honors program, many times doubts are expressed about the desirability of pursuing courses at this level, since the competition is usually very keen and higher grades are more difficult to achieve. By the same token if a student signs up for many difficult and demanding courses and does not do well (Withdraws and Incompletes included), this will be noted by the committee as well, and

may serve as a red flag to indicate that the student may have problems competing in the medical school program.

In addition to the detailed listing of cognitive and noncognitive aspects that a committee utilizes, there are several overriding considerations that schools must factor into their processes. Some of these include the following:

1. Desire to recruit state residents in order to provide maximum opportunities for students from that state.
2. Desire to emphasize recruitment of students who have indicated a strong interest in primary care.
3. Desire to recruit students who have indicated a willingness to practice in health-deficient communities.
4. Desire to recruit students who are interested in research or academic medicine.

The emphasis that the schools place on any of these types of goals will often characterize the "philosophy" of that medical school. In addition to these, there are Federal guidelines under which all schools must operate and include the following:

1. No discrimination on the basis of sex or age of candidate.
2. No discrimination on the basis of race or religion of candidate.
3. No discrimination on the basis of marital status of the candidate.
4. No discrimination on the basis of physical or health-related handicaps.

These Federal guidelines are oftentimes difficult to interdigitate in the process and assure equity in the consideration of all candidates. Currently, the two most difficult for medical schools to handle are the issues which relate to race and those which relate to handicaps. A short discussion on how schools handle the race issue follows.

Where, When and How is Race factored into the "Process"?

The Bakke case is now history, but the impact of this decision is certainly not. It has raised innumerable questions, and has brought unprecedented attention to the role of medical schools in assisting in the efforts to right past wrongs, whether they be right or wrong in this endeavor. Setting aside places for qualified minority students was indeed serving a goal, which was recognized as urgent and yet objectionable by those who opposed quotas. In many respects, affirmative action is the only means of increasing the absurdly small number of minority physicians, and such a means of devoting places exclusively is the only real promise of any significant change in the real numbers of minority health care providers. Since this goal has now come under scrutiny, it appears that the number of minority students who will enter medical school in the future is projected to total slightly over one thousand. In an article by Richard Margolis* entitled "Why 117 Medical Schools Can't Be Right," he states, "What Bakke's challenge has inadvertently accomplished is to reveal the medical colleges' embarrassing little secret: not that they are racist, but that they are capricious." He contends that Americans have developed their own medical priesthood with doctors as king of the hill. With many aspirants wanting to be kings, the old cliche "many will be called, but few will be chosen" certainly applies. Obviously Bakke perceived that he was a victim of a racial boomerang in which medical schools were attempting to rectify past injustices. The most important question now facing admissions committees is: how does a selection procedure operate which does not maintain a "double standard"? There are those who would contend that the subcommittee method is one which might be described as a "double standard" method. This might be true if one looked at the academic characteristics only in the narrowest sense, with little emphasis on other important guides to success. The one thing that is forcefully pointed out in the literature is that minority students do succeed in spite of lower MCAT scores and grade point averages. In the past decade, the *Journal of Medical Education* has carried numerous articles describing successful programs. For most schools which have had a substantial number of minority students, there is a definite recognition that since the early '70s the dropout rate has continued to decline as schools themselves become more cognizant of ways to predict success. The Association of American Medical Colleges played a significant role in this by providing extensive sessions for admissions officers, committee members, and premedical advisors in Simulated Minority Admissions Exercises.† In most schools today, minority students are being evaluated along with other

---

* Richard J. Margolis: Why 117 Medical Schools Can't Be Right. CHANGE, October 1977, pp. 26-33.

† See this section in Ch. 3.

students in the applicant pool, certainly at the voting procedure level. If subcommittees are utilized, they are considered more. in the realm of special resource people, and it is hoped would include those who might have received training through the AAMC Simulation Workshops. What has been recognized by committees is the importance of placing greater emphasis on the noncognitive data, with the recognition that many minority students have been disadvantaged in their educational opportunities, and hence may not have developed the academic credentials to the level found among majority students. As a consequence, minority students with lower MCATs and grade point averages than the majority population should be given serious consideration.

In addition, many schools also pay close attention to the student's study effort and the methods used by that student in learning large volumes of material.

What are some of the realities of the post-Bakke decision on admissions? This is a very difficult one to assess, since it is next to impossible to get a titer on all the groups who would need to be sampled to answer this question. One could look at the statistics at the beginning of this chapter and note the decline of minority students in the 1978 fall enrollment. This decline is unfortunately not a new phenomenon, and has been noted for the past three years. Several factors have been implicated in this, not the least of which is the high cost of education and the unwillingness of students, both majority and minority, to invest as much of their lifetime in the pursuit of a goal which may or may not be obtainable. Coupled with the known difficulties for all students to obtain entrance, there is further pressure on the admissions committees to be "more discreet" in the *how* of the selection process. There is evidence of a marked shift in societal commitment toward any affirmative action, particularly in a career area that is as competitive to enter as medicine is. These combined attitudes and reality factors not only dissuade students from selecting medicine as a career choice, but may more subtly thwart the good intentions of those on the admissions committees who wish to be a part of the "problem-solving group" in society, and who are interested in realistically providing for society a cross-section of care providers that is truly representative.

CHAPTER 14

Problems and Perspectives of Financing Medical Education

Frances D. French

The means of financing medical education impacts recruitment, retention, and career choice more profoundly today than ever before. The cost of medical education to students has increased remarkably and the cost of financing such an education is escalating daily as loan interest rates climb and grant dollars diminish or disappear. What does this mean to the economically disadvantaged minority student? It means that a barrier has arisen impeding the achievement of their hopes and aspirations. Is the barrier insurmountable? It may well be insurmountable unless we commit ourselves to achieving these goals:

1. A commitment to achieve the social goal that there should be equal access to medical education by all qualified applicants—there should not be a financial barrier.

2. A commitment to meet a societal need—providing equal access to health care by all United States citizens.

3. A commitment to preserve the very cherished right of all individuals: freedom of choice, with the final choice, the ultimate decision, based on solid information.

Frances D. French is Director of Academic Services, University of Michigan Medical School, Ann Arbor, Michigan.

What can we do to assist minority and economically disadvantaged students in surmounting the financial barrier? First, we must understand their special circumstances. Second, we must help them deal with reality. Third, together we must learn about the sources of financial assistance and their complexities. Fourth, we must become expert counselors, providing solid information so students can make informed decisions about choosing indentureship or indebtedness pathways to medical degrees. We must counsel these students on coping with personal and family crises that arise during medical school. Lastly, we must fully understand the importance of providing equal access to education, and work to achieve it. An amplification of these points might be helpful, if all of us are to work effectively to increase the number of physicians from under-represented groups and economically disadvantaged families.

DEALING WITH REALITY

All of us who work with economically disadvantaged students must help them deal with the reality that education costs money, that it is their responsibility to shoulder the burden of debt that results, that such debt is manageable, and that these facts should not deter them from pursuing a health professions career. The barrage of publicity today about the cost of medical education and the cost of money available to finance this endeavor has undoubtedly turned many young people away from aspiring for an M.D. degree. The reasons are obvious. It is our responsibility to tackle the problem head-on and discuss this with the pre-professional and science major undergraduate students at our own institutions. Medicine is a life-time commitment; eight years of investment in reaching the starting line is not too much. Our society needs physicians who are representative of all walks of life, all races, creeds and cultures, in order to provide the broadest spectrum of quality health care to our nation. A shorter term, less expensive educational investment in alternate fields may pay off quickly, but is not a trade-off for a place in the ranks of the most time honored profession, medicine.

When such students have entered the medical curriculum, efforts must continue to assure them that we understand their special problems and that we know that these result in a more stressful existence for them than it does for students who are not economically disadvantaged. The stress is even greater for students who are economically disadvantaged *and* also members of minority groups if they are attending schools with predominantly White student enrollments. Learning to cope with the White elitist is a culture shock which is compounded by financial stresses. We must help these students to cope.

SOURCES OF FINANCIAL ASSISTANCE

An in-depth analysis of the various sources of assistance is not appropriate for this publication; however, it is important to have a general knowledge of aid sources and their complexities. Students should be fully informed of the details of the options and should be encouraged to discuss them with their school's financial aid officer as early as possible. There are very, very few full scholarships which do not include provisions for repayment in service.

There are two so-called indentured service programs. The National Health Service Corps Scholarship Program and the Armed Services Scholarship Programs. Each pays a monthly stipend, all tuition, books, equipment, and other fees and stipulates that the student must serve one year for each year of scholarship support, with a minimum service period of two years.

The National Health Service Corps is designed to provide more family practitioners and place them in areas where physician shortages exist. The allowable internship-residency training period is limited to three years, with the intent to force students to enter a family practice residency training program. Priority for selection in the Corps is given to first year students, and the application deadline occurs in the spring, prior to the first year. This means that students must choose between an indentured service program or indebtedness before they matriculate. The early timing is most unfortunate because the choice affects the ultimate career pathway of the students. Career aptitudes and goals often change for students during their clinical training. This program either limits or delays exercising their options.

The application for the NHSC program constitutes a signed contract. If one is selected for the Corps, and subsequently decides not to participate, before having received aid or begun school, a $1,500 penalty is assessed, payable immediately, as a fine for breach of contract. Similarly, if the scholarship recipient later on wishes to buy out of the program, the cost is three times the amount of funds issued plus interest, payable in one year from contract termination. Students should be made aware that once the decision to enter the Corps is made, it is in most circumstances a binding decision. Students who are certain they wish to become family practitioners and who look forward to practicing medicine in rural or urban shortage areas happily participate in the Corps and gain a medical education repayable in time rather than money.

The Armed Services Scholarship Programs (Army, Navy, Air Force) similarly subsidize students; however, there is no provision for "buying out." Theoretically, a student may pursue the residency training program of his/her choice. Currently there is no assurance that these graduates will not be drafted into active service during that training period and for this reason the military programs are not popular. Many of the military training hospitals are excellent; students interested in military careers may wish to choose this as a means of financing their medical educations. Priority for selection in these programs is not necessarily given to students in their first year of medical school; the various options should be explored by interested students.

In summary, the indentured service programs provide full financing of medical education and restrict both residency training and location of practice. The numbers of available places in the programs are limited, so there is no assurance that students will be accepted. The alternative to these programs is indebtedness. Most students choose to finance their educations by borrowing money so they can maintain freedom of career choice.

Full information regarding the various kinds of loans, interest charges, and repayment options is available from school financial aid officers. There are loans guaranteed by federal and/or state agencies, disbursed by banks or other lending institutions (some states are direct lenders); Health Professions Loan funds are provided by the federal government to the schools for disbursement; the AMA-ERF has a loan program available to some students and the Robert Wood Johnson Foundation supports a loan program through the United Student Aid Fund. In addition, most schools have loan funds made available to them through alumni contributions. National Direct Student Loan funds are available to many, but not all, medical schools. All of these programs charge simple rather than compound interest; some have interest subsidies available while students are enrolled in school; all have ten-year repayment plans, and each has a different repayment system. School financial aid officers will select/recommend the appropriate source or combination of sources of loans appropriate for the individual student. Students may anticipate large amounts of indebtedness and a future commitment to repay a variety of different lenders.

A relatively new program is now operational called the Health Education Assistance Loan (HEAL). Students may borrow up to $50,000 through this program but it is enormously expensive. Interest is compounded semi-annually not to exceed 12 percent, and the interest payments may or may not be deferred at the discretion of the lender. If students of necessity must utilize this source of funds to its maximum, there is national concern that the repayment of $174,000 for a $50,000 loan will be unmanageable during the residency training program.

Historically, the Health Professions Loan has been the most desirable for medical students. Students who practice in shortage areas for two years may apply to the Secretary of HEW and request that 60 percent of the Health Professions Loan indebtedness be repaid to the school by the federal government. For a third, continuing year of practice, an additional 25 percent repayment could be made. During the past year only a portion of such applications were honored because of the lack of appropriated funds for this program. At every opportunity we should encourage the federal government to increase the appropriation for this very important program. An additional attractive feature of this program is that economically disadvantaged students who exhibit exceptional financial need and fail to complete their studies may have the entire debt cancelled if they exhibit hardship. Federal appropriations for this program have become limited and it is in some danger of being phased out by the federal government. Again, all of us should make every effort to encourage our elected officials to support continuation and funding for the Health Professions Loan Program.

Generally, the cost of loan money is increasing. It will not be unusual for students to graduate from medical schools with $20-$30-40,000 or $50,000 indebtedness. These amounts will exceed the parental incomes of students from economically disadvantaged families and will be very difficult for them to conceptualize. Thus it is important for us to depict for these students what these sums mean in terms of monthly payments over an extended period of time, the responsibility which rests on them to repay their debts so others might follow in their footsteps, and the long-term manageability of such indebtedness. Such counseling will place the proper perspective on indebtedness as an investment in their futures.

Free money used to be fairly plentiful, but now very little "free" money is available for students. Most medical schools have some grant money and it is usually issued to the neediest students. As a proportion of total aid issued, the role of grant money is minimal. This is troublesome because there is no doubt that our inability to commit meaningful scholarship support to minority/economically disadvantaged students throughout the duration of the medical education process has caused the enrollment of such students to decline. This opinion is based on my experience with the Health Professions Scholarship program which enabled schools to offer such support. During the period when that program was in operation minority enrollment did increase.

The health manpower legislation enacted in 1976 includes a program entitled the "Exceptional Financial Need Scholarship Program for First Year Students." Token funding for the program was first made available in the fall of 1978. Medical, dental, and osteopathic medicine schools received funds enabling them to issue from one to five such awards which paid full tuition, books, supplies, and fees plus a 12-month living expenses stipend. The intent of the program is laudable: to enable economically disadvantaged students to complete their first year of studies without financial jeopardy. The legislation also states that these students will be given priority consideration for places in the National Health Service Corps Program in their second year of school should they so desire. The funds authorized for the program were not fully appropriated by Congress for this academic year; total rescission has been proposed and this jeopardy will probably continue in the coming years until the legislation expires in 1980.

The only additional source of grant monies for economically disadvantaged students from groups underrepresented in medicine are those from National Medical Fellowships, Inc. This meritorious organization is dedicated to assisting the students we are discussing and through intensive fund raising efforts from private enterprise have made it possible to award grants to such needy students. The amounts vary with their fund-raising success. Earlier their awards to students were significant, but now only a fraction of the cost is met. First year students have priority for their grants; second year students receive awards if funds are available. These awards are to supplement grants from schools.

Sometimes students discover grant funds from private sources through their own diligent inquiry and resourcefulness. Students should be encouraged to explore such possibilities.

The financial assistance scene is currently in chaos because of the change in focus by the federal government, enacted in Public Law 94-484. At the present time the entire thrust of the legislation is geared to the National Health Service Corps as the only viable solution to the problem of maldistrubution. Loan programs and other potential aid sources are purposely made unattractive in order to enhance recruitment for the Corps. This approach has proven unrealistic and short-sighted because no consideration is given to financing medical education for students unable to secure a place in the National Health Service Corps. In addition the concept that all medical students will become rich doctors is rampant, albeit ludicrous, which reinforces the position of Congress to phase out programs such as the Health Professions Loan Progam and the Exceptional Financial Need Scholarship Program for First Year Students because they seemingly constitute a deal that is too good for someone who will one day be "rich." This position is untenable. Our only hope is that superceding legislation, which must be enacted for 1980, will reflect some semblance of the real world.

COUNSELING AND COPING

All of us who work with students will touch upon some aspect of financial counseling during their educational process, regardless of our titles or roles. A semi-sequential synopsis of the areas where financial counseling occurs may bring to focus those phases where you can assist directly or refer students to others for assistance. It is worth stressing that such counseling is especially important for minority and economically disadvantaged students, even though applicable to all students needing financial assistance to complete their medical educations.

Medical Education—Is It Worth It?

In the face of a publicity barrage that scares most young people in college (as well as those of us who have passed that age), pre-professional advisors and admissions officers who are working diligently to recruit minority and economically disadvantaged young men and women must place the cost and financing aspects of medical education in perspective.

One of the potentially effective ways to approach undergraduate students is by jointly presenting the views of pre-professional undergraduate advisors, the medical school admissions officers and/or recruiters, currently enrolled medical students, and students recently graduated who come from economically disadvantaged backgrounds. Presentations stressing that medical education is an investment of short duration when viewed in the long term are important for these young persons who wish to enter a helping profession. Counseling-recruiting sessions should occur perhaps as early as the first semester of undergraduate school, in order to attract the attention of these students before they get diverted from or disenchanted with medicine as a career goal. Reinforcement sessions should be arranged throughout the undergraduate education process, especially in conjunction with the semesters or terms where students are actually applying to medical schools. Questions will arise such as, "Should I even apply to a school where the beginning tuition is $10,000 per year?," "Should I apply only to the less expensive schools?" The panel of recruiters should be prepared to discuss these points.

Indebtedness or Indentureship?

Once students have been accepted to a medical school, they should be counseled about the options available for financing such education. As a general rule of thumb, students who are not absolutely positive about their desires to join a service commitment program should be discouraged from doing so, if they indeed understand that the alternative is indebtedness. Some have viewed these service commitment programs as a form of slavery while others view them as a means to an end. It is important to ascertain the thinking of your students and counsel them accordingly.

Budgeting

Most students have no experience in budgeting for the simple reason that they've never had to do it. Your medical school's financial aid program administrator should be qualified to assist students in this endeavor. Among other things, budgeting involves looking for the most economical ways in which to secure lodging, food, medical supplies, books, and equipment. Students who are not from the geographic area where your medical school is located need more assistance in this process than others who are accustomed to living there. Budgeting also implies establishing the framework within which these students will live in a given academic year, which brings us to our next topic.

Managing Money

Again, the school financial aid officer can assist students in this process. Most programs are geared to "first half and second half" funding which means that students will receive their entire financial assistance in two lump sums. Students with no resources who suddenly find themselves with several thousand dollars in the bank at the outset of a term often have difficulty in stretching these dollars over a several month period. One effective way of assisting them in this process, in addition to general counseling, is to urge them to use an "envelope system" where a week's food money is placed in an envelope and used only for food, the month's rent is similarly packaged, etc. It is never safe to assume that a student knows how to manage money. These students are trained in science and other liberal arts fields, not in business.

Planning Ahead

Almost without exception students receive financial assistance only for the period in which they are technically registered. This means that their funding ends as the semester ends, and they are left in limbo until another registration period commences. Students should be forewarned that this will occur so that they might early on arrange summer employment or save what they can to bridge this period of non-support. Planning ahead should also encompass the entire medical education period. Students should become accustomed to a projection of their total indebtedness levels at graduation from medical school.

How to Apply for Funds

Again, this is in the domain of the school financial aid officer, but generally it is helpful to know that very fact. With very few exceptions, the application process is initiated at the medical school financial aid office. Applying for financial assistance is onerous. The process requires a multitude of forms, many of which request the same information repeatedly. The forms are complicated, troublesome to complete, and where national needs analysis systems are used, cost the student money. The combination of factors is sometimes overwhelming to students; the financial aid office staff should be able to assist in this process. Students must become meticulous in this arduous endeavor because even one small error or omission can result in delays of several months in processing the funding application. If students are aware in advance that a bureaucratic hassle exists in completing financial assistance application forms, they are less likely to be astounded when greeted by the problem. Incidentally, this situation is not generated by the medical schools, but rather by the burdensome regulations and requirements of many of the available funding programs.

Part-Time Jobs During School

In the face of concern over indebtedness levels and meager cash resources, many students express the desire to obtain part-time employment while in school. Students should be encouraged, if possible, not to undertake employment during the first semester of their first year of medical school. The majority of students have difficulty adjusting to the curriculum, the environment, and the stresses of examinations. Coupling these problems with employment may precipitate unsatisfactory academic performance. Accordingly, it is better to wait until one is accustomed to the rigors of medical education itself before making a decision about whether or not to seek employment.

Personal and Family Crises

Students from economically disadvantaged families who pursue advanced educational degrees have a serious problem. The time spent in school precludes gainful employment. Historically these young men and women have been essential contributors to the survival of their families. Pursuing education not only halts that family resource but places an additional burden on the student because education costs money. When schools offer financial assistance to such students in amounts to cover the cost of education and related living expenses, it is not unusual for these students to share that financial assistance with their families and live marginally themselves. This is especially true when one considers that the foregone earning period needed to obtain an M.D. degree is usually eight years. Thus there is unusual jeopardy and stress for these individuals. The enormous cost of obtaining an M.D. degree is coupled with a fear of failure that is intense. Understanding this dilemma is a must, if we are to assist these students. Although generalizations are not always appropriate, it is possible to consider the generalization that students from economically disadvantaged families not only may have a closer relationship with their families, but also in a sense may become the family leader simply because of their new role as future doctors. In other words, these students tend to become responsible for handling their family's crises in terms of both moral and financial support. This new responsibility adds to the stress of the student when a crisis arises. Because acceptance of this responsibility adds to a student's feeling of self worth, the student may fail to recognize that the need to concentrate on education takes precedence over family needs. Before I understood this, many of our students jumped on an airplane every time a call came from home regarding illness or trouble. This unanticipated expenditure of funds created a financial problem and, in addition, in some instances the absenteeism created an academic problem. Prevention was the remedy and the preventive measure consisted of discussing the general problem with small groups of students, spelling out for them what happens when this course of action is taken. These students were urged to consult either the financial aid administrator or the student affairs dean or the academic counselor or the course director in advance of making a precipitous move. The students responded to this request. The results included instances of the student affairs dean calling the family's physician to ascertain the real medical state of the family member who was ill. This reassurance may have preempted a trip home. In other instances advance consultation resulted in planned external financial assistance when the expenditure of funds was deemed necessary. The small group discussion of the potential problems and results also generated an additional benefit: the students became aware they were not alone in assuming these roles and responsibilities and were reassured because their problems were not unique.

There is a vicious circle for some students where financial problems create academic problems which create marital problems which create psychological/psychiatric problems which create financial problems, etc. This necessitates a very close working relationship between student affairs deans, counselors, and financial aid administrators. If, through the financial aid system, students request funding to cover the costs of psychotherapy, the financial aid administrators should ascertain that the student did indeed see a dean or designated counselor in order to assure that the proposed therapy is of high quality and appropriate, as well as necessary. On the other hand, students who may not be aware that they could be helped by psychological or psychiatric counseling may be identified during the financial aid interview analysis process. These students should be encouraged to see the student affairs dean or counselor for evaluation and referral. It is important to continually urge students to avail themselves of these school support services if appropriate. The stress of the medical education process is immense and as mentioned earlier the stress is even greater for students from economically disadvantaged backgrounds, so the likelihood of their need for such assistance is great. Therapy is expensive; it is important to deal with this as an uninsured medical care cost that is a legitimate financial assistance expenditure.

Curriculum Counseling

In the majority of medical schools the clinical years' curriculum includes the opportunity for taking electives away from the school itself. Clinical electives can be arranged in other cities, in other states, and in other nations. The relative educational importance of arranging external electives should be weighed against relative costs in light of the student's cumulative indebtedness and the availability of funds for that particular student. Some students believe that curricular approval of such plans automatically assures funding, but this is not the case. Again, the curriculum counselor and the financial aid administrator must work closely together to assure that students who do not take a particular elective because of money are not impinging on their own career/success opportunities. Conversely, it is important that students who need not arrange such electives be counseled about the wisdom of keeping their debt levels manageable and arranging to stay at home base.

Travel for Internship-Residency Interviews

Students who are independently wealthy are able to arrange interviews for internship or residency programs anywhere they wish. This fact in itself is troublesome to students who do not have unlimited resources for travel, unless they have proper counseling. Counseling from deans and faculty members should include consideration of expense. There should not be financial barriers to career choices; however, funds available are limited and there are levels at which debt does become unmanageable, so it is necessary that realistic choices be made.

Debt Management

There are some projections that the *average* debt level of students needing financial assistance during medical school soon will be $50,000 at graduation. Some students are graduating with enormous debts at the present time. In the past most financial aid administrators did not assume any responsibility for loan collections or debt management plans. Now they must assume this role. As indicated in the materials regarding sources of loans, each program has a different repayment schedule. It is necessary for financial aid administrators to work with individual students and lay out for them the deferment options, the monthly payments, the total time involved, and estimate how much of their house officer's salary will be expended monthly to make these payments. Students who have debts verging on the unmanageable, should be counseled that it is possible to enter practice after one post-graduate year followed by licensure, in order to be able to meet their monthly loan payments. Some of our students have practiced emergency medicine for one or two years for this reason and then commenced with residency training of their choice. House officer salaries have not escalated at the same rates that indebtedness has, which creates hardship situations for some young physicians. At the present time, there is no viable way to consolidate one's debts and extend the length of the repayment period. Students who cannot manage all of the payments on their house officers' salaries should negotiate with the individual lenders to see if individual arrangements can be worked out. Although there is no certainty this will happen, most lenders have been very accommodating when such situations arise and have worked with these individuals on extended repayment arrangements. Lenders prefer this approach if the alternative is default. It is critical that students not default. Default not only endangers the livelihood of students who are following them through medical school but also damages the defaulter's credit rating. Graduates in training should be made aware of the federal programs which include forgiveness of loans from specified sources, incentive grants to set up practice in shortage areas, or sizeable bonus offers to licensed physicians who join the Public Health Service. The choices are complicated and every effort should be made to provide graduates with detailed information about their options.

HMO, Group Practice or Private Practices?

The almighty dollar will influence the choice for students with enormous debts. There is relatively little information available to students in medical school about the cost and rewards of these various options. Every effort should be made to obtain better information so students may become aware of the prospects and problems early on in their careers.

Credit Availability

At the present time, M.D.'s have very little difficulty obtaining credit. This will change. Most students have delayed getting married and/or having a family, buying a home, buying a car that runs, etc., until after they complete their medical education. Many bankers in the United States have indicated they are concerned about whether or not they will extend credit to students who approach them for home or other financing when they have educational debts of $50,000. The bankers' logic will prevail when they look at the annual income of a graduate in resident training and begin deducting all of the payments that would be necessary to manage such an arrangement. These individuals tend to come out with deficit balances. At the present time there is no resolution to this, but students should be aware that this is indeed a potential problem.

Inflation

Every cloud has its silver lining, and so does inflation. Specifically, at the present time from an economic view it is better to be in debt than not. The cost of education loan money today in the long-term economic view is a cheap investment, with a great return. A subsidized loan with a 7 percent interest at payout is essentially a gift when viewed by an economist. This is especially true when one considers that the interest payments on loans can be deducted from one's income tax when earnings are reported, which lessens even more the cost of the loan. It is worthwhile for students to be informed of this perspective.

In summary, it is no longer possible or appropriate to counsel students about only those things which affect them while they are enrolled in medical school. Counseling must take the life-time perspective into consideration and an attempt should be made to identify the options available to students as well as the pitfalls which may occur throughout their careers as physicians. Given today's situation, more and more doctors will be paying off their medical education indebtedness at the same time they are trying to finance the educations of their own children. There will be a domino effect of what is done today and those of us who work with students have a responsibility to communicate this point to them.

THE IMPORTANCE OF PROVIDING EQUAL ACCESS TO EDUCATION

All qualified students should have an equal chance of entering the medical professions regardless of their financial background. The financial barriers that exist must be surmounted for those students who are economically disadvantaged minority students. The nation needs to have these students enter the medical profession if we are ever to solve the long and chronic unmet health care needs of medically underserved minority populations. It is generally true that students tend to return to the geographic and urban or rural areas where they grew up when they establish their practice of medicine. If we are to solve the basic health care problems of this nation, these minority students must be recruited to medical school and every effort should be made to assure their success in obtaining the M.D. degree. We all have a role in helping to achieve equal access to education through communication and education of our colleagues, both at the local and national levels. A great deal is at stake and it is our responsibility to rise and meet this challenge.

The College-Medical School Interface
and Medical School Assistance

CHAPTER 15

Pre-Entry Summer Course for Minority Medical Students

Alonzo C. Atencio

INTRODUCTION

Prior to 1968, medical schools in the U.S. had shown relatively little concern and commitment toward students from racial minority groups. Since 1968, underrepresented minorities, Blacks, Chicanos, Native Americans and Mainland Puerto Ricans, have made some progress in increasing enrollment in medical school, but one need only to look at the data available to conclude that the effort has just begun. Admission to medical school has to a large extent relied heavily upon cognitive data. Non-cognitive evaluations have played only a minor role in the evaluation of students with low academic credentials. Non-cognitive evaluation as a rule has been used only to differentiate between those with equivalent high GPA's and MCAT scores.

This process has automatically excluded minorities from entering the competition for admission, since the educational attainment of minorities is substantially lower than for the White majority. This is evident from the reports of the Commission on Civil Rights and

Alonzo C. Atencio, Ph.D., is Assistant Professor of Biochemistry and Assistant Dean for Student Affairs, School of Medicine, University of New Mexico, Albuquerque, New Mexico.

the American Council on Education. A Civil Rights Commission report, "The Unfinished Education—1971," for example states that while 86% of the white students finish high school, only 60% of the Chicanos in the Southwest reach this goal. The American Council on Education report also indicates that the enrollment in college shows greater divergence (49% to 23%).

In 1971, more specifically, the American Council on Education reported that, of a total of 1,634,000 first year college entrants only 18,000 (1.1%) were Chicano, 14,700 Native American (0.9%), 3,300 (0.20%) Mainland Puerto Ricans, and 102,900 (6.3%) Black. The remaining 91.5% of entering freshmen were ethnic non-minority students.

The situation by 1974 improved somewhat. The majority representation in college dropped to 89.5 (1,499,100) while the Black and Chicano increased to 7.4 and 1.5% respectively. The remaining 1.6% accounts for the combined representation of Native Americans and Puerto Ricans.

From these data one would expect a concomitant increase in first year college enrollment. According to the statistics from the American Council on Education, the combined minority first year enrollment (1968-1974) increased only from 171,000 to 174,000 but dropped in percentage enrollment from 11.6 to 10.4%. In absolute numbers the non-minority enrollment increased from 1,063,000 to 1,495,200 compared to the Black enrollment increase from 58,200 to 102,700. There are no data available for the Chicanos, Native Americans, and Mainland Puerto Ricans.

These are cold hard figures and at best reveal trends in minority education. There are many sociological, economic, and racial factors which contribute to the educational attainment of minorities. The overall effect seems to be very little increase in the number entering and staying in college to meet the premedical requisites. Perhaps the reasons come about as a result of a combination of low confidence in their ability to reach the professional pinnacle, the cost of a college education, and a denial of opportunity to participate as an equal in our American society.

This problem becomes more serious when one also takes into consideration the increase in population under 18 years. From 1969 to 1973 the under-18-year-old white majority increased only 3.2% while the under-18 Black and Chicano population increased by 6.4 and 20.5% respectively.

Clearly the supply of academically prepared minority students for medical school was and is low, and in fact, lower than these figures above indicate, when one considers the attrition of minorities from college and includes those who graduate to participate in the labor force rather than continue to advanced degrees or medical school.

ADDRESSING THE PROBLEMS

This chapter will not attempt to review all of the various national efforts but will concentrate mostly on a very specific effort made by the University of New Mexico in addressing the problem of enrolling and retaining minority medical students. But I would be derelict in my duty if I did not mention some of the other attempts to increase minority representation by other U.S. Medical schools.

As of 1978 the AAMC compilation of summer programs indicates that 16 medical schools have secondary school programs, 27 address undergraduate students, and 29 have programs for new matriculants at their school. Five others provide opportunities to new matriculants from any U.S. medical school and a similar number have post-baccalaureate programs.

All these programs are aimed at strengthening the cognitive qualification of minority students by reinforcing their academic preparation for successful admission and completion of medical school. Perhaps another important aspect, though not necessarily by intent, of these programs is the non-quantifiable positive effect that results from the students' interaction with minority faculty and medical students, usually in a medical school setting.

No program will be successful without: (1) a sincere commitment by the medical school, (2) a sincere commitment to modify the admissions process by including non-cognitive data to determine the academic potential of the student, (3) a sincere commitment to develop an adequate support system for increasing retention in medical school, and lastly, (4) a serious recruitment effort to discover minority students with the academic potential and reserve to cope with the rigors of medical education and not the mere institution of a program for collecting minority names for the schools' statistical well-being.

THE ROLE OF MINORITY PROGRAMS
IN MEDICAL SCHOOL

The recruitment program should be a year-round effort to increase awareness of opportunities in the health sciences, and a realistic appraisal of the prerequisities for entering medical school. It should also include strong motivational aspects and should deal with the minority students as individuals, taking into consideration their culture, their environment, and realistic appraisals of their desires and motivations.

In the admissions process the staff of the program should play a strong advocacy role within the medical school setting, preferably in the actual admissions process itself. The program director should also develop and implement avenues for dealing with students labeled as high academic risks. These avenues may include adequate support, both academically as well as a personal counseling service to help students cope with their problems as they arise during their pre-medical and medical education. There is a wide range of problems which students encounter, varying from their own personal relationships to problems emanating from financial need due to unpredictable emergencies.

An adequate retention program should include a strong pre-entry basic science course along with test-taking skills studies and tutorial availability. With the increasing requirement that medical students pass National Boards Part I before being allowed to proceed to the third year, the school should also develop an adequate Board Review program. Unfortunately, many medical students are beginning to rely on the Kaplan type of reviews to fulfill this requirement. A medical school should have its own program.

Many problems encountered by minority medical students arise as a result of attitudes of faculty, non-minority students, and administration—attitudes arising from their perceptions of the minority student as a competitive student and colleague. Many view their entrance into medical school with suspicion and believe that they have not met the standards for admission.

Consequently, a minority program should also contain elements which allow for creating attitudinal changes through the process of interaction between minorities and non-minorities in order to clarify essential cultural differences between the two groups. Often well-intended individuals make remarks that are racially insulting, though this is not intended.

What is acceptable behavior in one culture is often viewed with suspicion in another. A simple example will serve to illustrate this point of view: In the Latin community male individuals hug and often kiss each other as a form of greeting and expression of friendship. In the Anglo-American culture such behavior between males is suspect rather than an acceptable form of greeting. Numerous other examples can be used but suffice it to say that the medical institution as well as the medical practice environment should recognize cultural differences in their interaction with minorities, be they patients or students. Thus the minority program should promote such interchange.

THE MEDICAL CAREER OPPORTUNITY PROGRAM AT THE UNIVERSITY OF NEW MEXICO

The medical career opportunity program (MCOP) at UNM attempts to address the elements outlined above—it includes (1) a Summer Basic Science Enrichment Program (BSEP), (2) an academic year-round involvement in recruitment and advisement, (3) a National Board Review component, and (4) an operational agreement for interaction with other medical schools, New Mexico high school and community organizations.

The Basic Science Enrichment Program

The BSEP is an eight-week summer pre-entry program for minority medical students. This component of the program addresses several primary and secondary objectives of MCOP. Among them are: (1) to increase the number of underrepresented minorities accepted to medical school; (2) to increase their ability to compete successfully within the basic science curricula; (3) to promote understanding between white faculty and administrators and minority medical students; (4) to expose medical students to the socio-medical problems in the nation's minority communities; (5) to encourage medical students to consider practicing in underserved areas after completion of medical training; and (6) to provide employment opportunities for minority students in the medical school setting.

The BSEP could be considered a remedial program but it is more of a reinforcement program designed to enrich the students' knowledge of the basic sciences, improve their study skills, refine self-evaluation skills, increase confidence, impart survival skills in medical school, and in general, promote minority medical student success and retention.

The BSEP curriculum is designed to simulate actual medical school environment. Three of the basic sciences required in the study of medicine are taught by medical school faculty in a traditional didactic method. During the first six weeks of the session, the students concurrently receive instruction in biochemistry and physiology. Gross anatomy is taught during the last two weeks of the session. All lectures and laboratory instruction are conducted in the medical school.

The participants also attend seminars, lectures, and panel discussions dealing with historical, political, and sociological aspects of medicine and medical education. Information on financial aid and post-graduate training is also provided. In addition, the students attend discussion sections and individual and small-group tutorial and informal counseling sessions conducted by minority medical students who serve as teaching assistants and confidants in the attitudinal problems encountered by minority medical students in medical school.

The participants in the program are drawn from all underrepresented minorities (Chicano, Black, Native American and Mainland Puerto Rican). Several factors enter into this selection for admission to BSEP. In general, students must: (1) be accepted by a medical school and recommended to the program by that school; (2) be considered a "high risk" applicant as determined within the admission process of that individual school; and (3) be considered "disadvantaged." During the past five years, students in the BSEP program have been recommended by 20 different medical schools.

The faculty and staff of BSEP for the summer session is under the direction of an assistant dean for student affairs who is also a tenured faculty member. Two other staff members, funded from state appropriations, are an associate director who is largely responsible for the day-to-day administration of the program and a program specialist whose major responsibilities occur during the academic year as a recruiter but who also assists with all general programmatic activities.

The faculty participants are drawn from the faculty of the school of medicine's basic science departments. Seminar speakers and consultants with expertise in specific areas varying from folk medicine to professors of sociology are drawn from other universities and community clinics. The teaching assistants are hired from currently enrolled first- and second- year medical students in good academic standing.

Efforts are made to hire individuals who will represent the ethnic representation of the BSEP student population and who demonstrate commitment to program goals and sensitivity to minorities.

Recruitment

The recruitment and motivational effort to increase the number of underrepresented minorities in medicine ranges from high school juniors and seniors, to undergraduate Chicano, Indian and Black students.

At the high school level the program includes lectures by minority medical students and faculty on-site visits in the high schools of the State of New Mexico. The program also provides tours of the School of Medicine and the University in general to high school students. More recently we have provided tours for sixth and seventh grade students.

In addition to the tours the students are shown films such as "Code Blue" and "What Can You Do?." These films provide visual evidence of minority students in medical schools along with the opportunity for the high school student to hear more on their background and how they achieved successful admission to medical school. One cannot overestimate the visual impact these films have on high school students and accompanying teachers. These films are also shown at high school assemblies when the recruiter makes visits to the high schools. The recruiter often finds that the films produce a greater response than "rap" sessions and panel discussion groups.

We also attempt to provide high school students with academic and career counseling and advice. This is done both by individual students' visits to the medical school office and on-site at the school. Our latest effort is to involve more high school counselors by meeting with them and showing these films. This is done in an attempt to sensitize more counselors to the situation confronting minorities as well as their participation in medical school. Our long range plan here is for counselors to identify students with academic potential who may be ignorant of what role they can play in health careers. Alternatively, we point out to them how they can prepare themselves adequately and provide them with sufficient information to make an educated career choice.

At the more advanced level we visit junior and community colleges as well as New Mexico universities. During the year we visit some thirteen New Mexico universities and their branch colleges along with three community colleges.

During these visits we provide information on premedical requirements, medical school application procedures, admissions policies, financial assistance, counseling, and academic advisement. In addition we collect the students' names and maintain files for follow-up purposes. The follow-up usually includes providing further information on AMCAS deadlines, MCAT test sites, and other information relative to the interview procedure and the admissions process.

The staff of BSEP also coordinates recruitment with the schools of pharmacy and nursing. We also provide assistance to and coordination with local and regional minority programs such as Health Career Recruitment of the All-Indian Pueblo Council Inc., the Navajo Health Authority, and Youth in School Employment Programs of the Albuquerque Public School system.

Admissions to Medical School

The admissions process at UNM is under the direction of the Office of Student Affairs and Admission and co-chaired by the two assistant deans. The committee consists of thirteen members of which five are minorities—the director of MCOP who is co-chairman, a BSEP staff member, two minority medical students, and a minority faculty member from the department of medicine.

The minority members of the committee not only provide advocacy for minority applicants, but in committee deliberation, non-minority members get to see how the minority views differ from their own interpretations. In short this is in part a process for sensitization of non-minority members. Efforts are also made to have minority students interviewed by at least one minority member of the committee.

The minority student's application is thus monitored from the initial contact by the recruiter through the process for admissions.

Although hard to quantify, we feel certain that such continued advocacy also helps sustain affirmative action efforts in other areas.

Advisement and Counseling

The MCOP staff is also available to provide counseling and advisement to medical students who find themselves experiencing academic, personal, or financial difficulties. Minority students are sometimes in need of low-risk counseling and seek sympathetic and empathic individuals whom they can trust to discuss personal and/or academic problems. This way the staff can intervene on behalf of the student at whatever level is necessary. Often a student experiencing academic difficulties does not reveal the source for fear that it may reflect on him and his family. Culturally the "extended family" is a reality to Chicano and Native American students. A death of an immediate member of the family makes demands on the medical student who is viewed as the one with knowledge to understand what to do. This can be demanding and the student is duty-bound to comply. Once this is known, a new dimension enters into the evaluation of the student. What was perceived initially as resulting from intentional neglect of studies now can be seen as arising from an emergency or other commitments. The array of problems confronting an extended family can also include births and baptisms which occupy a very important part in the culture. All these involvements are time-consuming and to the white faculty members often appear immature and irrational. They have difficulty understanding why an Indian student, for instance, suddenly returns to the reservation during school. The need of the family plays an important role in the minority community. This is why empathetic individuals are needed to understand the nature of the problem and to avoid making rash judgments and labeling the student. Without proper understanding, proper counseling cannot be provided.

Another part of the retention effort, of course, is academic reinforcement during the school year. For this the University appropriates funds for a peer tutorial program.

Students within a class are matched one to one, usually one in good academic standing becomes the tutor for the other one having difficulties. The tutors are reimbursed for their efforts and the tutee feels that he has the right to demand the services rather than feel he is imposing on his classmate's time on the volunteer basis.

Other retention services include study skills assessment and development, training to reduce test-taking anxiety and improve on test performance, and pre-examination review tests usually developed by the students themselves. Should a student require assistance beyond the test-taking, he is then placed in contact with the peer tutorial program or individual faculty, identified previously as sensitive to the minority students.

Other Related Activities

Any successful program has to go beyond its funded job description if it is to maximize the overall motivational and recruitment efforts. Thus, the staff of MCOP is involved in a number of local and national activities which have an impact on achieving the goals of increasing minority representation.

The MCOP director, for instance, is also the director of the Minority Bio-medical Science Program (MBS). This is an institution-wide research program for minority undergraduate and graduate students. There are a total of 40 faculty from ten science departments, all involved in providing research opportunities for 40 undergraduate and 18 graduate students. The MBS also has a recruiter who works closely with the medical school recruiter in identifying and recruiting minority students at all levels of education. The director, associate director, and recruiter also serve on several university committees, advisory councils, recruitment and selection committees, and other committees which assist in the administration of the University's minority and academic programs.

Other related activities, though not part of any specific program include: (1) assisting in developing proposals for a University-wide center for minorities in science and engineering; (2) participating in several loan and scholarship committees within the University; (3) serving on other academic committees concerned with promotion and evaluations as well as dealing with changes in medical education; (4) advocating the hiring of more minority faculty members; (5) strengthening the commitment of the University to serve in neighborhood minority community clinics.

National Boards Review Program

The National Boards Review Program addresses what has now become another very important objective of the minority retention program. In the past, passage of the National Boards Part I was not required for advancement into the third year of this medical school. This is now a requirement and students face the possibility of not advancing if they fail the Board Examination and after a third try and failure they may even have to leave the University. During the past nine years only 46% of minority students at UNM passed the National Boards on the first attempt. Results were similar at the University of Arizona and at the University of Colorado. The problem becomes serious if the students fail the second attempt. Consequently we have developed a summer Board Review program which starts on the last week of July and continues through August for students who have failed their first attempt. Neighboring schools will be invited to participate by recommending students. Majority students at UNM will also be participating.

The review program consists of an intensive review and an on-going assessment in the six major basic science areas. Students will be required to attend approximately seven hours of instruction and discussion followed by an examination in the topic covered that day. The examination will be Board type and computer-graded to provide accessibility and feedback readily to the student. Pre-test self assessment and review tests will be used and instruction in test-taking provided.

Several departments, faculty and medical students, along with the office of Biomedical Communications are involved in the development of the National Boards Review program.

Since this is the first year of operation we do not know how effective the program will be.

Operational Agreements Within The University of New Mexico

Various agreements among departments, committees at UNM, the Office of the Dean, the Office of Comptroller at the Medical School, the Office of Admissions, Steering Committees, the College of Nursing and Pharmacy and Biomedical Communications have been established.

Three departments, Biochemsitry, Physiology, and Anatomy have been supportive in developing curriculum and providing faculty for the 8-week summer program. As mentioned previously, representatives from the program staff serve on the Admissions Committee and work closely with the Office of Admissions staff in reviewing applicants to UNM.

The Dean of the School of Medicine is cooperative and has supported our efforts by providing financial support for salaries of office staff and the tutorial program. The Medical Center Comptroller has provided and continues to provide assistance in all financial and fiscal aspects of the program. Progress of first- and second-year medical students is monitored by the Steering Committee of which the director is a member and has served as chairman. This committee serves a very important function since promotion and evaluation policies emanate from this committee. The committee also has the responsibility in developing curriculum and examination policies.

There are some interinstitutional agreements developed also. In the past working arrangements have been negotiated with 20 other U.S. Medical schools and counselors at approximately 30 high schools, junior high, and elementary schools. Arrangements have also been developed with premedical advisors and professors from other New Mexico universities.

It should also be mentioned that all of the School of Medicine facilities, such as lecture halls, visual aids, multidisciplinary laboratories, study rooms, conference rooms, and a new modern well-stocked medical library are available to the summer program for instruction, meetings, seminars, and other functions necessary for successful implementation of the program.

DISCUSSION

Basic Science Enrichment Program

During the first three years, 1970-1972, the BSEP summer session was taught by volunteer faculty and concentrated on biochemistry and mathematics. Of the seventeen students who attended these sessions sixteen have graduated from medical school and are now either practicing medicine or finishing up their residencies.

Since 1973, we have had a total of 159 minority students participate in BSEP. Fifty-two of these students attended UNM, 103 enrolled at other U.S. medical schools, and four did not attend medical school. Most of these students have graduated but an accurate follow-up has not been done. Preliminary follow-up by communication with other U.S. medical schools indicates an excellent retention rate. To date we know of only three of the 103 who have left medical school.

At UNM, as shown in Table 1, BSEP students have a 96.2% retention rate. Perhaps the most glaring figure in this Table is the percent of students making irregular progress which averages out to 23.1%. Irregular progress results among these minority students for academic reasons.

On Table 2 the data of UNM for the period of 1964-1978 are shown. During this period 106 out of 129 minority medical students, or 82.2%, have made regular progresss. This figure includes BSEP students as well, but notice that the percentage of majority students making regular progress is 87%. Again, academic reasons are given as the primary reason for making irregular progress by minority students. The overall retention, however, is an excellent 96%, slightly better than the majority students who have a 93% retention rate.

These figures are indeed surprising when we compare the BSEP minority and majority students' performance in the MCAT. Table 3 shows that majority students score significantly better in the MCAT. Only 11.4% of the BSEP students scored above 550 in the old MCAT, and 16% above 8 in the new test.

Table 1. BSEP at the University of New Mexico School of Medicine, 1973-1978

	NON-CONTINGENCY ACCEPTANCES	CONTINGENCY ACCEPTANCES	ALL UNM BSEP PARTICIPANTS
Number of students enrolled	36	16	52
Number making regular progress	28	10	38
Percent enrolled students making regular progress	77.8%	62.5%	73.1%
Number making irregular progress	6	6	12
Academic reasons	4	5	9
Other (illness, fellowships, etc.)	2	1	3
Percent enrolled students making irregular progress	16.7%	37.5%	23.1%
Academic reasons	11.1%	31.3%	17.3%
Other (transfer, etc.)	5.5%	6.3%	5.8%
Attrition	2	0	2
Academic reasons	2	0	2
Other (transfer, etc.)	0	0	0
Percent attrition	5.6%	0	3.8%
Academic reasons	5.6%	0	3.8%
Other (transfer, etc.)	0	0	0
Retention	34	16	50
Percent retention	94.4%	100%	96.2%

Table 2. Progress and Attrition of New First-Year Students at the University of New Mexico School of Medicine*

	MAJORITY STUDENTS			MINORITY STUDENTS			TOTAL STUDENTS		
	MALE	FEMALE	TOTAL	MALE	FEMALE	TOTAL	MALE	FEMALE	TOTAL
Number of students enrolled	494	145	639	102	27	129	596	172	768
Number making regular progress	430	126	556	83	23	106	513	149	662
Percent enrolled students making regular progress	87.0	86.9	87.0	81.4	85.2	82.2	86.1	86.6	86.2
Number making irregular progress	30	8	38	15	3	18	45	11	56
Academic reasons	15	3	18	15	2	17	30	5	35
Other (illness, fellowship)	15	5	20	0	1	1	15	6	21
Percent enrolled students making irregular progress	6.1	5.5	5.9	14.7	11.1	14.0	7.5	6.4	7.3
Academic reasons	3.0	2.1	2.8	14.7	7.4	13.2	5.0	2.9	4.6
Other (illness, fellowship)	3.0	3.4	3.1	—	3.7	.8	2.5	3.5	2.7
Attrition	34	11	45	4	1	5	38	12	50
Academic reasons	21	5	26	3	1	4	24	6	30
Other (transfer, etc.)	13	6	19	1	0	1	14	6	20
Percent attrition	6.9	7.5	7.0	3.9	3.7	3.9	6.3	7.0	6.5
Academic reasons	4.3	3.4	4.1	2.9	3.7	3.1	4.0	3.5	3.9
Other (transfer, etc.)	2.6	4.1	2.9	1.0	—	.8	2.3	3.5	2.6
Retention	460	134	594	98	26	124	558	160	718
Percent retention	93.1	92.5	93.0	96.1	96.3	96.1	93.7	93.0	93.5

* Prepared by the UNM SOM Office of Admissions and Student Affairs.

249

Table 3. MCAT Profiles of UNM BSEP and Majority Students

PERIOD	SUBJECT	RANGE	PERCENTAGE BSEP	MAJORITY
1973-1977	MCAT	>550	11.4	89.7
	MCAAP			
1977-1978	Biology	> 8	26.1	95.0
	Chemistry	> 8	8.7	67.9
	Physics	> 8	13.0	66.1
	Science	> 8	8.7	81.4
	SA Reading	> 8	13.0	79.6
	SA Quant.	> 8	26.7	84.7

On the other hand, 89.7% of the majority students scored above 550 on the old test and well over 77% scored above 8 in the new. One would expect the student performance to be far below the actual number making regular progress if the MCAT is a valid index.

The GPA differential between the BSEP student, not shown in Table 3, is similar. Of the majority students, 65.5% have GPA's greater than 3.40 compared to 19% of the BSEP minority students. In fact, 33% of the BSEP students have GPA's less than 2.80 but greater than 2.20. While nearly a third of them have GPA's less than 2.8 only 3% of the majority students fall in this range.

The next question that arises is: Does BSEP help the minority student in the areas covered during the summer session? The results of these analyses are shown in Table 4. With the exception of the 1976-77 group, about 80% performed satisfactorily in biochemistry compared to 85% for the 200 majority students. Including 1976-77, 73% performed satisfactorily. Their performance in the areas of physiology and anatomy covered was excellent and comparable to the majority students. The majority students did not participate in BSEP. It should also be noted that these figures represent a first attempt; most of those who performed unsatisfactorily in the first try removed their unsatisfactory grade by make-up exam. The make-up examinations have been set up largely at the request of the BSEP director and UNM minority students. The make-up exam is constructed so that it measures an amount of knowledge equivalent to that tested in the first or initial examination.

As the first BSEP and other minority graduates from medical

Table 4.   UNM BSEP Students' Satisfactory First Year Performance in Biochemistry, Physiology, and Anatomy

YEAR	NO.	BIO-CHEMISTRY	PHYSIOLOGY*	ANATOMY†
1972-73	9	8	8	8
1973-74	11	7‡	7‡	11
1974-75	9	7‡	9	9
1975-76	4	4	4	4
1976-77	10	4‡	9	10
1977-78	8	7‡	7	8
Total	51	37	44	50
Percent	100	73	86	98
Non-BSEP (3 yr)	(200) 100	85	97	99

* Renal and Cardiovascular organ blocks.
† Gross, Morphology, and Head and Neck.
‡ Students failing course on first attempt pass by passing a make-up examination.

school begin their professional careers, we find that about 70% of them are practicing in New Mexico. Of the initial three BSEP students, one is an assistant professor of medicine, and the other two are practicing in their hometown areas.

Table 5 shows the trend in minority enrollment at UNM. Note that there is a dramatic increase in enrollment of minorities. Starting in the fall of 1970, minority enrollment has averaged about 20%.

These results, I believe, could not have been achieved without the programmatic effort described above.

At the high school level we have contacted well over 1000 minority students through these mechanisms. In reviewing some of the new college minority matriculants at UNM, we are beginning to see a more confident group emerging. Well over 35% of last year's 140 freshmen were chosen for the presidential scholarships given to New Mexico high school valedictorians. More minority high school students are beginning to test out of freshman university courses through the college level equivalent program. We would like to believe we have a role in helping to develop the trends. Clearly, the actual contributing factor is difficult to isolate.

Table 5.   Ethnic Minority Student Applicants
Matriculated By Class

YEAR OF ENTRY	CHICANO	BLACK	INDIAN	TOTAL MINORITY ENROLL- MENT	TOTAL 1ST YEAR CLASS ENROLLED*	ETHNIC MINORITY STUDENT AS PERCENT 1ST YEAR ENROLLED
1964	0	0	0	0	24	0
1965	0	0	0	0	24	0
1966	0	0	0	0	24	0
1967	1	0	0	1	24	4.2
1968	3	0	0	3	36	8.3
1969	1	1	1	3	36	8.3
1970	7	0	1	8	48	16.7
1971	10	1	0	11	56	20.0
1972	10	1	1	12	64	18.8
1973	15	0	3	18	68	26.5
1974	14	1	3	18	72	25.0
1975	15	0	0	15	73	20.5
1976	9	0	0	9	73	12.3
1977	13	3	1	17	73	23.3

* Does not include repeaters.

To reiterate, the two major obstacles confronting successful minority student enrollment are (1) a shrinking applicant pool and (2) a diminishing concern for minorities in U.S. society as a whole. Medical school faculty, in general, have always been reluctant to participate in special programs for minorities. They prefer to teach students who came well-prepared academically. The sensitivity to people becomes a concern in the clinical years, yet the student is expected to have an adequate fund of knowledge. But the minority student still lags behind in academic preparation.

We have to continue our efforts at all levels, creating awareness at the secondary schools, community colleges, and universities.

Summer programs are indispensible in carrying out this mission. They provide funds to help create avenues for encouraging and informing students of not only the need for more minorities in the health fields but also on the requirements toward achieving this goal.

Pre-entry summer and National Board Review support programs directly affect the retention of minority medical students and often serve to make the road smoother for majority students.

Needless to say the problem is multifaceted and complex, but with both institutional and program staff commitment we are beginning to address the problem.

CHAPTER 16

Orientation of Incoming Medical Students

Charles S. Ireland, Jr.

INTRODUCTION

With the advent of increased minority medical student enrollment beginning in the late sixties and the subsequent evolution of
activities to recruit, enroll, and retain them, the summer program
emerged as one means by which one or more of these ends could be
met.

There is no generic definition to encompass the range of
offerings that many medical schools established for minority students via the summer program. They have varied in setting,
clientele groups served, objectives, and outcomes.

Several summer programs sponsored by medical schools for
entering minority freshmen, frequently referred to as "pre-
enrollment" summer programs, came into being in the early
seventies. Although *they* vary in content, staffing, and philosophy,
most have sought to provide students with an early orientation to

Charles S. Ireland, Jr., M.S.W., is Assistant to the Dean; Director, Recruitment,
Admissions and Retention Program; and Assistant Professor of Social Work,
Temple University School of Medicine, Philadelphia, Pennsylvania.

the nature and expectations of the host school—particularly as they relate to the students' first year of professional training.[1]

It is clear, however, that most pre-enrollment programs were designed to offset the disparate retention and attrition rates that accompanied minority students' performances since their enrollment in the late sixties and which continue with as much disparity today—today at a time when the credentials of minority applicants for medical school acceptance are better than ever.

Why has the enrollment of minority medical students declined since 1974? Simply put, the vast majority of our nation's medical schools, with the exceptions of Howard, Meharry, and Morehouse, have not expressed the depth and extent of commitment to increase significantly the production of physicians from minority backgrounds.

According to Evans,[2] "This nation's medical schools—other than Howard University and Meharry Medical College—have never acted out of any real commitment toward increasing the numbers of U.S. minority students entering their doors. It is unfortunate, but nevertheless expected, that medical school officials are now pointing to the economic recession, a decline in scholarship money available for minorities, and increasing opportunities for Blacks, Mexican-Americans, American Indians, and Puerto Ricans in other fields such as law and business, as being mainly responsible for the drop in minority student recruitment. These factors probably are partly responsible, but it should be crystal clear that medical schools have always had some justifiable reason for excluding U.S. minority students."

Two words best describe what pre-enrollment programs for entering minority freshmen do—*they anticipate*—the worst and the best. The worst is found in the environment of the medical school and the best is within the student.

The tragedy at many medical schools, particularly in the predominantly white setting, is the absence of overall school commitment, real or perceived, to having minority students there in the first place—in atmospheres which cause minority students to feel different and unwanted. Another problem is that medical educa-

---

[1] Odegaard, C.E.: *Minorities in Medicine: From Receptive Passivity to Positive Action, 1966-76.* New York: Josiah Macy, Jr. Foundation, 1977.

[2] Evans, Therman E.: Editorial. *Washington Post*, January 28, 1976.

tion, while not much more difficult than some other educational processes, imposes a volume of work and a pace which dictates that academic success is always and must be favorably influenced by: the highest levels of self-confidence, self-discipline, determination, willingness to seek and accept help, and plain hard work.

While the unfamiliar atmosphere in the traditional medical school produces problems for many minority students, their own differences and their inner resources are sources of strength. Pre-enrollment summer programs—the successful ones—do anticipate the worst and the best. The overall background differences of minority medical students, indeed, do enter the picture.

The absence or inadequacy of career and premedical advising on college campuses has operated against potential medical school applicants.[3] Central factors operating particularly against most minority students are: the absence of sufficient numbers of visible and acceptable role models in their life's settings; myths, misconceptions, and informational voids about opportunities and pathways leading to a medical career; and the well known diversionary deterrents operating at the levels of secondary and undergraduate school counseling and course selection and scheduling. The result has been: lack of objectivity about career choices prior to and upon graduation; selection of major courses of study based on second-hand, "used" references; and charting career courses in secure, familiar waters.

The long-standing attitudes toward the occupational roles that women should traditionally occupy in our society have generally encumbered their career options and opportunities, and have been further reinforced by gender-based biases promulgated by counseling at all levels of their educational attainment.[4]

So, racism, sexism, and "the traditional way of doing things" have continued to operate to the disfavor of far too many "different" medical students.

The variety of special educational programs which have been directed towards solving the personal and group problems of many minority undergraduates has not always improved their chances for admission to and success in education. While the goals and aims

---

[3] Bruhn, John G.: The Ills of Premedical Advising. *J. Med. Educ.*, 52:676-678, 1977.

[4] Ireland, Evelyn C.: Attitudes Toward Women. MEd REP Conference, Biloxi, Mississippi, April 16-19, 1978.

of some of these kinds of college programs have been worthy, too many have been built upon models with underlying philosophies which are essentially negative. Many such programs have been based on the assumption that the individual comes to the program as a product of a deficient, deprived, disadvantaged cultural background and, thus, has certain defects which have to be corrected.

With the advent of increased representation of minority students in medical schools, similar interpretations can be made about the impact of *that* system on them. The "open door" policy approach has not meant success in medical education. More often than not, minority medical students are consciously admitted as unequal, and unconsciously left to discover equalizing opportunities for themselves.

The frustration, course failures, and attrition are dealt with as if there is something basically wrong with the minority student, rather than with the norm by which he is continually measured. For minorities, the perceived alien environment of the medical school asks for conformity or sameness among its total student population and, far too often, is unable or unwilling to entertain racial and cultural differences that occur as student strengths, particularly among minorities, and as resources to be recognized and reinforced.

BACKGROUND

In June, 1972, Temple University School of Medicine, as an extension of its earlier commitment to increase substantially the number of graduates from minority backgrounds representative of the region in which it is situated, conducted its first pre-enrollment summer program for entering minority freshmen.

Called SERA, the Summer Educational Reinforcement Activity emerged out of the confidence that the entering minority student had the scholastic ability and motivation to become a qualified physician. Many such students were committed to return to communities where the need for adequate quality health care is greatest. Often the roadblock that stood between them and their return to the community as M.D.'s was their limited familiarity with the setting and performance expectations of a medical school. Too often, the students did not know what was expected of them, nor did they have parents and/or other relatives who were physicians, and who could have instilled and nourished interests in medicine as a career from early childhood. Indeed, the minority student was and still is, in the main at Temple, the first one in the family to attend or graduate from college.

So, when nonminority medical students were occupied with learning course material, minority students who did not have the opportunity to participate in a program such as SERA risked the possibility of preoccupation with anxieties over appropriate ways of studying; how to take multiple-choice examinations; how to use a microscope; and with questions about why the other students seem to be so far ahead. The result was that self-doubt emerged, confidence waned, and failures occurred—failures from the anxieties and pressures of an alien environment, not from the lack of ability.

The incidence and significance of stress among many medical students is amply documented.[5] Minorities are not to be excluded from the overall medical student population in terms of their own vulnerabilities. Unfortunately, the intensity and complexity of stress among minority students in the predominantly white medical school setting, are considerably heightened when one considers their negative perceptions of such medical schools to begin with.[6]

SERA, from its beginning, sought to minimize the extent of trauma which occurs with minority medical students' entry into the predominantly white medical school setting, by attempting to better equip and perhaps "toughen" them to knowingly anticipate and cope with the academic and personal expectations of the medical education experience.

The concepts undergirding this seven-week program were heavily weighted by the recommendations of upperclass minority medical students that a comprehensive orientation to the setting and expectations of the School be provided to future incoming minority freshmen well in advance of their enrollment. This orientation, as they put it, might enable new students to go through an "early adjustment," thus reducing the risk of falling behind, not being

[5] Coburn, D., and Jovaisas, A. V.: Perceived Sources of Stress Among First Year Medical Students. *J. Med. Educ.,* 50:589-595, 1975.

[6] Johnson, H. C. Minority and Nonminority Medical Students' Perceptions of the Medical School Environment. *J. Med. Educ.,* 53:135-136, 1978.

able to catch up or, even worse, failure. As a group, small in number and having experienced an excessive rate of attrition and incidence of repeating portions or all of a year, they endured a burdensome stigma. As individuals, far too many lived with the constant fear of unsatisfactory academic performances and of being "unwelcome guests," despite their competencies and good academic standing. Their hue and cry was exemplified in the concern of the Student National Medical Association (SNMA) about the "real" commitment and responsibility of predominantly white medical schools to increase their production of minority physicians—particularly Black physicians.[7] Indeed, it was a local and national matter, and something needed to be done to establish "coping mechanisms" to resolve minority student/school differences.

THE SUMMER EDUCATIONAL REINFORCEMENT ACTIVITY (SERA)

Based on this backdrop, a description of the pre-enrollment summer program at Temple University School of Medicine that attempts to better equip, or give "a leg up" to selected entering freshmen follows below. This discussion exemplifies a shared program response that only a committed administration and a dedicated host of faculty, students, and staff could give to the evolution of one such successful program. As such, it reflects individual unit and aggregate interpretations of and alternatives to how Temple operates to increase the "holding power" of entering minority and disadvantaged freshman medical students. This result of several years of staff and faculty input to the present point of refinement of Temple's SERA makes for what we believe to be one of the most effective programs of its type in the nation.

SERA is a voluntary program aimed at ultimately retaining minority and disadvantaged students and enhancing their academic performances and quality of life as students. As of this writing, the 168 students who participated in SERA over the past seven summers were incoming freshmen who had fully met the

---

[7] The Dynamics of Communications: A Report and Evaluation of Solutions for Communication and Retention of the Minority Medical Student. Annual Conference of the Student National Medical Association, Philadelphia, April 1973.

requirements for enrollment in the Fall. SERA is a comprehensive effort by the School's faculty, staff, minority upperclassmen, and key community individuals to help new students obtain a realistic view of the medical school setting in general, and specifically to identify academic, social, and psychological patterns which will add to their success as medical students.

SERA is a program coordinated by the Recruitment, Admissions, and Retention (RAR) Program of the School of Medicine, which is funded by both Temple University and the Office of Health Resources Opportunity of the U.S. Department of Health, Education, and Welfare.

The short-range purpose of SERA is to give minority students first-hand exposure to and experiences in the nature and meaning of medical education at Temple before the actual commencement of the freshman year. Students are deliberately exposed to the demands and the pace which will be required of all medical students in the Fall. Helpful techniques and procedures for achieving success are examined. The student becomes acquainted with upperclasspersons and School faculty and staff who are available as academic, social, and emotional resources. SERA also familiarizes the student with the School's affiliated clinical facilities. Introduction of the student to the immediate community and its resident spokespersons is also an integral part of SERA.

Not all minority students need educational reinforcement services from SERA. Some benefit more from help with mobilizing their academic assets, while others use this time to make psychological and social adjustments to the School, the community in which they will live, and/or to their peer and family relationships. There's something in SERA for everyone!

SERA is a seven-week program conducted during the months of June and July as a "dry run" of what is involved in the first year of medical training. During the first week, students are acquainted with the overall setting of the School of Medicine. During the remaining six weeks, students take segments of courses in anatomy, biochemistry, and physiology offered during the regular academic year. At the same time, they are able to sharpen their learning skills, form study groups with other students, and avail themselves of the wide range of academic resources in the School. Each student receives a weekly stipend while attending SERA, in addition to receiving help with any pre-enrollment problems that might occur, such as housing, employment for a spouse, child care, and finalizing the financing of the cost of the first year of medical education.

The overriding objective of SERA is to increase the level of readiness of minority freshmen to complete medical education successfully and on time. The sub-objectives of SERA are: to assist entering minority freshmen in their acclimatization to their new learning experience by exposing them to the total environment of the medical school, the community in which it is situated, teaching facilities, faculty, and staff; to identify academic and related concerns for which supportive resources can be provided to resolve them; to provide opportunities for increasing the students' ability to master academic material, thereby decreasing the risk of academic drop-outs or recycling; to assist students in the early formation of sound learning and test-taking techniques; to increase their ability to negotiate the academic sector of the School; to assist students in the early identification and resolution of personal, family, financial, and housing problems which may interfere with academic pursuits; and to orient students to the use of the student support services of the School.

The two essential phases of SERA used to accomplish the abovementioned objectives are: a one-week orientation, and a six-week period of academic instruction accompanied with learning techniques activities and psychological/social counseling services.

Orientation Week

Orientation Week encompasses the following activities:

— introduction and interaction with administration, faculty and staff, minority upperclasspersons, teaching assistants (sophomores), recent minority graduates and key community leaders;
— tours of the other professional schools on campus, the hospital and other related facilities;
— "rap" sessions with key community leaders;
— discussion with recent minority graduates and upperclassmen on the meaning and nature of medical education;
— introduction and invitation to participation in Student National Medical Association, AMSA, and the Student Council;

— small "open" group sessions;
— introduction to the purpose and functions of the School's Retention Committee and its òther supportive services;
— introduction to the course areas of anatomy, biochemistry, physiology, and learning techniques; and
— initial formation of small study groups.

An average of fifteen hours of didactic and observational time is devoted to Orientation Week. The remaining schedule provides for individual student assessment and initial aid by program staff in the areas of personal (primarily housing and financial) and psychological readiness for maximum, uninterrupted participation in SERA.

Following Orientation Week, the six-week student services system of the Summer Educational Reinforcement Activity at Temple includes three interwoven activities units to specifically anticipate and address the social, psychological, cultural, and academic needs that many incoming minority freshmen might evidence during their adjustment to the realities of being medical students during the regular academic session. The three units are instructional activities, counseling services, and learning techniques activities.

Instructional Activities

The instructional activity of SERA provides the media by which students can be exposed to actual segments of first-year courses: anatomy, biochemistry, and physiology. The learning modules attempt to replicate formalized freshman classroom experiences as closely as possible. The instructional methods employed during these six weeks of the seven-week SERA are lecture, practicum, small-group review sessions, and one-on-one personal conferences between student and instructor. Learning techniques activities, to which approximately forty-three instructional hours are devoted, operate concurrently with the three basic science subjects. Learning techniques activities present various modalities for study habits such as: the advantages of group study, effective use of time, establishing priorities, and test-taking. That activity is more fully discussed later.

The academic content taught is at nearly the same pace and volume of the first year curriculum. The average time allotted to each of the three course segments is: anatomy (gross—40 hours, histology—8 hours, and neuroanatomy—23 hours); biochemistry—40 hours; and physiology—30 hours. This hourly distribution represents time provided for formalized instructional periods, as well as review sessions and examinations.

Many of the academic-year faculty and graduate assistants serve as summer faculty to SERA. Each department assigns a coordinator to define and implement instructional objectives by which students' academic performances and overall adjustments to the rigors of the educative experience at Temple can be identified and augmented by all components of SERA. Approximately twenty-five faculty and graduate assistants are involved in teaching the SERA students. This assignment of teaching personnel has remained relatively constant from summer to summer.

The summer sciences curriculum of SERA developed over the past seven years has attained its ultimate point of refinement. However, in order to insure the program's maximum impact on students in the noninstructional domain to rival the effectiveness of SERA's science instruction core, the variety and range of learning techniques activities and counseling services are periodically modified.

The noninstructional components of SERA—counseling services and learning techniques activities—utilizing the Counselor, the Program Director, the Learning Techniques Specialist, and teaching assistants, function continuously throughout SERA to promote early, independent, and successful student performances. To that end, they facilitate:

— individualized personal conferences with all SERA students, small group sessions with SERA students, upperclassmen, and teaching assistants;
— weekly problem-solving group sessions with teaching assistants for the duration of SERA;
— weekly consultation between faculty and program staff, as needs arise;
— individual evaluation conferences with each student at the termination of SERA;
— terminal evaluation meetings with faculty and staff involved in SERA;
— and follow-up contacts with SERA students during the month of August and into the freshman year.

The six members of the year-round professional staff of the Recruitment, Admissions, and Retention (RAR) Program, most of whom staff SERA, all possess the minimum of master's degrees in the disciplines of social casework, educational counseling, or reading psychology. Each member came to the program with significant prior experience, and was knowledgeable about the psychodynamics of student life in a higher education setting and about the life-style idiom of minority students.

During SERA, six teaching assistants augment the services and activities of the professional staff and faculty, respectively. They are academically successful entering sophomore medical students who participated in the previous year's SERA as trainees and meet the selection criteria of faculty and staff. The qualities of peer leadership, personal sensitivity, and academic success are carefully considered.

The noninstructional components of SERA—counseling services and learning techniques activities—are discussed separately below.

Counseling Services

Among the factors that tend to inhibit the educational process for minority and other differently-advantaged students in medical schools is the too frequent absence of professional counseling services. Yet, where such a service appears, it often incorporates traditional counseling methods. The advising services which faculty and staff have long used with nonminority students cannot do the job that needs to be done with the minority student. Dialogue between minority students and such personnel, where they exist, has shown that the language they use, the behavior they demonstrate, and the assumptions they make all operate to make the student feel put down. Minority students have had to deal with life in such a way that they have an immediate recognition of the philosophical and psychological stance of the person they are confronting. Thus, traditional counseling methods are ineffective for most minority students. Similarly, advising services spread among "interested" faculty and staff lack, in many instances, the personal experience and understanding of the life-styles of minority persons. The same holds true for some students. They often do not understand the pressures and expectations operating in the school's instructors and administrators. The channels of communication between such students, faculty, administration, and other staff, must always be open.

Counseling services provided during SERA impact upon a broad spectrum of student personnel needs. The primary objective of counseling services is to help develop a sufficient self-understanding by the students and appropriate perceptions of the medical school environment so that they can effectively navigate through the multi-faceted demands of the freshman year. Unlike traditional counseling methods and services, this activity must meet minority students head-on in terms of their negative school histories, the uniqueness of their life-styles, and the myriad of contemporary problems which confront most entering minority medical students.

The intent of counseling services is not to separate out social, economic, and psychological student personnel difficulties, but rather to understand and seek to offset the impact they can have on student academic performance. The cause of and solution to problematic academic performance cannot discount the importance of student motivation, goal direction, and clarity, nor the realities associated with a student's total life experience during the summer and subsequent academic year educative process. Counseling services must be outreach in nature, and staff must carry the responsibility for being aware and responsible advocates for the students in each area of their functioning in which counseling services are desired. The need areas serviced usually include the personal, academic, financial, and sociocultural dimensions of student life:

1. *Personal and Sociocultural*—the provision and/or development of concrete resources and guidance services directed toward problems related to personal adjustment, marriage, child care, housing, health care, socialization, and student group programs;
2. *Financial*—planning and development activities related to defining sources of student financial aid, including foundations, contributions, fellowships, and employment opportunities for spouses;
   a. dissemination of financial aid resources information;
   b. student money management, including explanation of terms and requirements of agreements undertaken; and
   c. assisting students in making applications for financial aid;

3. *Academic*—this dimension of counseling is critical, so critical in fact, that each student who is assigned to a Counselor meets regularly in individual, or small-group sessions or both, if warranted. The Counselor is the key operative who: advises students on their programs and general School requirements; facilitates any special tests or arrangements which need to be made; is the appropriate liaison with instructors and their departments of instruction; maintains process-recording on the progress of each student; and insures that students are provided with all that they are entitled to receive.

This service is intended to help bridge the communications gap between faculty and minority students, mentioned earlier. This includes serving as personal mediators for students and faculty members, and enhances the functioning of both parties, by avoiding some of the pressures and conflicts that arise out of misunderstandings. Thus, by working through problems, rather than letting them develop out of proportion, more students are able to become valuable contributors. Staff faces the problems that arise between minority students and the formal system; and attempts to work them through in a way that encourages the student and modifies the system so as to allow it to complement the potential of as many individuals as possible. The idea of later failing and/or dismissing the student who is different and who does not always easily fit into the system is not one which has been compatible with the commitment of the School and the aims of the Summer Educational Reinforcement Activity at Temple University.

Learning Techniques Activities

Medical schools follow rather precise screening procedures and assume that students admitted into such programs possess the skills needed to achieve at expected levels. These levels include proficiencies in both the traditional classroom skills and the concomitant achievement skills. Implied is that students know how to demonstrate learning on both the associative and conceptual levels. They are sufficiently intelligent, mature, organized, and task-oriented to perform successfully in the learning environment.

As the range of students entering medical schools broadened in the late sixties to include persons from minority backgrounds, the basic assumptions regarding students lost some of their validity. There was no longer a single modality for study habits, scheduling procedures, establishing priorities, and test-taking. Historically, those individuals who exhibited high achievement in the medical education setting mastered certain concomitant cognitive skills that have been identified as significant in successful movement through the training system. Minority and disadvantaged students frequently had not developed enough of these skills despite their demonstrated intellectual capacities, and therefore experienced many problems in competing. It was the lack of appropriate concomitant cognitive skills that indicated the need for their development to be included in a successful pre-enrollment summer program.

The fundamental objective that was derived for the learning techniques activities component of SERA is to expose minority students to selected learning experiences which facilitate their scholastic performances in medical school. In order to achieve that end, three sub-objectives must be met. They are:

1. to develop individualized learning skills which will enable the student to negotiate the training system;
2. to diagnose success deficiencies in the areas of personal attitude, experience, ability, and motivation; and
3. to generate a sense of community among such students through interpersonal problem-solving methods.

Consonant with the sub-objectives outlined above, three dimensions of learning techniques activities are discussed below.

The first dimension of learning techniques activities of SERA is designed to facilitate successful achievement of objective one. It has been shown that many minority students need help with developing strategies and patterns of behavior that will assure them successful and on-schedule movement through the medical school curriculum. These strategies and behavior patterns fall into three major operational domains. They include: informational gathering skills, negotiative skills, and manipulative skills.

Informational Gathering Skills—Students are taught methods for information accumulation so that they may more skillfully synthesize the data necessary to negotiate success. There are learning experiences provided to demonstrate alternative sources for gathering content material, as students prepare for test-taking and other evaluation mechanisms.

Negotiative Skills—Students are taught that the successes they seek are frequently disguised within their immediate environment. Often individuals can negotiate as much academic success as they can produce through test performances. Students are shown the interpersonal techniques of bargaining in the scholarly environment. They are also reinforced in the continued need for personal proficiency in their studies.

Manipulative Skills—Minorities and other special groups within our society have survived because of specialized coping behaviors which were responsive to the hostility of perceived environmental pressures. Essentially, they have had to deploy psychological defenses to exist in dire circumstances. Manipulation, circumvention, cunning, disguise, and dissembling are all corporate parts of their response patterns. These corporate parts are not only exhibited by special groups, but are present throughout our society as individuals move to achieve success objectives.

Many of the students who enter SERA have developed and exhibited functional manipulative skills to their background environments. Some have to be exposed to a process of retraining so that these skills may be transferred operationally to the alien environment of the medical education experience. A point of caution is to be noted. The area of conditioning and behavior modification may generate negative reactions on an interpersonal scale. The objectives in this instance are not to train "medical school hustlers" who achieve by "getting over," but to help students use their abilities to communicate and achieve, just as other students will be doing who come from frames of reference that are more similar to that of the medical school environment.

The second dimension of learning techniques activities is offered to meet objective two. Data derived from these activities facilitate the utilization of certain student skills that are necessary for success. These skills include: attitude, experience, and ability.

Attitude—Students are encouraged to adopt attitudes that are oriented towards a rigor and commitment required in high-stress learning situations.

Experience—Instructional activities provide the medium by which students have the opportunity to demonstrate the strength and effectiveness of their prior learning experiences, given the initial demands of medical education.

Ability—Quantitative assessment measures, such as psychological achievement and aptitude testing, are utilized to evaluate the ability of students to function in their planned training program. Intellective appraisal, learning skills, and knowledge appraisal are essential areas for measurement.

> *Intellective appraisal*—reading proficiency of technical matter which includes measurements of: speed, retention, comprehension, and the identification of critical concepts.

> *Learning skills*—associative skills which are measured by students' abilities to identify broad attachment units for new knowledge, and, through battery testing, to assess students' levels of science language skills and basic sciences information.

The third dimension of learning techniques activities of SERA provides for student skills development to include the tasks of:

> *test-taking*—objective (objective, including true/false, multiple-choice, and completion), and subjective (essay-type);
> *test-anxiety*—desensitization to test-taking anxiety;
> *note-taking;*
> *inquiry*—student analysis of course objectives and content;
> *budgeting of time and energy;*
> *utilization of resources*—student utilization of library, counseling, learning techniques, tutorial, advising, faculty, and/or health resources;
> *self-learning techniques;*
> *evaluation;* and
> *organization of study time and resources*—student body schedules and multiple modalities of learning.

This dimension allows for both skills development and deficiency diagnosis well before it occurs.

Motivation—While motivation is a difficult personal characteristic to identify and measure, every effort is made to determine the motivational level of each student and reinforce those that evidence significantly low levels.

In medical schools which host students representing the range of our society's racial and socioeconomic populations, it can be expected that minority and disadvantaged individuals will not be fully included in the milieu of the setting.[8] Specifically, many minority students are not exposed to or feel alienated from many of the helps, communications, and resources that are more readily available to nonminority students. They do not have the opportunity for leads, cues, and unofficial directives that complement the general study structure. As an alternative, SERA students are assigned to study groups while they function through instructional activities. This kind of group arrangement successfully serves to provide many sources of information, levels of learning, reinforcement, and confidence building, all of which contribute to a sense of community among themselves.

Coordinated Staff Services

The combined activities and services of SERA cannot be all things to all students. Therefore, the program is designed to utilize the diverse interests, skills, and backgrounds of all staff, as well as representatives from the faculty and administration of the medical school. As mentioned, the core of noninstructional services for students rests with counselors and the Learning Techniques Specialist, with skills in both disciplines (psychological/social and educational) essential for maximum effectiveness with students. It is important that they work closely together. Educational shortcomings affect emotions, and vice versa. Counselors and learning specialists working as a team can identify problems and help to find solutions.

Jointly supervised by the counselor and the Learning Techniques Specialist, the vital links between students, faculty, and program staff are six teaching assistants to each of whom is assigned a group of five to six trainees. Their basic task is to develop with the SERA students

---

[8] Baum, J. H., and Ireland, C. S., Jr.: Minority Student Performance on Pathology Examinations. *J. Nat. Med. Ass.*, 67: 324-325, 1973.

routes into the academic course content which will facilitate their acquisition and retention of scientific knowledge. They observe the students' classroom behavior; assist in the students' laboratories; facilitate the formation and conduct of study groups; serve as a referral agent to the SERA, other medical school, and community support services; promote the development of healthy interpersonal relationships; assist the students in the design of social/emotional outlets due to tension; provide the students with immediate feedback on a broad base of behaviors; and lend input based on student experiences to the other SERA staff and faculty in order to promote comprehensive services to the SERA student. They spend long and committed hours with their students during class, evenings, and on weekends to nurture the academic and personal growth of their new colleagues.

To achieve the service objectives sought by the SERA staff, the following basic organizational principle was established: a coordinated staff contribution to the students' repertoire of educational abilities. This may be viewed as the same type of commitment to students' welfare that exists in the concept of "family," as we understand it. By excluding any implication of paternalistic behaviors and by emphasizing the crucial quality of interpersonal trust and respect, the "family" approach avoids any strict role definition or unitary focus of accountability for inculcating academic survival skills into the SERA student. Each staff member has a reservoir of approaches to academic skill development from which students can draw in order to broaden their arsenals of academic and political tools in facing the medical educational survival test. In the same manner that a family is untiring in its effort to draw out and reinforce the strengths of each member, so does the SERA staff in a myriad of formal and informal ways serve to complement the positive efforts of medical students.

This information-gathering and service-distribution network complements the family responsibilities of the Learning Techniques Specialist. The participation of trainees in actual segments of first-year academic courses—anatomy, biochemistry, and physiology—facilitates the development of didactic and experiential learning modules which are consistent with formalized classroom experiences. The feedback from teaching assistants, the counselor, and faculty enables the Learning Techniques Specialist to discern by whom and in what mode the learning skill should be disseminated. It is not, therefore, a class-focused approach, but a family-type interaction which can be responsive to the specific needs of individuals or subgroups of the SERA population.

Another example of the value of this approach is in the multiple modes of students' performance evaluation which it encourages. The teaching assistants, almost daily, observe the students' laboratory responsiveness and their reasoning in classroom situations. The faculty evaluates their learning through periodic content examinations and discussions. The counselor listens to the students' descriptions of their own perceptions of their levels of academic preparation. The Learning Techniques Specialist may, through gross or particularized tests, measure the students' achievements in reading, study skills, or content retention. The administrative staff evaluates the students' approaches to handling their formal responsibilities, such as financial management and housing. This enables the family-style learning team to contribute to the design of a response to that specific modality in which the student evidences need. In short, academic skills-building encompasses much more than a "how-to-study" course. It is a comprehensive evaluation of a person's learning style as reflected in a variety of environments. This is then interwoven with a coordinated, concern-based, often student-initiated, process which seeks to build, with the students, effective options for problem-solving. SERA is not a seven-week "wonder course," but a developmental commitment to using the family's and the student's strengths to increase the student's successes.

A concrete example of the value of the team concept among the professional staff of the program would be the identification of a housing problem by a teaching assistant. The teaching assistant after assisting a student with finding appropriate housing, learns that the student's spouse is ill and the ensuing financial burden is interfering with his concentration in the class. The teaching assistant refers the student to the counselor who begins to work with him around his immediate concerns about the family situation. At the same time, the counselor requests the Learning Techniques Specialist to evaluate the student's ability to organize his study time and identify critical matter in the content of the course. In the days to follow, these two staff members share their findings and develop a unified strategy for aiding the student toward more effective functioning in both his personal and academic responsibilities.

At selected times during the final six weeks of SERA, students are assigned to direct clinical observation/participation experiences at the Emergency Room of Temple University Hospital. For many students, this is the first exposure to an acute health care setting. Every participant is given a minimum of two opportunities, 24 hours each and in groups of four, to work with physicians, physician's assistants, and nurses. Concurrently, one afternoon per week, classroom correlation discussions, preceded by live presentations of patients and/or suitable films, are conducted by physicians.

The clinical observation-correlation segment of SERA attempts to introduce the student to the interdependence of basic sciences knowledge and the application of clinical skills in the hospital setting. This first-hand and often "hands-on" experience of observing upperclassmen, residents, and staff physician in action serves to reinforce students' interest in medicine, as well as present a realistic projection of the tasks which lie ahead for them from the point of this beginning to that of graduating as a physician. At the conclusion of past SERA's, most students reported immeasurable benefits from these experiences and expressed strong desires that the time allotted for the clinical observation-correlation be extended.

SERA has been an orientation program for incoming minority freshmen for the past seven years. It has been the students themselves who, without fail, consistently rate its overall impact and helpfulness to them in highly positive terms. Not unlike the basic intent of SERA to provide a period for early school adjustment, with negligible exceptions, former students would encapsulate their summer experience in the way two of them did in 1975:

> "The program creates a sense of brotherhood among the minorities which is necessary to go through medical school. Minorities generally need this special program to make up for the things which a lot of White folks got naturally, such as first-hand experience in medical school and the hospital;" and

> "It informed me of the need for discipline, drive, and dedication that would be needed in order to obtain my degree in medicine. Being a minority student I was not aware of the fact that I could obtain an M.D. degree until my third year of college, so naturally I was not prepared psychologically for a medical career. The SERA program helped me prepare for this and alleviated many of my self-imposed fears."

SERA was originally intended to help students make an earlier adjustment by giving them a preview of some of the problems they might face during the academic year. Since it has gone beyond that, we should be heartened. In late 1977, an evaluation committee consisting of the SERA faculty coordinators, as part of their final report,[9] cited:

---

[9] Report of the SERA Evaluation Committee. Temple University School of Medicine, December 1977.

1. "The course grade received during the SERA program is a good predictor of course grades the student will receive during the regular medical school course. Students usually perform at about the same level in the summer and winter courses, and in many instances their performance improves;"
2. "A substantial number of the SERA students . . . perform at a respectable level in the regular medical school courses, i.e., their course grades range from the 70's to the 90's. This group of the SERA students compares favorably with the nonminority medical students."

The SERA program staff utilize the feedback from students' summer performances to focus on the development of other learning-related services between the closure of SERA and the beginning of the academic year. This bridge for summer pre-enrollment students further reduces or prevents the possibility of academic shock during the first year of their medical education.

So, SERA does not stand alone in the continuum of retention-related events that occur at the School of Medicine. It anticipates the continuity capabilities available from the full-time RAR Program staff and the faculty of the School. Once students begin the academic year, they are knowledgeable about and utilize the kinds of services described earlier, including the peer mechanism of a "buddy system" which pairs the attributes and background requirements of entering minority freshmen with the attributes and strengths of minority upperclassmen to best augment the adjustment needs of the former.

CONCLUSION

The Summer Educational Reinforcement Activity (SERA) is the initial and most meaningful impact that the resources of the School of Medicine at Temple University can provide minority and disadvantaged students in beginning their medical education. SERA simulates the quantity, quality, and tone of the School, by course demands made upon students. The student, in every instance, is given the opportunity to see potential problems at a time when encountering those problems, whatever they be, will not be punitive. The staff makes similar use of SERA, by observing the SERA students under "battle" conditions, and assisting them with whatever problems might arise during the program and possibly during the subsequent academic year. SERA is not, nor was it ever intended to be, a seven-week "wonder course." It is the means by which a committed school of medicine effects a substantive interface needed by both parties to realize common objectives—the increased production of physicians from underrepresented racial and social backgrounds.

As SERA is currently structured and operationalized, it is unfortunate that with the discouraging enrollment and retention rates of minority medical students across the nation, the sensitivity level of so many more schools of medicine is such that they have not established similar activities or programs which can anticipate and provide for the orientation needs of such persons to better insure their successes in dealing with the realities of the requirements of the medical education experience.

Roy Wilkins, the former executive director of the NAACP, expressed the dilemma another way in his syndicated column:[10]

> The argument over what kind of affirmative action is acceptable in the case of . . . admitting Black students by America's universities is proceeding apace. But any present-day formula has got to make provision for catching up. It has got to realize that regardless of the blame (the legally unequal schools for the races in the South or the administratively unequal schools in the North), [what] President Johnson called "a hundred unseen forces" shape ability. Perhaps LBJ said it best in a speech at Howard University on June 4, 1965: "You do not take a person who, for years, has been hobbled by chains and liberate him, bring him up to the starting line of a race and then say, You are free to compete with all the others."

Pre-enrollment summer programs for minority and other disadvantaged medical students are "interim evils" which impose an unwanted, special status and, in doing so, lower self-esteem and incur the resentment of nonminority classmates, faculty, and administrators, as we are seeing now so much more vividly. But with the pool of minority medical school applicants across the nation being static, if not diminishing; when fewer minority stu-

---

[10] Wilkins, Roy: "The Game of Catch-Up." *Philadelphia Evening Bulletin,* April 29, 1975, p. 7.

dents are being accepted to medical schools than in the recent past; and where their grades in the majority are higher than ever; it would seem that pre-enrollment programs can and should be the means by which many more schools can accept many more "reasonable risks"—risks that, in all likelihood, will materialize into successes and aid in increasing our nation's production of minority physicians.

CHAPTER 17

The Medical Education Interface

Maxine E. Bleich

INTRODUCTION

Twelve years after the onset of the "Minorities in Medicine Movement," it is clear the minority students have met with success. Against social/cultural, financial, and academic odds that sometimes have seemed insurmountable, the applicant pool has grown, the minority student enrollment has increased, and most important of all, at least 90 percent* of the students are graduating to become practicing physicians.

The success of the minority medical students is a reflection of their ability to meet the challenges. However, the current limited applicant pool, the faltering enrollment, and the academic problems of minority medical students are a reflection of the nation's educational institutions' inabilities to meet the challenges.

Maxine E. Bleich is Program Director of the Josiah Macy, Jr. Foundation, New York, New York.

* In 1973, 89 percent of the minority students had graduated from medical school, 91 percent of the students were expected to graduate after taking additional time to complete their work, and "first-year retention of Black Americans has risen from 91 percent of 1971-72 entrants to 95 percent of 1974-75 entrants." Data taken from Waldman, Bart: "Economic and Racial Disadvantage as Reflected in Traditional Medical School Selection Factors." *J. Med. Educ.*, 52:961-970, 1977.

Many minority students come from families with limited financial incomes. In the Black colleges more than 90 percent of the students require financial assistance. A recent survey conducted by the United Negro College Fund reports the median income of students enrolled in the Fund's member colleges to be $6,815, less than 40 percent of the median income of students enrolled in predominantly White, private colleges.

Although some financial assistance is available, often the minority students must work to support themselves. Many graduate from college with a fairly high level of indebtedness. These financial responsibilities interfere with some students' efforts to prepare themselves for medical school, causing them to get poor grades or drop the premedical program. Others might not even consider medicine for they feel an obligation to earn a living upon graduation from college.

Table I demonstrates the downward trend since 1974-75 in the percentage of minority students enrolled in the first-year classes of the nation's medical schools. Further, the data demonstrate that the absolute numbers of minority students enrolled as first-year students has been stagnant.

Table 2 demonstrates that since 1972 there has not been growth in the minority student applicant pool.

The drop in the percentage of Black applicants accepted to medical school is clearly observable in Table 3. Interestingly, however, the percentage of accepted Black applicants remains higher than the percentage of acceptances of all student applicants. It is also noteworthy that the percentage of acceptances of all student applicants shows a downward trend.

In summary, there is a downward trend in the percentage of minority admissions; no growth in the minority applicant pool; and a drop in the percentage of minority applicants accepted to medical school.

The reversal of these undesirable trends is a major challenge to the nation's educational institutions, particularly the colleges and medical schools. However, minority students have made advances in general at the undergraduate and professional school levels, which suggest a positive future.

Today minority students represent 17 percent of the nation's college-age populations; 12 percent of the nation's undergraduate students; and between 8 percent and 9 percent of the students

Table 1. Selected Minority Group Enrollment in First-Year Classes in U.S. Medical Schools (1968-1979).

ACADEMIC YEAR	BLACK AMERICAN*		AMERICAN INDIAN		MEXICAN AMERICAN		MAINLAND PUERTO RICAN		TOTAL SELECTED MINORITY GROUP		TOTAL FIRST-YEAR ENROLLMENT
	NUMBER ENROLLED	% OF TOTAL ENROLLMENT	NUMBER ENROLLED	% OF TOTAL ENROLLMENT	NUMBER ENROLLED	% OF TOTAL ENROLLMENT	NUMBER ENROLLED	% OF TOTAL ENROLLMENT	NUMBER ENROLLED	% OF TOTAL ENROLLMENT	
1968-69	266	2.7	3	0.03	20	0.2	3	0.03	292	2.9	9,863
1969-70	440	4.2	7	0.1	44	0.4	10	0.1	501	4.8	10,422
1970-71	697	6.1	11	0.1	73	0.6	27	0.2	808	7.1	11,348
1971-72	882	7.1	23	0.2	118	1.0	40	0.3	1,063	8.5	12,361
1972-73	957	7.0	34	0.3	137	1.0	44	0.3	1,172	8.6	13,677
1973-74	1,023	7.5	44	0.3	174	1.2	56	0.4	1,297	9.1	14,124
1974-75	1,106	7.5	71	0.5	227	1.5	69	0.5	1,473	10.1	14,763
1975-76	1,036	6.8	60	0.4	224	1.5	71	0.5	1,391	9.1	15,295
1976-77	1,040	6.7	43	0.3	245	1.6	72	0.5	1,400	9.0	15,613
1977-78	1,085	6.7	51	0.3	246	1.5	68	0.4	1,450	9.0	16,136
1978-79	1,064	6.4	47	0.3	260	1.6	75	0.5	1,446	8.7	14,074

* Black Americans at Howard and Meharry medical schools accounted for 120 of these 1969-70 freshmen and 195 of these 1974-75 freshmen.

Source: Data taken from AAMC enrollment data.

Table 2. Applicants to First-Year Classes in U.S. Medical Schools (1970-76).

ACADEMIC YEAR	BLACK AMERICAN	AMERICAN INDIAN	MEXICAN AMERICAN	MAINLAND PUERTO RICAN	TOTAL NUMBER OF MINORITY GROUP APPLICANTS	TOTAL NUMBER OF APPLICANTS
1970-71	1,250					24,987
1971-72	1,552					29,172
1972-73	2,382					36,135
1973-74*	2,227	240	349	233	3,049	40,506
1974-75	2,368	131	437	170	3,106	42,624
1975-76	2,286	128	434	204	3,052	42,303
1976-77	2,486	123	452	209	3,270	42,155
1977-78	2,487	122	487	203	3,299	40,569

* Data for American Indians, Mexican Americans, and Mainland Puerto Ricans was not collected prior to 1973.
Source: Data taken from AAMC and adapted from *The Journal of The American Medical Association,* December 27, 1976, Volume 236, No. 26, Index Issue, p. 2961, Table 8.

Table 3. Percent of Applicants Accepted to Medical School for Selected Years

	% OF ALL STUDENTS ACCEPTED	% OF BLACK STUDENTS ACCEPTED
1971-72	42.3	52.2
1972-73	38.1	36.0
1975-76	36.3	41.3
1976-77	37.4	39.1
1977-78	39.4	38.8

Source: Association of American Medical Colleges.

enrolled in graduate and professional schools. The similarities in their level of participation in graduate school and in law and medical schools are striking (Table 4).

Since 1967 there has been a significant increase in minority participation in undergraduate education (Table 5). The rate of increase in minority enrollments in four-year colleges has not been

Table 4. Summary Comparison of Graduate, Law, and Medical School Enrollment Representations (in Percent) of Blacks, Spanish-Surnamed Persons, and American Indians for 1969 and 1976.

GROUP	GRADUATE SCHOOLS	LAW SCHOOLS	MEDICAL SCHOOLS
		1969		
Blacks	4.0	3.8	4.2
Spanish-surnamed	1.1	1.0	0.5
American Indian	0.3	0.1	0.1
Total	5.4	4.9	4.8
		1976		
Blacks	6.4	5.4	6.7
Spanish-surnamed	1.5	2.3	2.1
American Indian	0.4	0.3	0.3
Total	8.3	8.0	9.1

Note: Total representation of these minorities in 1976 was about 12 percent for undergraduate schools and 5 percent for graduate management schools.

Source: *Selective Admissions in Higher Education*, Report of the Carnegie Council on Policy Studies in Higher Education. San Francisco: Jossey-Bass, Inc., Publishers, 1977, p. 149. Used with permission.

matched in the two-year institutions. Further, in the fall of 1978 it was reported that 40 percent of the Black students enrolled in higher education were enrolled in four-year colleges: 20 percent in Black institutions and 20 percent in White.

In 1973-74, 3,531 minority students received baccalaureate degrees in the biological sciences; 1,399 in the physical sciences; and 1,764 in mathematics (Table 6). Although education and the social sciences continue to be the most popular undergraduate majors for minority students, the biological and physical sciences and mathematics that year graduated almost 6,700 minority students. Interestingly, a little more than 3,000 minority students applied to medical school in both 1973-74 and in 1974-75.

In addition to these positive trends, it is anticipated that minority representation at the undergraduate level will continue to increase (Table 7). Although the overall number of 18-year-olds is projected to diminish, the percentage of minorities in this age group is anticipated to grow.

The real challenge to the colleges and medical schools is how to capitalize on the positive developments that have taken place in the past decade. The interface between college and medical school is a crucial link.

POST-BACCALAUREATE PREMEDICAL FELLOWSHIP PROGRAM SUPPORTED BY THE JOSIAH MACY, JR. FOUNDATION

In the 1960's many were stirred to afford opportunities for the nation's minorities to become active participants in all aspects of society. The nation's medical schools were no exception.

One of the first efforts was the Post-Baccalaureate Premedical Fellowship Program, which began in 1966, financed by the Josiah Macy, Jr. Foundation. It was designed to demonstrate to the medical schools that Black students, particularly those who had graduated from traditionally Black colleges in the South, could be competitive candidates for admission.

Students who wanted to study medicine, but who either had not applied to a medical school, or had not been accepted, were selected. After attending a special summer session at Haverford College, or, in later years, at Oberlin, the students enrolled for a

Table 5. Percentage of Nonwhites in Different Types of Institutions

Institution	1967	1970	1973	1976
Two-year colleges	12.3	17.1	14.2	14.7
Four-year colleges	10.9	9.9	12.7	15.2
Universities	6.4	5.4	5.0	9.7
Total	10.1	11.4	11.5	13.8

Source: ACE/UCLA Freshman National Norms Studies, Astin and others, 1976, p. 47; 1973, p. 39; 1970, p. 37; 1967, p. 32.
    Taken from: *Selective Admissions in Higher Education.* Report of the Carnegie Council on Policy Studies in Higher Education. San Francisco, Jossey-Bass, Inc., Publishers, 1977, p. 154. Used with permission.

full academic year in one of seven participating colleges—Bryn Mawr, Haverford, Knox, Kalamazoo, Oberlin, Pomona, and Swarthmore. They took courses in chemistry, biology, mathematics, English, and occasionally other subjects, according to their particular needs.

The program was sponsored for five years. In that time seventy-six students were accepted and seventy-two completed the post-baccalaureate year; a total of fifty-seven, or 79 percent, were graduates of Black colleges. Of the seventy-two students who completed the program, sixty-six, or 92 percent, were accepted to medical school, and sixty-five enrolled.

In response to the financial problems the Post-Baccalaureate Premedical Fellows faced when they got to medical school, a grant-in-aid program was established, also by the Macy Foundation. Since the first year of medical school was felt to be the most critical, each fellow who needed it was awarded $2,500 for the first year; $1,500 was awarded for each of the following three years.

As of the Spring of 1977, of the 65 Fellows who had enrolled in medical school, 52 had graduated, one was still in school, and twelve, or 18 percent, had withdrawn. Thirty-five of the 52 graduates were enrolled in residency programs and 17 were in practice, including two with academic appointments.

Table 8 includes a breakdown, as of July, 1978, of the fields of training/practice of the Post-Baccalaureate Premedical Fellows. For comparison, Table 9 gives a breakdown of all Board-Certified Specialists and Black specialists in 1967.

Table 6. Percentage Distribution of Minority Baccalaureate Recipients Among Fields of Study.

FIELD OF STUDY	TOTAL NUMBER OF RECIPIENTS[a]	PERCENTAGE OF MINORITY RECIPIENTS				
		SUBTOTAL	BLACK	SPANISH-SURNAMED	ASIAN	AMERICAN INDIAN
Arts and humanities	139,900	6.1	3.3	1.8	0.7	0.2
Biological sciences	53,500	6.6	3.6	1.1	1.7	0.1
Business and management	133,300	7.6	4.9	1.2	1.2	0.3
Education	177,800	9.6	7.9	1.1	0.3	0.3
Engineering	62,500	5.1	1.8	1.4	1.5	0.4
Mathematics	24,500	7.2	4.6	0.7	1.7	0.1
Physical sciences	26,400	5.3	2.7	1.3	1.1	0.2
Psychology	52,100	7.4	4.8	1.4	1.0	0.3
Social sciences	158,800	9.7	7.2	1.4	0.8	0.3
All other fields	158,400	7.9	5.2	1.1	1.2	0.4
Total, all fields	989,200	7.8	5.3	1.3	0.9	0.3

Note: The above figures represent population estimates based on a stratified sample of all institutions that confer a bachelor's degree. In view of variations in response rates among institutions and other factors that affect the accuracy of the survey findings, caution should be exercised in interpretation of these data.

[a] Includes U.S. citizens and foreign nationals holding permanent visas.

Source: National Board on Graduate Education (1976, p. 236)

Taken from: *Selective Admissions in Higher Education*. Report of the Carnegie Council on Policy Studies in Higher Education. San Francisco: Jossey-Bass, Inc., Publishers, 1977, p. 158. Used with permission.

Table 7. Census Projections of 18-Year-Old Black and Other Nonwhites in the United States Population by Admission Years from 1976 through 1994 (in Thousands).

ADMISSION YEAR	TOTAL NUMBER	BLACK NUMBER	BLACK PERCENTAGE	OTHER NONWHITES NUMBER	OTHER NONWHITES PERCENTAGE
1976	4,253	560	13.2	72	1.7
1977	4,244	573	13.5	76	1.8
1978	4,229	573	13.5	78	1.8
1979	4,292	583	13.6	83	1.9
1980	4,211	581	13.8	85	2.0
1981	4,145	580	14.0	87	2.1
1982	4,087	579	14.2	89	2.2
1983	3,917	569	14.5	92	2.3
1984	3,703	548	14.8	96	2.6
1985	3,604	525	14.6	96	2.7
1986	3,521	519	14.7	97	2.8
1987	3,567	530	14.8	101	2.8
1988	3,653	539	14.8	107	2.9
1989	3,733	566	15.2	117	3.1
1990	3,426	533	15.6	121	3.5
1991	3,240	514	15.9	122	3.8
1992	3,168	496	15.6	125	3.9
1993	3,247	506	15.6	127	3.9
1994	3,199	495	15.5	125	3.9

Source: U.S. Bureau of the Census (1977, pp. 28, 37-54).

Taken from: *Selective Admissions in Higher Education*. Report of the Carnegie Council on Policy Studies in Higher Education, San Francisco, Jossey-Bass, Inc., Publishers, 1977, p. 154. Used with permission.

**Table 8.   Macy Post-Baccalaureate Premedical Fellows:
Fields of Training/Practice as of July, 1978.**

	NUMBER	PERCENT
Internal Medicine	24	45%
Family Practice	7	13%
General Surgery	6	11%
Pediatrics	4	8%
Obstetrics/Gynecology	3	6%
Radiology	3	6%
Psychiatry	2	4%
Anesthesiology	1	2%
Pathology	1	2%
	53	100% (approx.)

The Post-Baccalaureate Premedical Fellows clearly were successful pioneers in the "Minorities in Medicine Movement." They
demonstrated to the medical schools that students from colleges
not well represented in medical school could be successful candidates, as well as competent medical students. The students had an
opportunity to strengthen their backgrounds in fields important to
the work in medical school.

OTHER POST-BACCALAUREATE
PREMEDICAL PROGRAMS

There have been a number of other post-baccalaureate programs for minority students interested in medicine. One, sponsored by a medical school, enrolls minority students who have been
unsuccessful candidates to the medical school. Each year ten such
students are selected for a one-year program to demonstrate they
will be successful medical students.

Beginning in 1972, Connecticut College has conducted for
several years another type of post-baccalaureate program which
enrolled minority students who had graduated from college without taking the required premedical courses. A similar program was
conducted by National Medical Fellowships in 1973-74 and 1974-
75. The Connecticut College program has been financed by several
foundation and federal grants; the National Medical Fellowships'

Table 9.   Comparison of Specialty Preference of
Black Doctors vs. all Doctors in the United States, 1967.

BLACK SPECIALISTS		ALL BOARD-CERTIFIED SPECIALISTS	
General Surgery	27%	Internal Medicine	25%
Obstetrics/Gynecology	20%	General Surgery	21%
Pediatrics	19%	Pediatrics	16%
Internal Medicine	14%	Obstetrics/Gynecology	13%
Psychiatry and Neurology	11%	Radiology	13%
Radiology	9%	Psychiatry and Neurology	12%
	100%		100%

program was supported by the Van Ameringen Foundation. As a result of these programs a number of minority students are, or soon will be, doctors in spite of a late start.

The post-baccalaureate approach to prepare students for medical schools is not unique to minority students. In recent years Bryn Mawr College and the School of General Studies at Columbia University have sponsored such programs. The Bryn Mawr program is limited to students who have not applied to medical school; the Columbia program does not have such a limitation. Both programs provide the students with the science and mathematics courses necessary for admission to medical school. The graduates of the programs have had an 80 percent or better acceptance rate to medical school.

RESPONSIBILITIES OF UNDERGRADUATE COLLEGES

Background and Preparation of Premedical Advisors*

Premedical advisors are of significant importance to both the premedical students and the medical schools. Usually they are members of departments of biology or chemistry; most often departments of biology.

---

* See also Chapters 4 and 5.

Stability in the position of premedical advisor is crucial, as well as the support of an active, well-informed premedical advisory committee, made up of representatives from the departments of biology, chemistry, physics, mathematics, and the humanities.

The advisors have many responsibilities: they must be knowledgeable about medical school admissions requirements, the admissions process, the Medical College Admission Test (MCAT), and the biology and chemistry courses necessary to prepare a successful medical school candidate.

They must be thoroughly knowledgeable about the science and mathematics courses offered by their own institutions. If, for example, the biology courses do not provide the material at the appropriate quantitative level, the advisors should be able to explain the deficiencies and help the students arrange to supplement their program. Further, they should try to deter students from enrolling in a section of a course not appropriate for premedical students.

In relation to the medical schools, the advisors must have first-hand information about them, particularly the medical schools that accept the majority of their students. Also, it is important that members of the Admissions Committees of those medical schools get to know the advisors.

It is critical to the success of the advisors that their institutions support them. This support might take the form of a limited teaching responsibility, secretarial assistance, and a budget to attend meetings at both the local and national levels.

Faculty Development—The Teaching of Biology and Other Sciences Basic to the Preparation of Premedical Students

In the past twenty years there have been great advances in the biological sciences that have resulted in their development from a purely descriptive science, to one that is quantitative at both the molecular and cellular levels. Unfortunately, the biological sciences offered at many small colleges, particularly at the Black colleges, were unable to develop at the same pace. As a consequence the programs have remained at a descriptive level.

During the initial success of the "Minorities in Medicine Movement," a higher proportion of Black medical students were graduates of Black colleges. Because of the descriptive nature of their preparation they were considered to be "at risk" by the medical schools. As a consequence, as the number of minority students graduating from non-Black colleges increased, the percentage and actual number of Black college graduates accepted to medical school declined.

However, as was reported this Fall, 20 percent of the Black students enrolled in four-year colleges are enrolled in the Black colleges. The Black colleges continue to be a unique resource. It is crucial that the current programs to broaden the academic backgrounds of their faculties and redesign the science curricula are advanced. The groundwork has been laid by the Federal Government through the Minority Biomedical Support Program (MBS) and the Minority Access to Research Careers Program (MARC), as well as efforts sponsored by the National Science Foundation. Private philanthropy has also participated in these efforts, and State legislatures have assisted in the financing of modern science buildings, laboratories, and equipment.

The administrators of the Black colleges and other minority institutions must encourage and support their faculty in these efforts to modernize.

**Special Academic Support Programs and
Services Basic to the Success
of Undergraduate Students Preparing for
the Study of Medicine, Including
Research Opportunities, Clinical Experiences,
and Financial Assistance**

During the twelve-year period of advances in the "Minorities in Medicine Movement," the academic quality of many public high schools, particularly those that have been educating minority students, has deteriorated. Too often minority students are graduating from high school with, at best, an eighth grade reading level, and perhaps with only two years of algebra.

As a result of this inadequate preparation, many students must use the freshman and/or sophomore years in college to strengthen their mathematics preparation, as well as their reading abilities. Many are unable to take calculus before their junior year. As a result they find themselves enrolled in calculus, organic chemistry, and physics at the same time.

The resolution of this problem is a great challenge to the colleges. It is critical that the students' academic deficiencies be overcome before they undertake course work in preparation for the study of medicine.

One approach might be summer programs prior to the first year of college. These sessions could be diagnostic in nature, assessing the students' strengths and weaknesses in mathematics and reading.

If necessary, the students might spend five years in college. The first year might be spent in developing the background in mathematics and reading necessary to be successful in the subsequent science and mathematics courses.

The expansion of the pool of undergraduate minority students prepared for medical school depends, in great part, on what the undergraduate colleges can provide. In many colleges the undergraduate science curricula must be revised, and at the same time the students must have a broad, rigorous high school background in mathematics, reading, and quantitative problem-solving.

If the appropriate courses are not available, arrangements might be made for students to enroll in such courses at nearby colleges, or in summer schools that provide them.

In addition to providing academic assistance upon entry into college, tutorial assistance might be made available throughout the four years. Although the tutorials might be provided by students, the faculty should play an active role.

Also, student and faculty participation in research projects is important. Programs like MBS and MARC provide such opportunities. The Scholars Program at the Woods Hole Marine Biological Laboratory provides research opportunities and courses for Black college faculty and students during the summer and the month of January. Many laboratories in major universities and medical schools provide research opportunities for both faculty members and students during the summer.

For those large universities and academically superior small four-year colleges which do not need to modernize their science programs, greater success on the part of minority premedical students might be ensured. Often, after the sophomore year, these schools determine whom they will recommend for medical school. It is at this point that many minority students give up their intentions to study medicine. However, with the appropriate academic assistance and encouragement, many of these students might be retained as premedical students and successful medical school candidates.

Out of a concern for a high grade point average, students often select courses designed for non-majors or for students not preparing for professional education. Courses in physics and organic chemistry especially fall into this category—courses necessary as preparation for medical school. Counseling must be provided to deter students from making such choices. If, for the sake of the grade point average, students do enroll in the less rigorous courses, they should be urged to take the appropriate courses in a sufficiently demanding summer school.

There are numerous summer programs, both at colleges and at medical schools, that attempt to strengthen the academic backgrounds of minority premedical students. They provide specially designed courses in biology, chemistry, mathematics, and biochemistry; review sessions for the MCAT; research experiences; and clinical experiences in cooperating hospitals. Premedical advisors have the responsibility to learn about the summer programs and assist the students in applying.

Some states have established programs to provide greater opportunities for minorities to study medicine. These programs have included scholarship monies at the undergraduate level, as well as at the medical school level. Also, there are private scholarships for minority students in good academic standing for undergraduate and medical school fees. Programs such as MBS and MARC provide stipends for students. Often science departments will give premedical students priority for the work-study jobs that are available.

It is important that those minority premedical students with financial need have an opportunity to obtain assistance in the form of scholarships, stipends, loans, or work-study funds. It is equally important that, if possible, whatever employment they may seek be in a setting that will strengthen their background and motivation, i.e., in a college or medical school science laboratory; in a science department; perhaps in a hospital.

Further, it is important that the premedical advisors keep the students well informed about the financial assistance available to medical students. As early as possible minority premedical students should know about the National Medical Fellowships, the National Health Service Corps, and military programs; loan availability; state incentives and private scources. Although the amounts available in each program are limited, the advisor must discuss their possibilities in a realistic manner without discouraging the student.

RESPONSIBILITIES OF MEDICAL SCHOOLS

Setting Academic Standards and Assisting Colleges to Prepare Students to Meet the Standards

Many Black colleges are located near a medical school. Committees of faculty members from both the Black colleges and the medical schools might be formed to discuss the academic experiences of minority medical students. Those medical school courses, such as biochemistry and physiology, that most frequently pose problems might be reviewed. The medical school faculty members might detail the principles that are included in the courses and what might be necessary undergraduate preparation for success. The medical school might provide faculty to help the colleges with teaching and curriculum redesign.

Setting Admissions Requirements and Assisting Colleges to Prepare Students to Meet Them

The medical schools should clearly state their admissions requirements, and work with the colleges to prepare the students for acceptance. If, as an example, the MCAT is important to admissions it should be so clearly stated. Those areas in which the minority students do poorly should be identified. The academic reasons for the students' difficulties should be shared with the college faculty members.

On the other hand, members of medical school admissions committees might become knowledgable about the growing literature concerning minorities and standardized examinations, particularly the MCAT. Although there have been significant scoring differentials, most minority students, at least 90 percent, have been successful medical school graduates.

Further, medical school admissions committees might become familiar with the academic progress of their minority students. They should know at what academic level students consistently are "at risk," and explain to applicants what it means to be considered "at academic risk."

Preparation and Development of Leaders* of Offices of Minority Affairs

One of the most significant developments in the "Minorities for Medicine Movement" has been the establishment of Offices of Minority Affairs. Although they have contributed greatly to the success of minority medical students, some of them have posed administrative problems for the medical schools.

The Offices of Minority Affairs serve many functions. They need to have a staff that can recruit; develop and administer the necessary academic support programs; actively participate in the admissions process as well as the promotions process; provide guidance and counseling for minority medical students; be an advocate for the minority students within the medical school; develop and maintain an active professional relationship with the undergraduate institutions that prepare the minority students; develop and administer academic programs with colleges and public schools to prepare a pool of minority candidates; and last, but not least, find the appropriate financial assistance to support its programs.

A small number of Offices of Minority Affairs have been directed by minority clinical and basic science faculty members. Although such a background has credibility with the medical school faculty and administration, the Director's professional standing is soon placed at risk. The pressure and demands are all-consuming, difficult to deny. There is little time for the teaching and laboratory work traditional to a faculty member.

On the other hand, most medical schools have appointed Directors who have not had the academic background traditionally respected by medical school faculties and administrations. This has caused serious limitations for some programs. However, because of their importance, the medical schools must support Offices of

---

* See Chapter 18.

Minority Affairs, and foster the development of their leaders. At least the Director's salary, the salary for a secretary, along with office space should be part of the medical school's budget.

The Director should have a background in science teaching and/or counseling. At least a Master's Degree should be required, and some background in mathematics and/or science. This last requirement is important, for the psychological and social problems of medical school are exacerbated by academic deficiencies. The Minority Affairs Director must understand the academic demands placed on the students.

Further, the Office of Minority Affairs should be sponsored by the Administration of the medical school, perhaps through both the Associate Deans for Student Affairs and Academic Affairs.

Preparation of Faculty to Be Sensitive to the Unique Academic and Cultural Needs of Minority Students

For the past fifteen years the medical schools have been able to enroll some of the best prepared students in the nation; students who, for the most part, have had broad academic experience in the biomedical sciences. At the same time the overall attrition rate in medical school declined from 5 percent to 1 percent.

As a consequence medical school faculty members have developed as teachers of professional-level students and researchers. Academic support programs for less prepared students are thought to be inappropriate in a medical school setting. Often such efforts are poorly regarded, and the students who need the assistance are not respected. It is important that the administration of the medical schools set an example by developing incentives for faculty members, particularly basic science faculty members, to become aware of the unique academic and cultural needs of the minority students.

Preparation and Development of Minority Faculty Members

Medical schools must be careful not to exploit unduly the few minority faculty that exist. They must be allowed to achieve as professionals, in spite of the great demands placed on them to help integrate the medical schools; their professional careers must be paramount.

One expeditious way the medical schools might augment the ranks of minority faculty members is to appoint minority physicians from the community to be members of the clinical faculty. These physicians may help to build good relationships with the minority community, and may serve as role models for the minority medical students. They may also provide insights and assistance to the medical schools' efforts to increase the number of minority medical students.

Only a small percentage of all medical students select careers in academic medicine; the percentage of minority medical students selecting academic medicine is even smaller. One reason for the small number of minority medical students selecting academic medicine relates to their high level of indebtedness upon graduation from medical school. Their financial responsibilities inhibit them from the further training necessary for good academic positions.

Another factor is the perception, on the part of some minority students and many medical school faculty members, that minority physicians are trained for the main purpose of providing medical care to minority communities. As a consequence of this attitude minority students who demonstrate potential for academic medicine are not nurtured and encouraged.

Minority medical school faculty members serve as important role models to minority medical students and to other students contemplating a career in medicine.

Programs might be developed to provide financial assistance at the residency and fellowship levels to prepare minority physicians for careers in academic medicine. Medical school faculty members might encourage outstanding minority medical students to pursue research careers and academic medicine.

CHAPTER 18

A Minority Affairs Office in a Medical School

Althea Alexander

What is a Minority Affairs Office? How should it function? What are its goals? Who does it serve? Perhaps the answers to these questions are as many and varied as there are people concerned with and committed to minority medical education. This section will deal with the essential requirements of such an "office" and convey our ten-year experience. In so doing, it is hoped that others may avoid our mistakes and utilize our success in shaping their programs.

ON COMMITMENT

A Minority Affairs Program must have both ideological and financial support of the medical school which it is to serve. Clear-cut quantitative and qualitative goals must be established, and once embarked upon, the necessity of ongoing commitment is self-evident. Expanding minority medical education is not an easy

Althea Alexander is Research Associate, Division of Research in Medical Education and Director, Office of Minority Affairs, School of Medicine, University of Southern California, Los Angeles, California.

task, but it is rendered impossible without the full support of the respective Boards, Presidents, and Deans.

One should assume that there will be "factions of resistance" within any medical school embarking on a program designed to increase recruitment and retention of minority medical students. Establishment of an "Office of Minority Affairs" is a highly visible action that is more likely than not to generate criticism from some faculty and students. Why do minorities need a special office? Does this not usurp the role of the Dean of Students? Why should minorities get special help and counseling? These and a variety of other questions, many of which will be antagonistic if not outright hostile, represent the expected response. A minority program not protected by an "umbrella of commitment" at the highest level of authority will find itself jeopardized by these detractors. Conversely, with the needed support, many programs have been and will continue to be successful despite these detractors. It is not the purpose of this chapter to present the merits of minority medical education, but in light of recent dialogue vis-a-vis Bakke and the vestiges of racism that still remain, one would be naive not to anticipate "anti-minority sentiment" when going about the business of establishing a minority office.

It has been our experience that a successful office not only serves the needs of minority students, but presents a format for constructive interaction with non-minority students. Our office has grown into this and now serves in such a manner. Often there are more non-minorities present than minorities. Students in general view the office as a supportive place where they can ventilate anxieties in a relaxed, informal setting. We have, by design, established an informal office which by its nature provides a non-threatening environment away from the pressure of classes, exams, labs, and grades. Our staff projects a non-authority-figure role. We arrange our work schedule so that it does not conflict with student breaks. This and a full coffee pot, as well as our close proximity to lecture halls and labs, has made the office a natural refuge from the day-to-day constraints of academics.

This format has served us well. We find that many student problems are resolved before they become serious, by simple listening and support. Many times the student only needs reassurance or direction to an available university resource that can help.

ON DEFINITION

An efficacious minority office will, out of necessity, involve itself with all aspects of student needs. As such, it should transcend and expand on the roles of other medical school institutions, including:

1. Admissions
2. Financial Aid
3. Promotions
4. Basic Sciences
5. Clinical Medicine
6. Personal Counseling
7. Postgraduate Training

Admissions

Since admissions is the crucial function on which minority medical education is based, it is obvious that a successful program must involve a role in the recruitment and selection process. This should entail actual voting representation on admissions committees and contact with candidates prior to selection.

Given the complexity of evaluating candidates by predicting which ones are qualified to complete the medical curriculum and become competent practicing physicians, it is imperative that cultural, as well as educational backgrounds, be considered. Who is more qualified to evaluate the Black or Brown candidate than a Black or Brown student or faculty member? Moreover, since an Office of Minority Affairs is held accountable for the success of minority students, it is only logical that it play a role in selection.

Our goal is to speak with all minority candidates. This is not in lieu of their interviews. It is informal and non-structured. Candidates are introduced to other minority students and are shown around the medical center. They visit the office and "converse" with students, thereby gaining insights into our program which are not obtainable through routine interview.

In no way should the role of the Minority Affairs Office be considered as a substitute admissions office. Some may mistakenly do so or express the view that minorities are given special considerations, whereas in fact, it is simply a matter of adding another productive, useful dimension to the process of selecting good candidates. Both grades and MCAT exams are objective criteria which do not offer predictive value as to which candidates will make good physicians. These screening devices simply reflect the likelihood of satisfactory performance during the first two basic science years. Admissions committees consider many subjective elements such as maturity, outside interests, experience, and commitment. The minorities office simply helps in this assessment.

Financial Aid

Once admitted, the next concern of the new students is how they will finance their medical education. Compared to ten years ago, there is now a paucity of grant-in-aid monies available. Students must rely more and more heavily on loans. This coupled with the increased costs of tuition, living expenses, books, and supplies may result in significant debt on completion of medical school. If the student is married and has dependents, debts of enormous proportions will accrue.

Our efforts are directed towards softening this financial burden. We maintain a close day-to-day working relationship with the financial aid officer. We keep abreast of the relative needs of each student. Significant effort is expended to insure that all grant monies are used appropriately. Students are helped toward securing low-interest, long-term loans. My advice is of a general nature. More importantly, our financial aid officer goes over the student's budget step by step.

A Minority Alumni fund has been established. We are soliciting and securing monies from earlier graduates now in practice. We have found a local private individual source which will match on a two-to-one basis every dollar given by Alumni. It is our hope that this fund will help significantly to reduce the total debt incurred by our students.

Promotions

It is essential that close liaison be established and maintained between the Office of Minority Affairs and the Promotions Committee of the Medical School. Ideally, this can best be done by securing a seat on this committee, but having close contact with its members may suffice.

Because of our relationship with students, we are on many occasions able to detect academic difficulty early. Usually these problems can be resolved by simply determining why the student is in trouble and then directing the necessary effort towards correction. Of the students who encounter academic difficulty, most attribute their situation to personal problems. Usually these can be resolved by personal counseling. If needed, academic help is available in the form of tutoring or special "review sessions". Most students simply need to talk to someone who is supportive and will listen. This is often easier said than done. Many students are reluctant to talk to other students or authority figures such as "Deans" concerning their problems. They need to know that whomever they speak with will not misinterpret or misuse the information. Also the counselor must be readily available to avoid delays of several days or weeks, since academic problems have a tendency to enlarge rapidly. The counseling role of the Minority Office also assumes responsibility for a knowledge and appreciation for cultural patterns represented by each student.

If indeed the student continues to do poorly, despite counseling, tutoring, and a supportive ear, he or she may have to appear before the promotions committee. The role of the Minority Office in this situation is to provide the committee with insight into how the student may be helped to correct the deficiency. It is imperative that this process be non-punitive.

Basic Sciences

It is important that the Minority Office establish a working relationship with the basic science faculty. If a student is going to have problems, it is usually due to one or more of the basic sciences, since this part of the curriculum is usually the most stressful simply because of the enormous amount of material that must be learned and assimilated in a very short period of time.

We have had a summer program for entering first-year students. It is four weeks in duration and taught by basic science faculty. Material covered includes Basic Biochemistry, Histology, Gross Anatomy, and Physiology. The purpose of this program is not remedial, it is designed to give the student a feeling for the volume and degree of difficulty encountered in the first two years. You might consider this a "trial run" since the student is subjected to the same pressures, including exams, that he will need to deal with successfully over the following two years. This approach has been successful in helping the student make the necessary adjustment.

Participation was based on the evaluation of the Dean of Students and Dean of Admissions. During the last few years of its existence, the program was cross-cultural (Blacks, Chicanos, Whites). Though we no longer have a summer program, it is my hope that it will be reinstituted if only for the importance of the experience.

Clinical Medicine

For the most part, minority students do extremely well in the clinical aspects of medicine. At the risk of generalizing, it seems that the background experiences of our students serve them well in acquiring the skills necessary for an effective "doctor-patient" relationship. Perhaps this is a result of increased empathy, insight, or simply an expression of communality of experience since most patients in our "teaching institution" are themselves minorities.

Our emphasis has been to build on this strength through a system of "Big Brothers and Sisters" whereby each entering freshman is assigned an upperclass student to help make the transition from the first two years of academics to the second two years of clinical medicine. This involves such things as scheduling of clerkships, selection of attending physicians (where possible), and general advice regarding functioning in a large medical complex with its hierarchy of students, interns, residents, fellows, and staff.

Many of our minority alumni are now on staff as full-time, part-time, and volunteer attending physicians. They take an active role in both teaching and counseling students, especially with respect to the selection of what medical field they wish to enter. Several sit on the admissions committee.

It is indeed rewarding to see minority physicians whom we began working with as high school students now serving their respective communities as well as making a contribution to minority medical education.

Frederick Douglass said in 1866, "Peace between races is not to be secured by degrading one race and exalting another, by giving power to one race and withholding it from another; but by maintaining a state of equal justice between all classes."

There is no debate as to the responsibility of an institution to include the greatest possible level of diversity in its student body. Establishing that diversity with compassion, sensitivity, and understanding at least attempts to understand cultural differences and the importance of their viability. Without such understanding and commitment, no institution which claims to produce health care deliverers can consider itself viable. It is the only way we can move our society closer to its full potential. To ignore this glowing opportunity would be like casting ourselves into an endless tunnel.

CHAPTER 19

Student Academic Support Services and Retention

Miriam S. Willey

INTRODUCTION

The first priority for student academic support services is to improve student retention and thereby increase the number of graduates in each class. Since problems with retention can have a demoralizing effect on any group of students, particularly if the retention rate for one subgroup is lower than that of their classmates, another benefit associated with improved retention is improved morale. The second priority for academic support services is to raise the overall level of student academic performance by making the services available to all students, with the expectation that they will be more competitive in their professional standing at graduation.

An understanding of the historical development of student academic support services in American medical schools provides one important basis for understanding the current needs for these services. Retention has been, and continues to be, the primary purpose for providing academic support to students. During the

---

Miriam S. Willey, Ph.D., is Assistant Professor and Director, Office of Medical Education, Howard University College of Medicine, Washington, D.C.

past twenty-five years, three factors have particularly affected retention of students in American medical schools: (a) size and quality of the pool of students applying for admission to the medical schools; (b) amounts and targets of existent outside funding programs for medical students and for medical education, and (c) options available to medical students for subsequently obtaining licensure to practice as physicians. These factors typically have been outside the control of medical schools and determined largely by contemporary social values and political policies. An examination of how these factors have affected concerns of medical faculties about academic performance of their students in general, and minority students in particular, helps explain many recent developments of student academic support services in medical school in the United States.

In the 1950s and early 1960s, the number of applicants for each available seat in the medical schools decreased and the retention rate of medical students also decreased.[1,2] However, little pressure was felt by medical schools to increase the overall number of physicians or to increase the number or proportion of minority physicians. Prior to the late 1960s, neither direct financial aid to students nor funding of medical education programs was designed to bring about any significant change in the number, proportion, or distribution of minority students in medical schools.[3-5] Attention to retention of medical students was directed at improving academic performance in general[1] rather than at increasing the retention rate of specific students (e.g., minority) who could be identified at the time of admission. Consequently, efforts to increase retention were aimed mainly at (a) improving recruitment and admissions procedures for better student selection, (b) extending counseling and advisory programs, and (c) initiating changes in teaching programs and curricula.[1] During this period, medical school graduates had two ways to obtain licensure: National Board Examinations (NBE) administered by the National Board of Medical Examiners, and licensing examinations developed and administered by individual state medical boards. Although geographically limited, licensure by state board examinations frequently was easier than by national examination (i.e., NBE), and in some states licensure was virtually assured for medical school graduates.[6,7]

By the late 1960s, the average number of applicants for each available seat increased and the retention rate also increased.[2]

Pressure had developed, not only to increase the number of physicians in general,[4,8] but also to increase the number and proportion of minority physicians.[5,9,10] Increased funding became available for direct financial aid to minority medical students,[11] as well as for programs designed to recruit and improve the retention of these students.[12]

During the 1970s, concern over attrition was increasingly directed at improving academic performance of specific students designated at the time of admission as minority and/or disadvantaged. Thus, efforts to improve retention dealt with (a) recruiting and preparing minority students prior to enrollment, and (b) providing academic support directly to these students during the regular school year.[2,13,14] However, in this period options for licensure were reduced because state board examinations were gradually replaced by the new Federation Licensing Examination (FLEX) developed by the Federation of State Medical Boards of the United States.[6] Some medical schools attempted to assure licensure of their graduates by requiring them to pass one of the national examinations (NBE or FLEX) as a condition for promotion and/or graduation.[15]

This chapter presents a variety of student academic support services and programs used by medical schools to improve the academic performance, retention, and ultimate licensure of all students. Although medical schools usually introduce these support services for the benefit of minority and/or disadvantaged students, experiences at these schools confirm that their entire student bodies take advantage of the services.[10]

TYPES OF STUDENT ACADEMIC SUPPORT SERVICES

All students who appear to need academic support services will not voluntarily take advantage of them. However, students will be more likely to make appropriate use of available services if no stigma is attached to, and no isolation results from, participation in these services. In a predominantly White institution, it is particularly important to avoid having need for service associated with a minority group. One way to make sure that such an association does not occur is to make all services available to all students. However, if resources are limited, those students who appear to need academic support most may be encouraged to participate, and given priority for receiving service and financial assistance for those services.

The attitudes of the persons who provide student academic support services toward the function of those services and the students whom they serve affect the quality of the services and programs. In order to help develop and maintain constructive attitudes toward academic support services, the following four basic principles have been found especially useful: (a) Each individual medical student is admitted by a medical school with the expectation of graduation. (b) Within the resources of the school, it is appropriate to provide the academic support services necessary for all students to have a reasonable opportunity to graduate. (c) Academic support services, therefore, need to be designed to provide solutions to problems as defined by those being served—both the school and the individual students. (d) Regardless of the extent of academic support services, however, a medical school also must convey to all students that they have the capabilities and responsibilities to achieve a satisfactory level of academic performance. In applying these principles, a number of medical schools have found that the closer the relationship between the services and the curriculum, the easier it is for students to utilize those services in improving academic performance.

Services for Pre-Enrolled Students

Although the services are described separately, many summer programs combine elements of two or more types of services and have the following features in common.

Purpose of Programs. Within a premedical curriculum, students do not have to cope with individual courses taught by several faculty members, heavy scheduling, and the rapid pace of academic assignments that typify first-year medical curricula. Most medical students can adjust to changes in one of these areas. However, they often have to adjust to changes in more than one area and also cope with other problems such as catching up on prerequisite information, developing maturity, getting back into habits of studying after a period out of school, adapting to a different racial environment, developing new learning skills, and solving other problems of housing, finances, family, or health that may impinge on their academic performance. Students who have to deal with several of these changes and problems simultaneously during the first year may find it very difficult to achieve satisfactory academic performance.

Most of the programs for pre-enrolled students are carried out during the summer, and may have any of these purposes. First, summer programs can help students (a) to become more effective and independent as learners, (b) to make appropriate use of academic support services that may be available during the regular school year, and (c) to solve some of the other problems mentioned earlier, before they begin the first semester. Therefore, such programs should be considered "preparatory," not "remedial." Second, summer programs are helpful to students who have demonstrated the potential for success in medical school, but who may be expected to encounter difficulty in making the transition from undergraudate to medical education. For this reason, these programs are not designed to develop or create that potential in students.

Selection of Participants. One of the major pitfalls in selecting students for a summer program is to choose students whose needs are too similar to each other's. In order to avoid this, two types of students could be encouraged to participate: (a) students who are young and immature but who have strong academic backgrounds, and (b) students who are more mature but who have academic backgrounds that are less competitive. In addition, a few places might be made available to other students who request to participate. Such a mix of students not only provides stimulation within the group, but also avoids the possibility of a stigma being attached to the program and identification and isolation of the participants.

Another difficulty may occur as the number of participants approaches twenty. Subgroups and cliques are likely to form among the participants which may have a negative influence on the program unless handled appropriately. For example, members of a subgroup can be assigned to different laboratory groups. A third problem lies in determining the basis on which students are allowed to continue in the programs. Whether students attend on a voluntary or required basis, they should be allowed to continue in the program only as long as they fully participate in all aspects of the program, meet all requirements for attendance, and complete all assignments on time. Otherwise, such students will not fully benefit from the program and, perhaps more importantly, they will have an adverse effect on the morale of the other students.

Priorities for Content and Activities. One of the temptations in designing a summer program is to try to cover too many areas of weakness observed among medical students, including some areas relevant to professional competence but not necessarily critical for retention. Within the resources of the school, programs should be designed to cover those areas that are most important to assuring student retention during the first year—the period of maximum attrition. Four such areas which typically need to be considered include attitudes, experiences, skills, and topical information. A few comments on each area follow. (a) Attitudes—students can be encouraged to assume responsibility for their own learning by including a few test items on content described in objectives but not covered in class, and by requiring full participation in the program even though no grades will be entered on transcripts. (b) Experiences—clinical and research experiences may not be as important in preenrollment programs as in pre-admission programs when recruiting and familiarization with the field of medicine are important. Nevertheless, a useful type of experience is to provide the necessary training for students to become paid, classroom assistants in their freshman courses (e.g., anatomy dissector, laboratory assistant, classroom projectionist) during the regular school year or in a summer program the following year. (c) Skills—assignments and scheduled class time should approach the pace of the first-year curriculum so that students have an opportunity to identify problems they are likely to encounter in the regular medical curriculum, and to develop skills necessary for managing their time and coping with the anticipated academic workload. (d) Information—both medical faculty and students can be helpful in rating the importance of topics in preparing students for the first-year curriculum.

The question of speed reading arises so frequently in discussions of summer programs that it warrants special comment. Although most students can increase their reading rate with directed effort and practice, the basic limitation is the rate at which they can "think about" the information presented in the text material. An important factor affecting both reading rate and comprehension is familiarity with basic science and clinical terminology. To meet this need, a number of summer programs include a self-instructional course in medical terminology. A major problem in addressing reading skills as a separate area of study occurs when the teaching is done .by reading specialists who are not familiar with the medical curriculum and who do not adapt their methods, attitudes, and materials to the needs of medical students. Even though the application of speed reading to medical texts may be limited, some students find the skill is worthwhile for recreational reading.

Schedules for Programs. One difficult aspect of planning summer programs is establishing a daily schedule that is not beyond the abilities of students to complete assignments at the beginning, but increases in pace so that students can develop their own ways of adapting to the pace of the first year. Except for those few medical schools that offer courses on a self-instructional basis, most first-year schedules include 30 to 35 hours of lectures and laboratories each week. If full participation in all scheduled activities is required, students will find a summer program on a similar schedule an exhausting experience. Therefore, such a program should end early enough in the summer to allow participants a few weeks in which to recover so that they can return with as much energy for the fall semester as those students who did not participate in the program.

Another area for careful consideration in planning summer programs is estimating the time students will require to cover each topic. When student coverage is slower than expected, a key question is whether students' efforts are adequate or expectations for them are excessive. On the other hand, when student coverage is more rapid than expected, back-up assignments need to be ready to use. This type of planning removes pressure from program personnel to maintain original schedules which may turn out to be inappropriate for a particular group of students.

Grading and Evaluating Student Performance. Some schools use the successful completion of a summer program as a basis for conditional admission. This procedure will pose a problem if the criteria for such conditional admissions are not applied consistently in requiring attendance. Otherwise, only those students who participate will run the risk of *not* being admitted on the basis of unsatisfactory performance. It is generally easier for program personnel to remain objective in assigning grades and making evaluations of student performance if they are not aware of the conditional admission status of participants. Frequent grading throughout a program is not only necessary for assessing conditional admissions, but also useful in helping students to develop a more realistic self-appraisal of their academic performance, and to seek appropriate support services should they need them during the regular school year.

Financial Resources. Summer programs require substantial financial support, although the level of support depends on which components are funded by the school. Costs to be considered include salaries for faculty and staff, consultant honoraria, and wages for medical and graduate student tutors; student travel, stripends, room and board; materials and supplies, and other costs related to the administration of the program. In addition to outside grant/contract funding, some costs may be offset by tuition, scholarships or fellowships, and financial aid. It is usually considered better to have a program for entering students, even though limited to students who can pay some or all of their own expenses, than to have no program at all. In order to establish eligibility for financial aid, some schools define their summer program participants as regular medical students by giving elective course credit for the program.

Unstable funding of basic program components can pose a serious logistics program. For example, the number of potential participants may be reduced when program announcements are delayed pending funding of program personnel. Moreover, stability in funding salaries and wages will significantly reduce the stress frequently associated with administration of academic support services for pre-enrolled students.

Types of Services and Programs

1. Reinforcement of Prerequisites

The primary function of this type of summer program is to reinforce prerequisite knowledge and skills. Although the focus is on knowledge and skills typically taught in the undergraduate curriculum, applications should be made to problems likely to be encountered in the medical curriculum. For example, mathematics skills can be applied to biochemistry problems, and communications skills can be applied to describing gross anatomy structures and histology slides. Student activities might include taking diagnostic tests, using self-instructional materials, attending lectures, completing independent reading assignments, preparing reports, working with tutors, taking frequent quizzes and using results to improve performance. The teaching staff should be drawn from among persons who are familiar with the undergraduate curriculum, including undergraduate faculty and graduate teaching assistants.

2. *Preview of the First-Year Curriculum*

The primary function of this type of summer program is to lighten the academic load during the first year by covering selected topics during the summer. Although students may participate in similar types of activities as in a program based on prerequisite information, the content should focus on the first-year medical curriculum and the teaching staff should be drawn from among those who are familiar with first year courses. Medical students who have just completed their freshman year and graduate students who have taken courses with medical students are more likely to be available to teach than medical faculty who usually are busy with research during the summer. However, it is important to foster faculty consultations with student tutors. Most entering students are better prepared for learning from lectures and textbooks than from gross and microscopic laboratory work. For that reason, laboratory facilities need to be obtained to help prepare students for learning in those facilities.

3. *Medical Course for Credit*

The primary function of this type of summer program is to lighten the academic load during the first year by teaching a freshman course during the summer. One of the courses most frequently taught is gross anatomy. All aspects of the course should be comparable to the course as it is taught during the regular academic year, including the faculty. Four potential problems that may arise when courses are offered for credit include: (a) Pace—the effect of intensive coverage of an entire course during the summer. (b) Isolation—see Chapter 19 for a discussion of the potential for, and possible effects of, isolation on students who are identified as participants because they are not enrolled in all freshman courses. (c) Grades—it is difficult to assign test scores and course grades that are comparable to those assigned to other members of the class during the academic year. (d) Failure—although the overall course load should be lighter for students who must repeat the course during the academic year, students may find the course boring and/or underestimate the amount of work they must do to complete the repeated course successfully.

4. Learning Skills for a Medical Curriculum

The primary function of this type of summer program is to help students to become more effective in meeting the academic requirements of a medical curriculum. Learning skills are transferable from one course to another and should allow students to become more independent in all learning activities.

Four types of learning problems that students frequently encounter with learning skills include: (a) studying information covered in an examination but performing poorly on the examination in spite of their effort; (b) performing relatively well on an examination, but not recalling the information shortly afterwards; (c) knowing information covered on an examination, but performing poorly because they are confused by the formats of the test items; and (d) failing to find enough time for those activities that are necessary for good academic performance. Learning skills which may be combined to overcome such problems deal with reading textbooks, lecture notetaking, organizing information, memorizing, exam-taking, and time management. Materials should be appropriate for medical students both in style and examples and provide structured presentation and practice of skills with frequent feedback on how to improve performance. Practice assignments need to be made on textbook passages, video-tape lectures, released examination items, and syllabus and handout materials from recent medical courses.

One of the most effective ways to present the learning skills is during a three-day workshop at the beginning of the program, with frequent follow-up to provide suggestions on an individual basis for further development of the skills. Persons who work directly with students on learning skills should receive both training in the specific skills and an intensive orientation to the nature of a medical school, its curriculum, students, and faculty.

5. *Workshop on Learning Skills*

The primary function of this type of service, usually scheduled during orientation week, is essentially the same as for summer programs based on learning skills. Although the goals are more modest due to the limited time, the effectiveness can be enhanced by the availability of trained persons to assist students in further development of skills during the academic year. The entire entering freshman class should be invited to participate on a voluntary basis as part of the routine services offered by the medical school. The materials need to be very structured to allow rapid, systematic presentation with feedback and examples of applications to first-year courses. Workshop activities must include limited opportunities for practice in order to avoid the less effective process of a "spectator sport." Scheduling a skills workshop over a three-day period, with no competing orientation activities, seems to be adequate to cover most skills. The question of effectiveness of a workshop arises often enough to warrant a comment. Student reactions regarding effectiveness tend to fall into three categories: (a) "Ahha, so that's what I've been doing," which serves to be reinforcing; (b) "Oh, I think I'll try that," which opens up another option for study; and (c) "I don't think I need to do that," which may be followed up later, if the student experiences academic difficulty, by a request for help in developing skills.

Services for Enrolled Students

Although the services are described separately, two or more types of services can be combined into a coordinated program of academic support, and have the following features in common.

Purpose of Services. In general terms, the purpose of academic support services for enrolled students is to help students assume responsibility for their own learning, facilitate that learning, but avoid dependency on the services or personnel as a permanent crutch. Frequently persons directly involved in support services are tempted to make value judgments about which students do not have the potential to become physicians and to reflect that judgment, although perhaps unintentionally, to students. Experienced personnel overcome this temptation by adopting the attitude that each student who is admitted to a college of medicine is expected to graduate, and that the function of support services is to assure that each student will fulfill such an expectation.

Selection of participants. As with pre-enrolled students, those students who are enrolled and appear in need of academic support services are more likely to make appropriate use of available services if there is no stigma or isolation connected with participation.

Components (Materials, Activities, Schedules). Medical students who experience academic difficulty usually feel that they do not have enough time to do what is necessary to meet course requirements. Therefore, all components of services provided directly to students during the academic year must help students to meet their immediate course requirements. The effectiveness of all academic support services will be enhanced by integrating the services, as much as possible, into the ongoing curriculum.

Resource requirements. A few of the services described in this section can be implemented with no additional funding, training, personnel or space—the major requirement being the desire or commitment of personnel in place to provide academic support for students. For other services, student participation may be affected by the way in which services are funded. As with programs for pre-enrolled students, medical schools can cover the cost of services for students selected on the basis of academic and financial needs when resources are limited.

Types of Services and Programs

1. Curriculum Adjustment

The reason for adjusting the curriculum is to lighten the academic load during the basic science years, thereby improving student academic performance and retention. Curriculum adjustment is usually accomplished by omitting electives and/or rescheduling the two years of preclinical courses over a three-year period. Questions which have been raised about this type of program include: (a) Should participation be voluntary or a condition of admission? (b) How great is the risk of isolation and stigmatization? (c) How might the loss of identity with one's entering class affect participants?

These and other questions pertaining to curriculum adjustment are discussed in Chapter 19.

2. *Notetaking Service*

Two functions of this type of service are: (a) to assure students of a complete and accurate reference regarding the information presented in lecture, and (b) to provide models of good notes for students who need to develop skill in this area. Participation depends, in part, on the way the service is funded. For example, with full funding by the medical school, copies may be distributed to all students; with partial funding, a limited number of copies may be placed on reserve in a library; with no funding, students who want the service must pay for it, although costs may be covered for some students on the basis of academic or financial need. Lecture notes, usually taken by students, should be distributed within 24 hours to be of most value. The quality of lecture notes seems to improve when the notetaker is identified on each copy. Some of the better services have considerable student involvement. However, two problems may occur when students are involved: (a) there may be a delay each year in initiating the service while the class decides how to manage the service, and (b) students may spend too much time on notetaking at the expense of their regular academic responsibilities. Ways of dealing with these problems include encouraging students to organize the service during orientation, and then monitoring their academic performance during the school year. Faculty often express concern that students will use the note service as a substitute for attending lectures. Since so little is known about the relative effectiveness of auditory or visual presentations for learning in individual students, a reasonable assumption is that all students should be expected to attend all regularly scheduled lectures and laboratories.

3. *Tutorial Service*

The function of this type of service is to provide personal assistance to help students understand topics which they find difficult. Students may be self-referred or referred by faculty, other students, or other medical school personnel. Tutorial service in preclinical courses may be provided by medical students, graduate teaching assistants, or basic science faculty. When medical students are chosen to tutor, two methods of selection which have been used successfully are: (a) students identify the person whom they prefer for tutoring, and/or (b) medical school personnel select and assign tutors.

When students provide tutorial service, three potential problems and related precautions need to be kept in mind. First, a tutor's personality may interfere with the ability to be helpful to students who are under academic pressure. Therefore, tutors should be selected not only on the basis of academic competence (no failed courses a minimum), but also on the basis of personality characteristics appropriate for the helping role of a tutor. Second, a tutor may inadvertently encourage the dependency of students rather than encourage them to become independent learners. For this reason, all tutors should participate in an orientation to tutoring and report regularly, though informally, on their work with students to the faculty or staff member who supervises the tutorial program. Third, the more enthusiastic tutors may spend too much time tutoring at the expense of their own academic responsibilities (although sophomore tutors may use their tutoring as one way of reviewing first-year courses in preparation for the National Board Examination, Part I). To deal with this problem, the academic performance of all tutors should be monitored so that they do not jeopardize their own academic record.

Tutors should have access to current course schedules, textbooks, syllabi, released examinations, and a copier for sharing materials. One factor which undoubtedly contributes to the relative success of one-on-one tutoring over group tutorials is the very limited amount of free time in the typical medical curriculum. Students frequently find that a large portion of this limited time spent in group tutorials may be "wasted" on discussions of topics which are too simple or too complex to meet their individual needs.

4. *Academic Monitoring Service*

The function of this service is to identify students who are experiencing academic difficulty early enough to take some kind of action that will improve their current performance. This service is the key to the effectiveness of any other services that can be improved by early identification of potential problems. In turn, the ultimate value of a monitoring service is dependent upon other institutional resources that may be helpful, directly or indirectly, in improving academic performance. Because predictions of student success and failure in courses are seldom 100 percent correct, a basic monitoring service is valuable for all students. Such a service can be useful, not only in tracking academic performance of individual students, but also in establishing an audit trail for assessing the effectiveness of subsequent action.

A monitoring service can be carried out by any responsible faculty or staff member who is permitted to have access to student scores and grades. Early access to scores and grades through department representatives or central scoring records can speed up the process of identifying students who are experiencing academic difficulty and make recommendations for immediate action.

5. *Academic Counseling Service*

The functions of this service are to help students (a) identify problems contributing to poor academic performance, (b) apply appropriate resources for corrective or supportive action, and ultimately (c) improve academic performance. Students may be identified through an academic monitoring service, other referrals, or self-referral. To avoid stigmatizing this service, it should be available to all students who wish to improve their academic performance regardless of whether attrition is threatened. In order to bring about changes in student behavior that will result in improved performance, academic counselors have found the following principles to be especially useful. First, emphasize action that changes behavior to improve performance and curtail or minimize discussions which may unduly delay constructive changes. Second, coordinate contacts with students to prevent students from (a) feeling overwhelmed by contacts from too many persons or (b) failing to solve problems by not making any changes suggested by different personnel. Third, require students to accept responsibility for their own learning by choosing which changes they will undertake in order to improve their own academic performance.

6. *Learning Skills in a Medical Curriculum*

The function of this service is essentially the same as for preenrolled students; differences occur in accommodating time constraints imposed by the curriculum. One of the first activities in implementing a learning skills service is to avoid stigmatization by announcing, during orientation week, that it is available for all students as one of several services provided by the school. Sessions on learning skills can be held as weekly seminars for interested groups of students or as weekly appointments for individual students. The more free time students have, the more appointments a skills counselor can make each week. When more students request individual appointments than can be scheduled, appointments can be made according to the priorities of the medical school regarding academic needs. Although some skills such as memorizing and exam-taking lend themselves to group sessions, students who continue to experience difficulty will benefit from individual sessions in which a skills counselor will assess the student's skills and provide an opportunity for controlled practice during the session.

7. Re-examinations to Remove Deficiencies

The function of this type of program is to provide a means of removing deficiencies so that students can be promoted with members of their entering class. Two scheduling requirements that have to be met for successful use of re-examinations are: (a) re-examinations should not compete with student responsibilities in other courses, and (b) time should be made available for additional study prior to the re-examination.

8. Directed Review for Re-examinations

The function of this type of program is to help students to prepare for re-examinations to remove deficiencies. Some schools find that student performance does not improve significantly on re-examinations; a directed review program during the summer is one way of improving that performance. The key to the credibility of the program is the extent to which the re-examinations are comparable to examinations administered during the regular school year. All review materials and tutorial activities must be closely coordinated with the re-examinations. If medical or graduate students are employed as tutors for the review sessions, faculty should be responsible for close supervision of the content presented in the review sessions.

9. *Repeating or Substituting Courses to Remove Deficiencies*

Perhaps the most common means of removing deficiencies is through repeating selected courses, substituting summer school courses,* and repeating an entire year's curriculum. Students who substitute courses frequently need assistance in planning how to maintain their financial aid status, meet additional costs, and assess the comparability of courses.

10. *Preparing for Licensure Examinations*

Preparation for licensure examinations becomes important for retention only in schools which require the passing of licensure examinations for promotion and/or graduation. Methods of preparing for licensure examinations are described in Chapter 9.

CONCLUSION

This chapter has presented a variety of student academic support services and programs used by medical schools to improve the academic performance, retention, and ultimate licensure of their students, including minority students. This information should be of value in meeting the goals of the 1978 Report of the AAMC Task Force on Minority Student Opportunities in Medicine,[16] for one of its six major goals is to "strengthen programs which support the normal progress and successful graduation of racial minority students enrolled in medical schools."

Recently, the pool of applicants to medical school has started to decrease.[17] If this recent decrease becomes a trend, then, on the basis of past trends, the rate of student retention also can be expected to decrease in the 1980s. In that event, more medical schools may turn to formal student academic support services and programs to counteract student attrition.

---

* For a listing of summer school courses, see "Medical School Summer Makeup Courses" which is published annually by the AAMC Division of Student Programs. It is distributed each spring to medical school dean's offices and also is available on request from the AAMC.

REFERENCES

1. Johnson, D. G., and Hutchins, E. B.: Doctor or Dropout? A Study of Medical Student Attrition. *J. Med. Educ.*, 41:1099-1269, 1966.
2. Johnson, D. G., and Sedlacek, W. E.: Retention by Sex and Race of 1968-1972 U.S. Medical School Entrants. *J. Med. Educ.*, 50:925-933, 1975.
3. Quality and Equality, New Levels of Federal Responsibility for Higher Education (A Special Report and Recommendations of the Carnegie Commission on Higher Education, December 1968).
4. Higher Education and the Nation's Health: Policies for Medical and Dental Education (A Special Report and Recommendations by the Carnegie Commission on Higher Education, October 1970).
5. Curtis, J. L.: *Blacks, Medical Schools and Society.* Ann Arbor: University of Michigan Press, 1971.
6. Evaluation in the Continuum of Medical Education: Report of the Committee on Goals and Priorities of the National Board of Medical Examiners, June 1973.
7. Medical Licensure Statistics for 1964. J.A.M.A. 192:855-904, 1965.
8. A Bicentennial Anniversary Program for the Expansion of Medical Education: Report of the AAMC Committee on the Expansion of Medical Education. *J. Med. Educ.*, 46:105-116, 1971.
9. Nelson, B. W., Bird, R. A., and Rogers, G. M.: Expanding Educational Opportunities in Medicine for Blacks and Other Minority Students. *J. Med. Educ.*, 45:731-736, 1970.
10. Odegaard, C. E.: *Minorities in Medicine: From Receptive Passivity to Positive Action, 1966-76.* New York: Josiah Macy, Jr., Foundation, 1977.
11. Johnson, D. G.: OEO-AAMC Grant (Editorial). *J. Med. Educ.*, 44:1082-1083, 1969.
12. Johnson, D. G., Smith, V. C., Jr., and Tarnoff, S. L.: Recruitment and Progress of Minority Medical School Entrants, 1970-72: A Cooperative Study by the SNMA and the AAMC. *J. Med. Educ.*, 50:711-755, 1975.
13. Nelson, B. W., Bird, R. A., and Rodgers, G. M.: Educational Pathway Analysis for the Study of Minority Representation in Medical School. *J. Med. Educ.*, 46:745-749, 1971.
14. Minority Student Opportunities in United States Medical Schools, 1978-79. Washington, D.C.: Association of American Medical Colleges, 1977.
15. AAMC Curriculum Directory, 1978-79. Washington, D.C.: Association of American Medical Colleges, 1978.
16. Report of the Association of American Medical Colleges Task Force on Minority Student Opportunities. Washington, D. C.: Association of American Medical Colleges, 1978.
17. Medical School Admission Requirements, 1979-80. Washington, D. C.: Association of American Medical Colleges, 1978.

CHAPTER 20

Accelerated and Extended Programs

Eleanor L. Ison-Franklin

INTRODUCTION

Tutorials, reinforcement programs and similarly titled activities at U.S. medical schools are recent additions to teaching responsibilities. Their advent is in large part a response to the increased enrollment of minority students during the past two decades. The basis for this is not the minority student per se, but in the fact that most medical schools, with the exceptions of Howard and Meharry, had little experience in the recruitment and admission of minorities. In an attempt to admit reasonable numbers, medical schools were immediately faced with the products of poor and inadequate educational systems in which the majority of minority applicants had been trained. Federal incentives allowed little time for the inexperienced schools to gather better data for their decision-making. As a consequence, schools admitted a disproportionate number of these students with credentials below those historically regarded as acceptable for entry. It is not unexpected, therefore, that medical educators would tend to identify, as causally related, a need for

Eleanor L. Ison-Franklin, Ph.D., is Professor of Physiology and Associate Dean for Academic Affairs, College of Medicine, Howard University, Washington, D.C.

certain non-traditional aspects of the teaching programs with the increase in numbers of non-traditional medical students.

With the passing of time, certain generalities were drawn to the extent that practically all minority students were believed to be in need of special remediation if they were to be successful medical students. Individual test scores and premedical data, of course, deny this generality. Clearly, not all minority students need special treatment.

Curriculum alternatives in medical education in the United States have appeared in a variety of forms over the past twenty years. Major modifications were stimulated in response to both internal and external challenges to the standard curriculum sequence and content. The milieu which permitted the evolution of these alternate programs will be briefly described since these factors have influenced both form and content. On the whole, these were not developed with the minority student in mind. A characterization of the general types of alternate curricula will also be made as a point of departure toward a discussion of features in honors and accelerated programs involving minority students.

The objectives of this chapter, in summary therefore, are:

1. To alert the medical educator to the need for distinguishing those minority students who do not require remediation from those who do;

2. To describe the aggregate of socio-professional forces which influenced the revisionary process in medical education;

3. To describe the three general categories of alternate curricula in medical schools; and

4. To identify those features in the planning and management of honors, accelerated and dual-training extended programs which are facilitating to the typical student whose educational preparation was gained at a predominantly minority school.

EFFECTS OF GENERALIZING PRESUMPTIONS

Because of the widely publicized differences in average quantitative admissions data between minorities and the typical White male applicant to medical school, a number of schools have set in place entire administrative structures and academic programs exclusively to serve the minority student. These efforts to provide beneficent support systems for the academically disadvantaged student have been very important in bridging the gaps in premedical preparation. At the same time, they have introduced a new stigma or exclusionary atmosphere in which the minority medical student perceives himself or herself to be "different" from, or worse, "inferior" to the majority student. The presumption (or perceived expectation) that the minority medical student who neglects to take advantage of available special programs is doomed to failure is often a self-fulfilling prophecy. The key word here is "presumption." Implicitly, the only requirement for access to the special programs is that the student be a minority student. Too often only secondary consideration is given to the actual premedical credentials presented by the student upon admission. Generally ignored also is the successful performance by the student during the initial term in medical school since continued participation in the special programs is expected.

The point to be made here is that admission and monitoring processes should aim toward early identification of the minority student who can be expected to matriculate successfully. This prerequisite step is the first to be taken in designing alternate medical curricula with the minority student in mind.

FACTORS INFLUENCING CURRICULUM CHANGES IN U.S. MEDICAL SCHOOLS

Beginning in the 1950's, medical education was to experience a period of high drama when Case Western Reserve introduced a totally interdisciplinary professional educational program. Close onto this daring departure from the traditional lock-stepped, four-year sequence, Jefferson Medical School implemented its abbreviated curriculum. As might be expected, reaction to these initiatives was varied. The conservatives were gravely doubtful of the wisdom of these innovations (without benefit of supporting data, it should be added). At the other end, medical educators with adventurous spirits were stimulated to try varying degrees of curriculum modifications at their institutions. Newly formed medical schools were liberated from the need to demonstrate their stability and credibility through standard educational programs and created entirely new types of educational organizations.

The environments within and without the academic medical

community were to contribute significantly to the flux which began in those earlier years and continues today. The elements of the major influences described here will also characterize the period during which minority enrollments increased in medical schools, even though those increases were not considered in the plans for curricular modifications.

Questions were raised within academic medicine by both faculty and students as to the "need," "relevancy," and "appropriateness" of the educational scope of courses for the practice of medicine. As well, questions were raised as to the effectiveness of pedagogy or modes of teaching in medical schools. These stirrings from within medical schools resulted in partial or entire changes from territorial disciplinary control to interdisciplinary teaching formats. The use of student-operated teaching equipment, self-instructional materials, computerized courses and testing were to become more and more commonplace (although not without serious misgivings amongst medical school faculties).

Federal support programs have been the strongest external influence on curricular changes. Among these were incentives for abbreviating the undergraduate medical training period (as one approach to reducing the cost of medical education); for increasing the numbers of physicians trained per year, although more recently for improving physician distribution and primary care specialty choices; and for increasing the representation of minorities in the physician manpower pool.

Of the external factors, it is perhaps the focus on minorities that has spawned the broadest range of complex introspections and modifications in academic medicine. Heightened concern for reevaluation of admissions criteria and test scores as indices of potential success in medical school *vis-a-vis* the practice of medicine lay at one end of the spectrum effecting change. At the other end lay the concern for artificial barriers to specialty choices, postgraduate education, and practice patterns which are believed to restrict maximal participation on the part of minorities. In between were the multiple concerns for student retention, optional curriculum sequences, quality control of the educational product, financial aid, public access to medical care, and the like. All of these have been compounded by the recognition also that inconsistent attention is given to subjects such as genetics, nutrition, geriatrics, interpersonal and interprofessional roles and relationships, health care cost containment, and the legal-ethical issues raised as a consequence of advancing medical technology and research.

It is the Brownian movement of these societal and professional particles which seeks to equilibrate into a new level of educational creativity in medicine. The human element involves the expansion of the educational boundaries to include those groups which until now, have been generally excluded.

EXTANT CURRICULUM ALTERNATIVES

There are two general categories of alternative medical school curricula which have evolved in addition to the *traditional* four-year sequence: the *accelerated programs*, and the *extended programs*. In some instances more than one option is available at a single medical school. In others the alternative curriculum has, at least for a time, supplanted the more traditional form. Some of the characteristics of each of these are briefly presented here.

Traditional Curriculum. The general format of the traditional curriculum as defined here is a four-year program during which the preclinical basic sciences dominate the first two years of instruction followed by two years of primary clinical training. The large majority of medical schools adhere to this general format as their basic curriculum even though innovations of interdisciplinary courses, clinical correlations with early clinical experiences in the first two years, and elective opportunities appear in varying degrees from institution to institution. Except for elective options, all students at a given level are required to take the same group of courses and examinations, including in some instances, the National Board Medical Examinations. For the most part, courses tend to be discipline-oriented although several schools have significantly softened disciplinary demarcations by the use of modular and computer-assisted instruction. The primary feature, therefore, of the traditional curriculum is its four-year duration (36 to 38 months of instruction), of prescribed courses for students at each level with focus on basic science disciplines followed by clinical science disciplines.

Accelerated Curricula. The basic principle of the accelerated curriculum involves either earlier entrance into the professional program (abbreviation of premedical training), earlier exit from the professional program (abbreviation of medical school curriculum), or a combination of these. The students who enter these programs are highly selected by faculty committees in most instances, although in the Howard University experience they are self-selected. This will be described further under Special Comments toward the end of this chapter.

Shortening of the educational process has been accomplished by one or more of the following: (a) reduction in length or elimination of certain courses considered to be nonessential from the traditional sequence, (b) telescoping of the traditional sequence by use of summer teaching primarily in the premedical and/or preclinical courses, (c) installation of multiple self-tutorial courses and/or computer-monitored unit instruction, and (d) specially designed shortened curricula which are offered instead of or run concurrently with traditional programs where more than one curricular option is available.

No attempt will be made here to discuss in detail the different forms of curriculum attenuation which exist. There appears to be a persistent resistance to the concept on the part of portions of medical faculties, however, despite the overall successes of the large majority of students completing such programs. The experiences of medical schools which have attempted such programs have essentially benefitted the faculties in their ability to consider more flexibility in curriculum planning. Most shortened programs range from 30 to 35 months of instruction.

A distinction between the accelerated program and an "honors" program is appropriate here. The title "honors" program is more likely to be applied where the student negotiates a large portion of the content mastery independently from the usual faculty controlled classroom. Learning under this condition may occur in any of the three forms of curriculum described in this section. The title "accelerated" or "shortened" program is more likely to indicate a somewhat structured, faculty-supervised learning situation. If it is both shortened and studied at an independent rate by the student, it should then be titled an "honors accelerated program."

Extended Curriculum. As the title implies, the schedule for this sequence allows for a period of up to 50 months of matriculation for the professional program. One form of the extended curriculum is based on the "reduced load" concept in which the medical student pursues the same courses as in the traditional or basic curriculum, but somewhat fewer courses within a given term, thus requiring longer to navigate the total. No other requirement is placed upon the student in this type of extended program. The reduced load programs in most instances have been specifically created for minority students. While the availability of a part-time medical education program should be viewed as a potential advantage for students who must work to pay for their education, or for students who need special schedule flexibility in order to accommodate family responsibilities, it has to some extent provided an opportunity for minority students who otherwise might not have had access to a medical education.

A second form of the extended medical curriculum is one designed to allow the student to pursue simultaneously the M.D. degree and research or other health-related training. These are usually combined degree programs with the second degree or special training opportunities in biomedical research, public health, health administration, behavioral science and similar complementary pursuits more related to the students' career plans. In instances where no formal sequence is in place, many medical schools have accommodated such career aspirants on an individual basis. The efficiency of this curriculum is that the total time for achieving the combined training is markedly reduced despite the longer period spent leading to the professional degree.

PLANNING CURRICULAR OPTIONS WITH THE MINORITY STUDENT IN MIND

Perhaps the most important outgrowth of the recent activity in medical education is the challenge to the imagination for designing curricula for a more heterogeneous student population than previously enjoyed by medical school faculties. A common planning error in schools where more than one program is in place is the resultant partitioning of student groups along racial, ethnic and/or economic lines. While this may be unavoidable in some instances, the program options should provide clear opportunities for movement across the partitions. At the least, each student should have the assurance that the options are available to him or her.

Aside from the feature of accessibility of the alternate curriculum, certain other features of the programs are more facilitating for minority students than are others. It ought to be recognized that a major resource of the Black applicant pool, for instance, continues to be the traditionally Black colleges, although this situation is rapidly shifting. Similarly, other minority groups characteristically come from specific regions of the country. In the majority of their premedical experiences, college programs have been carefully structured with well defined expectations and sequencing of the premedical education. Preprofessional counseling serves to reinforce the stipulated prerequisite preparation announced by medical schools. The minority student (as well as the majority student) who comes with such experiences is likely to function more comfortably in a somewhat structured medical curriculum than in one in which he or she is expected to study independently.

In this regard, the following are particularly recommended.

Statement on Eligibility and Program Requirements. A clear description of the criteria on which eligibility for the alternate program is based should be available to all students. If these are not different from the criteria for the regular curriculum, it should be stated as such. Where there are both advantages and disadvantages to the student, the description should include these (e.g., cost savings versus loss of opportunity to take electives). Information regarding schedule and time period differences among the available curriculum choices will be important to making practical decisions on the part of the student.

The student should know who besides himself will participate in the decision on whether or not he meets all eligibility requirements. Implicit in this suggestion is the prerogative of the student to accept or reject the optional course although final authority in the admission process must be retained by the appropriate faculty committees and deans.

Statement of Performance Expectations. Consistent with the value of the structured alternative program is the need for a statement of expected performance levels on the part of the student. Faculty and curriculum managers should carefully define expected outcomes based on the program purpose, and establish student performance objectives in relation to these. Achievement of the objectives should be staged such that they coincide with fixed time periods. Thus, the student is made aware of *what* is to be accomplished by him as well as *how much time* is allotted for each phase. The methods by which they will be evaluated are usually of major concern among medical students. This is all the more true for most minority students. Of special concern are the judgmental evaluations characteristically made during the clinical training. The quality of expected performance *and* interpersonal interaction codes should not be presumed to be known by the student.

Statement on Student Advancement. Where practicable, designated steps in the program should be identified as points at which the student will be "promoted" to the next stage. In the standard four-year program, these are usually at the end of a term and/or of the academic year. Such points are not easily identified in the accelerated or extended curricula because of their irregular time blocs. More important than the actual selection of such end-stages is the need on the part of the student to receive frequent advice with respect to progress. The occurrence of such intervals is important also to faculty as a means of assessing the group progress for all such students pursuing the same phase of the curriculum. The consequences of failure to fulfill performance expectations or of student withdrawal from the program must be included in the planning. Furthermore, the student should be apprised of these prior to any final decisions regarding entry into the program. In schools which offer more than one optional curriculum, it is prudent to publish a single document on conditions for advancement which includes those established for all available curricula. In this way, all students and all faculty will have easy access to the policy. In a later portion of this chapter, publishing of a single policy statement for purposes of promotion will be shown to have additional advantages.

Role of the Student in Planning and Evaluation. There is significant value to be gained from the student's perspective during the curriculum planning process. While it may necessarily be narrower in terms of the essentials of course content, it is invariably broad in reflecting student response to the performance expectations, time periods, and consequences of failure or withdrawal. To a great extent student proposals are useful in the temporizing and refinement of faculty goals with respect to curriculum. The more heterogeneity of student involvement in the planning process, the more likely the suitability of the curricula to the needs of the student population. These are not, however, intended to be met at the expense of program quality. The optional nature of the curricula suggests only that there is program flexibility and that the different alternatives can be designed to achieve the same professional product. The student's choice of program (or of a school offering such choices) will in part be influenced by his or her career plans as much as by any personal preferences.

IDENTIFICATION AND SELECTION
OF THE STUDENT

The process of selection of students, especially for accelerated programs, has taken two forms: one in which the student is preselected by the admissions committee prior to matriculation, and the second in which the student is admitted following a specified period of matriculation. For the most part, particularly during the earlier years, the decision as to which student should go into the accelerated program was initiated by faculty. The criteria were based principally upon high preadmission test scores and college grades. As a result, minority students were almost entirely excluded from participation in these programs. In part, this was due to the lack of minority selection experience within the admitting committees. In part, too, in the planning process, faculty foresaw the accelerated programs as somewhat elitist and thereby excluded the majority of the student body.

The inability of educators and psychometrists to ascribe quantifiable attributes to certain noncognitive characteristics (reliability, motivation, resourcefulness, competitiveness, self-esteem) is a recognized failing in the assembling of preadmission data. The personal applicant interview continues to provide the only clues to these personality traits, and it is admittedly unreliable in its success rate.

These two factors—faculty selection on the basis of high preadmission scores and unreliable indices of noncognitive traits—have served to frustrate minority student access to special medical curricula.

Self-selection by the student appears to be a reasonably successful method of identifying minority student prospects. The success, of course, is dependent upon whether the criteria for eligibility are clearly understood and whether the performance expectations are well defined. The success will also be affected by the time at which the student enters the program. The Howard shortened medical program admits students only after the completion of the first year. During the first year, both faculty and students are able to assess the capability of the student to enter the program. The noncognitive elements involved in the decision-making process are reflected in the individual student's initiative and interest. With increasing experience and opportunity to observe the student, the faculty committee is better able to predict probable success of the student. An important feature not to be overlooked is the fact that the student takes the first step in applying for the accelerated (or extended) program. Faculty response to this initiative is guided by the criteria of eligibility which were established in the plan of the program.

The selection process must be related to the purpose of the program. The question should be answered regarding whether the shortened curriculum, for example, is designed as an "honors track" or as an option for early completion of the medical education. It may be the decision of the faculty that it is both. However, it may be either one or the other. The obvious distinction between the two is the limiting criteria of eligibility. If the second instance is the aim of the program, i.e., shortening of the training period, then a set of minimal academic criteria, available finances, age, previous professional training and other factors might play a role in the selection of students. If the program is designed as an honors program, then academic credentials will very likely be the determinant in the selection. For extended programs (not for remedial support), the purpose of the program should also be linked to the selection process. To a large extent, justification for acceptance into a dual-training experience should rest with the student, although approval authority remains a faculty responsibility.

The fundamental principle to be recognized in the selection process is the quasi-contractual agreement into which the student and the medical school enter. On the one hand the student agrees to fulfill the aims of the program and to maintain acceptable performance and reporting standards. On the other hand, the faculty agrees to objectively assess the suitability of the student for the requested program, to provide counselling and instruction, and to introduce whatever support systems that will facilitate the matriculant.

INTEGRATION OF MULTIPLE CURRICULA

An ideal arrangement in a total medical education program is one which offers more than one option to students. One of the first concerns which faculties must resolve is the matter of cost effectiveness of such a venture and the efficient management of time for the teaching faculty. Concurrent parallel programs are both expensive and time-consuming. The process of program design should include identification of courses and clerkship entities which can be shared simultaneously by students from the several programs. This will involve not only the distribution of instructional assignments, but also classroom space requirements, availability and diversity of clinical teaching material, and sophistication of student support systems (academic counselling, financial aid, on-call hospital facilities, and the like).

The interaction of students between multiple programs within a common instructional setting is perhaps the major benefit to be gained as a result of these considerations. This additional spin-off is usually an unexpected value from intentional interlocks between curricula while resolving the concerns for economic and manpower efficiency. Complementary degree programs (leading also to the M.P.H., M.B.A., and Ph.D. degrees) which are available in extended medical curricula add a special dimension to student interactional benefits. In the course of the resulting distribution of students having diverse interests, abilities and experiences, a substantial amount of peer instruction and stimulation seems to occur which frequently is absent in the locked-step programs such as the traditional or parallel sequences. These latter forms of the curriculum tend to group students somewhat in isolation from other groups.

A specific example of the type of interlock referred to here is as follows: A shortened program may involve a year in which the second year students take basic science courses with traditional second year students for one part of the year and clinical clerkships with traditional third year students for the other part of the year. If the sequencing of the accelerated program is such that the clinical experience precedes certain basic science courses, the traditional second-year students will invariably benefit from the hands-on experience and applicability of the basic sciences to clinical situations already gained by the accelerated students. Similarly, the traditional third year students can impart benefits to the accelerated students during the clinical clerkship phase of the year. If at the same time, dual-degree students in clinical pharmacology are simultaneously enrolled in either the basic science or clinical clerkships or both, considerable mutually beneficial exchange among the three categories of students will occur.

ORGANIZATION FOR STUDENT MONITORING IN MULTIPLE PROGRAMS

There are three levels of organization for optimum monitoring of student performance in multiple programs at a single institution. These are (a) the faculty and/or student advisor(s) (b) the faculty committee on academic review or student promotions, and (c) the administrative personnel (deans and administrative staff). At all levels, a thorough understanding of the features of the programs must be mutually shared by faculty and administrators. The minority student, like other medical students, may rely on one resource for information and guidance rather than selectively seeking help at each of the levels. It is therefore extremely important that any discrepancies in the information received be held at an absolute minimum. No single phenomenon can destroy the confidence in or commitment of the student to fulfillment of program requirements more than conflicting information.

The ability of the student to use institutional advisory resources in pursuing a given program will be determined on the basis of personal preference and easiness of access to these resources. Some students are infinitely more comfortable in using informal, one-on-one relationships such as those which are formed between the student and the advisor, who may be a faculty member or another student or one of each. In a variety of settings within this relationship, the student can seek at one time both personal and academic advice. Faculty interest and encouragement are often more easily supplied by individual faculty to individual students. With regard to minority students, there appears to be a preference to identify with individuals who can serve as resource persons for a variety of services. It is all the more crucial where this form of support system is available that the faculty (and student) advisors be appropriately oriented and thus can be most effective in carrying out these responsibilities. The most frequent hazard in these relationships is that of "dependency" of the student. This should be strongly cautioned against in the advisor orientation process. At best, there should be a cooperative understanding between the advisor and the faculty committee and administration.

The faculty committee on academic review (student promotions) is the body which acts to authorize the change of status of the student based on academic performance. In addition to the performance data reported, it is advisable that this committee receive any additional information which will aid in its decision. Non-academic factors are especially useful for the report of the committee's decision to the student. The advisory report may sometimes suggest that the student consider leaving the accelerated program for reasons other than academic. The judicious incorporation of personality or extenuative circumstances received from the advisor should be based entirely on whether the decision is of benefit to the student and to the program. The interaction between the faculty committee and the faculty advisor which is recommended here will reduce the likelihood of conflicting advice or guidance to the student. The existence of a published policy statement regarding program expectations and conditions will be reinforced by such cooperative support of the student.

As often as not, deans will be sought out by the student for guidance (academic deans, student affairs deans). The image of "final authority" with which deans tend to be invested represents a potential mediating agent between the conflicting actions of the faculty committee for academic review and those of the faculty advisor. The role of arbiter-judge is unavoidable in specific situations. However, care should be taken by the deans to minimize the opportunity for situations in which these two—the committee and the advisor—may become adversary in their roles.

To give a specific example, faculty advisors sometimes unconsciously begin to develop a sense of responsibility for their advisee's total welfare. They will regard the student's failures, sufferings, losses etc. as a failing on their part to adequately support the advisee. When the student's record is reviewed by the committee, such an "involved" advisor will feel compelled to act on behalf of the student as an advocate or champion. Quite obviously the result of such encounters serve neither the student nor the program needs. Variations on this form of interaction among the three levels of the student monitoring system can be anticipated whenever the guidelines are not clear.

From the foregoing, it can be seen that the three-tiered arrangement of the student monitoring system must be constituted as a team effort, organized to meet student needs (academic counselling, program guidance, progress review) through more than one channel. Coordination of this system should preferably be the responsibility of a dean but may be carried out by others. The interface between the student, advisor, and faculty committee would seem to require the perspective of a dean. The essential principles to be kept in mind in establishing the monitoring system are (a) the availability of the system to the student, (b) the availability of program performance expectations to the student and to all elements of the monitoring team, (c) the existence of a cooperative relationship among all levels of the monitoring system, and (d) the coordinating role of the dean(s).

OTHER CATEGORIES OF STUDENT SUPPORT REQUIREMENTS

More than in any of the other curricula, students in the accelerated or shortened medical programs will require special attention or special considerations in the following:

A. Early counselling in the selection of a *postgraduate training program*. The shortened program sequence will very likely require the student to begin planning for postgraduate training before he or she has been exposed to all of the clinical sciences. For the student whose specialty preference has not been decided, there is a natural reluctance to do so in the absence of this exploratory opportunity. All students, and especially accelerated students, should be apprised of the usefulness of the flexible PGY-1 programs and their applicability to requirements for categorical specialties. Such counselling should be coupled with either formal or informal discussions with residency program directors and/or recruiters in order to permit a thorough introduction to the panoply of program possibilities.

Basic ground rules to be followed in selecting a training program ought not to be avoided in the counselling process. Minority students tend to have somewhat limited experience or information regarding what to look for in selecting a residency training program (as do any students whose professional exposure is limited prior to coming to medical school). Some of the factors which may enter in making their choices are geographic region, preferred practice locations, spouse preferences, house staff salaries, quality of housing for house officers and the like. These are sometimes given equal weight with such factors as quality of the training program and training faculty, patient load and variety of available clinical material, opportunities to interact with trainees at other hospitals, house staff schedules, libraries, research activity, and similar attributes which will affect their professional growth and development. While the final selection of the postgraduate training program ultimately rests with the student, the decision should not be based on limited criteria and at least a knowledge of those factors which *should* go into his or her decision-making.

Of special importance is the interview. It is interesting that premedical advisors are far more active in preparing the applicant for the premedical interview than are medical school officers in preparing the medical student for the residency interview. No intention is meant here to suggest that medical students should be coached. At this stage of their training they should be adequately prepared academically should such clinical testing be used in the applicant evaluation process. In addition to the test of medical knowledge, judgment and application, other characteristics which enter into the subjective evaluation of the person should be pointed out—especially to those students who tend to neglect these in their day-to-day preoccupation with clerkship duties.

B. The *Dean's Letter,* notably in institutions with more than one medical education program, should not overlook the need to provide an assurance comment regarding the adequacy of the non-traditional program. The suggestion here is perhaps simplistic. On the other hand, the medical school may feel that, on the face of it, such statements will tend to "beg the question." The reason for making this point is twofold: the statement allays any questions which may come to the mind of the reader who, otherwise, will mentally diminish the student's competitiveness in the first place; and in the second place, it should be assumed that the specific residency program director (or director of postgraduate medical education of the hospital) may have had no previous house staff from non-traditional programs. The inclusion of the statement thus cuts a swath through any doubting clouds of the reviewers. The ultimate beneficiary, of course, is the student. The accuracy of the individual student's evaluation by the dean will enhance both the credibility of the program and of the student.

C. Apart from the above facilitating activities related to post-graduate training for students in non-traditional programs, one of the most acute considerations to be remembered is that of *financial support*. Budgeting of financial aid funds in anticipation of the special needs of students in both the accelerated and extended programs is frequently overlooked. Most accelerated programs will make use of summers, thus eliminating one of the opportunities for students to earn money toward their educational expenses. Minority students tend to plan their medical training with summer work as one of their financial resources. The need for summer academic support should be anticipated for these students, else this alone will reduce their access to the accelerated programs. The financial aid may be offered in the form of loans or a combination of loans and scholarships. Participation in the accelerated program will not affect the support received by students on the Public Health Service or Military Service Scholarships. However, those students in extended or dual-training programs will be affected because of the three- or four-year maximum support offered through scholarships. Financial aid budgeting officers will thus need to anticipate strategies for easement for these students.

It is worthwhile to consider noting such financial aid resources (including the range and forms of available aid) in the offering document since this information will certainly influence the decision of the student in selecting the program which is both practicable and career satisfying.

SPECIAL COMMENTS

Interwoven in the above discussion is a composite of personal experiences at the Howard University College of Medicine and of experiences of academic programs reported by directors at other medical schools. The advised procedures and features of special medical education programs are necessarily focused here on the minority student, although most of these considerations would be of value to any medical student. Any semblance of the recommendations which appears to view the responsibilities of the medical school from the student's point of view was intentional. The common thread which can be detected throughout the chapter is that of insuring availability of resource documents and informed persons to the student, without stigma and without masking the student's own responsibility for his or her decisions, program obligations, and learning. Admittedly, it is not always easy to recognize the line separating "enough" from "too much." Institutional resources frequently determine the limits of the types of academic programs and student support systems. More often, faculty commitment (or lack of it) will be the limiting factor.

As curricular alternatives offer options for flexibility in the professional educational program, they also allow the medical school the freedom to adjust the curriculum to the student rather than the student to the curriculum. By and large, student response to these opportunities is usually very positive (though not always perfectly so) and, surprisingly, faculty enthusiasm for teaching is heightened. If one were to try to identify the prominent advantages of the multiple curriculum programs at a given institution in which the student population is relatively heterogeneous, they would likely be (1) that of the self-selection to a given program, thus minimizing the need for consideration of noncognitive characteristics by admission committees, and (2) the interaction between the students in the several programs.

ACCELERATED AND EXTENDED PROGRAMS

Bibliography

1. Association of American Medical Colleges. *1976-77 Curriculum Directory.* Washington, D.C., 1976.
2. Association of American Medical Colleges. *1975-76 Curriculum Directory.* Washington, D.C., 1975.
3. Association of American Medical Colleges. *1974-75 Curriculum Directory.* Washington, D.C., 1974.
4. Association of American Medical Colleges. *1973-74 Curriculum Directory.* Washington, D.C., 1973.
5. Beran, R. L., and Kriner, R. E.: A Study of Three-Year Curricula in U.S. Medical Schools. Association of American Colleges. Washington, D.C., 1978.

6. Fogel, B. J.: New Programs of Medical Education and the Basic Medical Sciences. *J. Nat. Med. Assoc.,* **68:**170-171, 1976.
7. Garrard, J., and Weber, R. G.: Comparison of Three- and Four-Year Medical School Graduates. *J. Med. Educ.,* **49:**547-552, 1974.
8. Trzebiatowski, G. L., and Peterson, S.: A Study of Faculty Attitudes Toward Ohio State's Three-Year Medical Program. *J. Med. Educ.,* **54:**205-209, 1979.
9. Kettel, L. J., et al.: Arizona's Three-Year Medical Curriculum: A Postmortem. *J. Med. Educ.,* **54:**210-216, 1979.

The Future Perspective

CHAPTER 21

Affirmative Action: Impact on the Future

Herbert O. Reid and Lezli Baskerville

I want to make certain that, in the aftermath of Bakke, you continue to develop, implement and enforce vigorously affirmative action programs.[1]

President Carter

Affirmative action as a public policy has been in existence since the 1960's. It became this country's pronounced policy of attempting to erase the present effects of past discrimination at a time when this country had before it overwhelming evidence that Blacks and other minorities throughout the country were the victims of systematic invidious discrimination in education, employment, housing, and virtually every area of American life.

Herbert O. Reid, LL.D., is Charles Hamilton Houston Distinguished Professor of Law, Howard University School of Law, Washington, D.C.

Lezli Baskerville is Faculty Research Assistant, Howard University School of Law, Washington, D.C.

[1] *New York Times,* July 22, 1978, p. 9.

Faced with studies which revealed that discrimination based on race was the rule rather than the exception, it became evident that a "color-blind" remedy would not achieve equality of opportunities. The government therefore required that affirmative steps be taken to achieve parity. What was required was the deliberate undertaking of measures to "make whole" the victims of discrimination and to place them in their "rightful place" in American society. Judicially approved affirmative steps to "make whole" victims of invidious discrimination include, but are not limited to, setting goals and timetables for increasing the number of Blacks in schools and the American labor force, requiring employers and public education institutions to advertise in Black publications and on radio stations with predominantly Black listening audiences. Affirmative steps are required to remove any artificial or arbitrary barriers which might operate to keep Blacks disadvantaged. The ultimate goal of affirmative action is to achieve fair representation of Blacks in all areas of the American mainstream.

NEED TO TRAIN AND DEVELOP BLACK MEDICAL TALENT

Perhaps more than in any other area, affirmative action is needed to increase the enrollment of Blacks in the medical profession. This is because, historically, Blacks have been grossly underrepresented in participation and membership in this highly specialized field. (See Odegaard, *Minorities in Medicine: From Receptive Passivity to Positive Action, 1966-1977* (1977).)

A recent, yet unpublished statistical study prepared by Dr. Elizabeth Abramowitz of the Institute for the Study of Educational Policy is most illustrative of this theory.[2] This study reveals a well-known fact that the need exists for "more doctors as health providers sensitive to the needs of Black patients and as medical researchers studying health problems related to social class and race." Notwithstanding medical research, federal involvement with medical schools has centered around providing financial assistance

---

[2] Abramowitz, E.: Black Enrollment in Medical Schools. In *More Promise Than Progress.* Institute for the Study of Educational Policy, Howard University, Washington, D.C.

for the training of those persons promising to work in underserved rural and urban communities. In spite of this attempt, however, the number of Black doctors in the United States falls short of being described as negligible.

In 1974, for example, Black doctors comprised 2 percent of all practicing doctors in the U.S., while at the same time, Black citizens comprised 11 percent of all citizens. Keeping these figures in mind, if the only means of health service accessible to Blacks emanated from the 6,000 Black doctors, there was only one Black doctor for every 3,400 Black persons. In comparing this situation with the then existing 330,000 White doctors, there was one White doctor for every 557 White persons. The result: the Black doctor continues to be a limited resource in the medical delivery system for Black and White patients, similarly.

The American Medical Association, hoping to alleviate this "supply" problem, endorsed the remedy of increasing the number of Black medical students to a figure roughly proportional to the Black population. The goal set in the late 1960's, by the AMA, was to have 10 percent Black enrollment in medical schools by the mid-1970's. In 1969, however, Blacks totalled 2.8 percent of the 37,669 medical students, and by 1974, Blacks totalled only 6 percent of the 53,554 medical students. Granted, that in this time span Black enrollment in all medical schools increased 223 percent (from 1,038 in 1969 to 3,355 in 1974), however, Black enrollment in all medical schools has not reached, and is not even near reaching, a comparable degree of similitude with the Black population.

In 1969, only two historically Black medical schools existed in the U.S., Howard University and Meharry Medical College, and these schools enrolled slightly less than one-half (46 percent) of all Black medical students. However, by 1973, Black enrollment in historically Black medical schools accounted for only 21 percent of all Black medical students. In other words, between 1969 and 1972, the most significant increase in Black enrollment in medical schools occurred on the campuses of historically and predominantly Black medical schools.

This racial isolation in the field of medicine is indicative of the racial isolation and non-access of Blacks to other professional and highly technical fields.

An additional factor to which Blacks need to keep ever alert is, that as medical scientific knowledge increases, it becomes more important to insure that Black technicians are trained and participate in the new areas of scientific decision-making. The developing medical expertise in personality modification, population control, organ transplants, and test-tube child births are a few of these areas.

To have talked about race genocide a few years ago would have appeared paranoid or influenced by foreign ideology. Americans are justly proud of their advance in medical knowledge and technology. But the advancements in these areas pose serious problems to the survival of Blacks and the poor in America.

Personality modification had its incubation within the prison system and among the poor. The real problem is who and by what standards will "normal behavior" be determined. This obviously will impact on the poor and unwanted in the society.

In the area of population control, of great concern are the circumstances and conditions under which consent to sterilization had supposedly been given; there is a conscious effort in this country to control the numbers of the poor by sterilization. This is an ominous threat to Black survival.

Organ transplantation raised the serious threatening prospect that Blacks and the poor will become the junkyard for "parts" or "spare parts" for the majority. New definitions of death and the need for good organs already pose issues essential to Black survival.

Thus we must continue to emphasize a new dimension to equality—the need for Black presence in medical and scientific decision-making.

AFFIRMATIVE ACTION—BAKKE TO WEBER

The anticipated decision by the Supreme Court of the United States was heralded as a "landmark" in the struggle for the advancement of civil rights. Now that the Court has rendered its decision, the *Bakke* case may still signal a "landmark" in the civil rights progress or retrogression.

The progress made during the leadership of the White House from Presidents Truman to Nixon, was possible because of the affirmative leadership which the Supreme Court and the rest of the judiciary gave to the realization of long deferred dreams of equality.

Bakke may mark the end of that Presidential leadership, as well as a clear and positive judiciary prepared to move this Republic into a leadership role in the international struggle for Human Rights.

Though the Court concluded that race could be used as a factor in shaping remedial activities by public officials, the vacillation and indecision of the Court will give comfort and support to those who would destroy the affirmative action thrust of the civil rights struggle.

It is of the utmost importance for the American public to keep clear what the Supreme Court held in its *Bakke* decision and to distinguish that from what the various Justices stated as rationale for their respective positions.

Mr. Justice Brennan, joined by Justices White, Marshall, and Blackmun, while concurring and dissenting in part of the judgment, succinctly summarized the holding of the Court:

> The Court today, in reversing in part the judgment of the Superior Court of California, affirms the constitutional power of Federal and State Government to act affirmatively and to achieve equal opportunity for all. The difficulty of the issue presented—whether Government may use race-conscious programs to redress the continuing effects of past discrimination—and the mature consideration which each of our Brethren has brought to it have resulted in many opinions, no single one speaking for the Court. But this should not and must not mask the central meaning of today's opinions: Government may take race into account when it acts not to demean or insult any racial group, but to remedy disadvantages cast on minorities by past racial prejudice, at least when appropriate findings have been made by judicial, legislative, or administrative bodies with competence to act in this area.

> The Chief Justice and Brothers Stewart, Rehnquist and Stevens, have concluded that Title VI of the Civil Rights Act of 1964, 78 Stat. 232, as amended, 42 U.S.C. § 2000d et seq. (1970 ed. and Supp. V) prohibits programs such as that at the Davis Medical School. On this statutory theory alone, they would hold that respondent Allan Bakke's rights have been violated and that he must, therefore, be admitted to the Medical School. Our Brother Powell, reaching the Constitution, concludes that, although race may be taken into account in university admissions program used by petitioner, which resulted in the exclusion of respondent Bakke, was not shown to be necessary to achieve petitioner's stated goals. Accordingly, these Members of the Court from a majority of five

affirming the judgment of the Supreme Court of California insofar as it holds that respondent Bakke is "entitled to an order that he be admitted to the University." *Bakke v. Regents of the University of California,* 18 Cal. 3d 34, 64, 132 Cal. Rptr. 680, 700, 553 P.2d 1152, 1172 (1976).

We agree with Mr. Justice Powell that, as applied to the case before us, Title VI goes no further in prohibiting the use of race than the Equal Protection Clause of the Fourteenth Amendment itself. We also agree that the effect of the California Supreme Court's affirmance of the judgment of the Superior Court of California would be to prohibit the University from establishing in the future affirmative action programs that take race into account. See *ante,* at 2738 n. Since we conclude that the affirmative admissions program at the Davis Medical School is constitutional we would reverse the judgment below in all respects. Mr. Justice Powell agrees that some uses of race in university admissions are permissible and, therefore, he joins with us to make five votes reversing the judgment below insofar as it[3] prohibits the University from establishing race-conscious programs in the future.

It is interesting to note Mr. Justice Stevens, joined by the Chief Justice and Justices Stewart and Rehnquist, while concurring and dissenting in part of the judgment reacted to this summary of the legal and constitutional effect of the Court's judgment in footnote 1 of their opinion in the following language:

Four members of the Court have undertaken to announce the legal and constitutional effect of this Court's judgment. See opinion of Justices Brennan, White, Marshall and Blackmun, ante at 2766-2767. It is hardly necessary to state that only a majority can speak for the court or determine what is the "central meaning" of any judgment of the Court.[4]

The Court's holdings are relatively narrow. What must be added is that the opinion of Mr. Powell was not joined in by other Justices in a manner to justify the public emphasis which has been placed on his views as the "views of the Court." They are not the views of any Justice except Mr. Justice Powell.

Nathaniel Jones, General Counsel, National Association for the

---

[3] Bakke, *supra,* 2766-2767.
[4] Bakke, *supra.*

Advancement of Colored People, has concluded the state of law as to affirmative action to be:

1. If any employer, school system, or other public agency is sued in court and the court finds that illegal racial discrimination has existed, the court has the authority to order affirmative action including goals and timetables, quota hiring and promotion, and teacher and pupil assignments, based on race.

2. If a racial discrimination lawsuit is settled without going to trial, as part of the settlement (consent decree) the court may approve goals or quotas.

3. If a federal, state, or local legislative body determines that racial exclusion has existed in some program and passes a law requiring affirmative action plans using race factors, that law will be held constitutional.

4. If an administrative agency (such as HEW, Department of Labor, or HUD) investigates a program or an industry and has reason to believe racial exclusion has taken place, its affirmative action requirements including goals and timetables based on race will be upheld.

5. If an employer, union, or public agency decides to adopt an affirmative action plan for the purpose of bringing racial and cultural diversity to its workforce or program, it may base its decisions concerning employment or admissions partly on race provided:

   a. All qualified applicants have a chance to compete;
   b. minority race may be considered "a plus" or can be given extra weight, but it cannot be the exclusive, controlling factor;
   c. the use of race must be part of a "flexible" evaluation system;
   d. race must be used in a way that genuinely includes minorities in, not as a subterfuge for racial exclusion.

It is important to understand that the qualifications listed above apply only when there is *no* finding or evidence of past racial exclusion. If there is evidence of past exclusion on the basis of race, greater reliance on racial factors to remedy past illegal conduct is appropriate.

The decision of the Court is being read as outlawing quotas and affirming "reverse discrimination." Mr. Justice Powell's views give some credence and comfort to the enemies of affirmative action.

The impact of the *Bakke* decision on the destiny of affirmative action remains unclear. Several indicators imply that affirmative action and its constituent goals and timetables remain a viable remedy to combat discrimination.

In the area of employment, the Supreme Court refused to review a twenty-five percent non-White hiring consent decree ("quota") for the entry level positions of the Rochester, New York police department. To facilitate the decree the city established a 90 point passing score for White applicants who take the entry exam and Black applicants need only score 75 points (*Prate* v. *Freedman*, 90 S.Ct. 2274 (1978).

One week after the Court announced *Bakke, supra,* the Court upheld a 1973 affirmative action consent decree for American Telephone and Telegraph Company in *Communications Workers of American, et. al.* v. *E.E.O.C.,* 98 S.Ct. 3145 (1978). Three unions petitioned the Court to review certain provisions of the decree which provides for promotional preferences and seniority "override" for classes of women, Blacks and other minorities.

Another area where the *Bakke* decision has impacted is the minority preference provision of the "Public Works Employment Act of 1977" (Public Law 95028), the 10 percent set-asides. The Act appropriates $4 billion to cities and states as grantees through the U.S. Department of Commerce Economic Development Administration. The particular set-aside provision under attack provides that 10 percent of each local grant be business given to qualified minority businesses. The provision, authored by Congressman Parren J. Mitchell (D. - 7th Md.), states in part: "No grant shall be made under this Act for any local public works project unless the applicant gives satisfactory assurance to the Secretary that at least 10 per centum of the amount of each grant shall be expended for minority business enterprise."

To date a total of twenty-three cases have been brought in various federal district courts seeking to enjoin the states from letting the funds under the Act. Of the sixteen cases decided, fourteen upheld the set-aside provision and in two the court found the provision unconstitutional. Mention of these two cases illustrates the judicial attacks.

The district court of Western Pennsylvania in *Constructors Association of Western Pennsylvania* v. *Kreps*, 573 F.2d 811 (1977), found that a 10 percent minority business provision was enacted pursuant to the compelling governmental interest of remedying past and present effects of discrimination suffered by minority entrepreneurs. The Court reasoned that evidence of existing programs which offer alternatives to this type of provision in government contracts have not produced considerable minority participation. The case views the 10 percent figure as reasonable and not a limitation. The Act intends not to create a numerical requirement, nor to assure that minorities receive 10 percent of existing contracts, but to stimulate the construction industry by allocating extra funds to an aspect of the industry.

On the contrary, the district court for Central California found a 10 percent provision to be unconstitutional and violative of Title VI in *Associated General Contractors of California* v. *Secretary of Commerce*, 441 F. Supp. 955 (1977). This court issued a declaratory judgment determining that the provision as applied violated the Equal Protection Clause, was invidious, and an impermissible race quota. The order restrained the local defendants of the City of Los Angeles from implementing the provision from and after January 1, 1978. The court found that the 10 percent provision failed to sustain the compelling governmental test because "no discrimination against minority business enterprises sought to be assisted by this legislation is alleged," and "since underemployed minorities in the industry could be aided by racially neutral legislation having less of a detrimental impact." On appeal to the U.S. Supreme Court, the District Court decision was vacated and remanded as moot for the funds under the program had already been allocated. (See, *Los Angeles County* v. *Associated General Contractors.*) However, White contractor associations are going back to court challenging the 10 percent set-aside provision on the merits as an unlawful racial quota analogous to the *Bakke* situation. Whether the contractor associations will be successful in their suits on the merits remains uncertain.

The foregoing cases illustate the conflict of laws with respect to contractual set-asides for minority entrepreneurs. The case of *Weber* v. *Kaiser,* 563 F.2d 216 (6th Circuit 1978) illustrates the predicament of the employer, who seeks to correct an imbalance in work-force by setting aside training opportunities for minorities. Such was the situation with the Kaiser Aluminum Corporation in Gramercy, Louisiana. Weber, a White, alleged that by preferring Black employees with less seniority for admission to on-the-job training, Kaiser and the United Steel Workers Union were guilty of "reverse discrimination."

The District Court and Sixth Circuit Court of Appeals found that the preferential treatment afforded minorities, where there was no judicial determination of prior discrimination by the employer, violated Title VI of the Civil Rights Act. The Court held that in the absence of prior discrimination, a racial quota ceases to be an equitable remedy and becomes an unlawful racial preference. The Court also held that Executive Order 11246 could not justify such a preference. (The training program resulted from an agreement in 1974 between Kaiser and Steel Workers Union, calling for on-the-job training for minorities on a 1-to-1 ratio with Whites.)

The U.S. Supreme Court will decide this term whether this type of voluntary affirmative action can sustain judicial scrutiny.

America Loses Its Zeal for Affirmative Action

We the National Medical Association, the National Dental Association and the National Bar Association hold with Justice Marshall that it is necessary to take race into account so that the status quo will not be frozen at a point where equality has not been reached. It is not enough to prohibit further racism. Affirmative steps must be taken to assist those who have been affected by discrimination.

It is important for all Black groups, particularly professional organizations, to apply pressure to insure that affirmative action programs continue. The fear of our Associations is that the net effect of Bakke can be a negative one. The Bakke case dealt with medical schools, but dental and law schools with programs similar to the one at the University of California are in jeopardy, if the case is improperly interpreted.

In an effort to increase the number of qualified Black applicants entering professional schools, our Associations will monitor foundations, agencies and programs with respect to these admissions. The retention of admitted students will also be a crucial consideration.

The Supreme Court decision says that affirmative action programs can lawfully use race as a factor in the admissions process. Indeed, it is our position that the Bakke decision represents a green light to continue and creatively expand the opportunities available to minority students.

Equally, the Bakke decision reaffirms our insistence upon equal educational opportunities in elementary, junior high and high schools. It is only when our basic educational programs are dramatically improved during the developmental years of the child that there will be no difficulty meeting the legitimate requirements of professional schools.

The Bakke case must not signal an end or a decrease of affirmative action. It rather reaffirms our commitment to end all traces of slavery, discrimination and racism. Financial as well as political assistance must be generated so that students can receive aid in meeting the ever increasing costs of today's professional schools.

Our Associations are committed to using our resources to help write the next chapter in our quest for equal education opportunities. Affirmative action in no way means a lowering of standards. Significantly, the valedictorian of the class to which Allan Bakke was denied admission was a Black student. Finally, as organizations, we will speak out to elected officials and the national population about the long range urgency of our view on this issue.

We wholeheartedly endorse the NAACP call for a White House Conference on Affirmative Action.[5]

Despite the fact that the National Medical Association and other organizations met Bakke with this resolve, nevertheless there has been a decline in this country's commitment to affirmative action. One manner in which the government has succeeded in undermining affirmative action is by redefining "minority." Initially enacted to "make whole" Blacks and minorities who were the victims of systematic invidious discrimination, affirmative action plans have now become a means of preferring the majority. A recent Washington Post article tells us that "minority" now includes all females; all those of Spanish, Asian, Pacific Island, American Indian or Eskimo ancestry, and Vietnam-era veterans; all present or formerly handicapped; all workers between the ages of 40 and 64 (and most between 65 and 70); and members of various religious and ethnic groups . . . such as Jews, Catholics, Italians, Greeks and Slavic groups.[6] The expansion of the minority class clearly undermines the

---

[5] Joint Press Statement from the National Medical, Dental, and Bar Associations. *NMA News*, Sept./Oct. 1978, p. 10.

[6] Reid, I. R.: Rules to Protect Minorities' Rights Guard a Majority. *Washington Post*, March 18, 1979, p. 1.

statutory goal of affording affirmative relief to victims of systematic invidious discrimination. Blacks are faced with a new type of discrimination when they discover that not only are they entitled to "preferential" treatment, but a majority of their competitors, clearly not victims of systematic invidious discrimination, are entitled to preference also.

Slippage in this country's zeal for affirmative action is further evidenced by what happened to "busing" when Judge Sirica recently upheld from constitutional attack the Eagleton-Binden rider in *Brown* v. *Califano*. The sentiment which allowed this to happen is apparent in the field of affirmative action with such amendments as the Walker Amendment which prohibits the use of quotas and numerical requirements in school desegregation efforts. Further evidence of efforts to undermine affirmative action is the legislative assault and constant judicial attack on the validity of Minority Set-Aside.

More illustrative of the extent of legislative attempts to undermine affirmative action is a bill introduced by Senator Hatch on March 7, 1979, the "Freedom From Quotas Act of 1979." This proposed piece of legislation proscribes the enforcement of goals, quotas, time-tables, or ratios of any kind absent of a judicial determination of an individual act of discrimination. Section 4 of the proposed act states:

Prohibited Practices

> Section 4. No department or agency of the Federal Government may enforce any provision of Title VI (*sic*) of the Civil Rights Act of 1964; Executive Order 11246, as amended; Executive Order 11625, as amended; or any other statute, order, regulation or procedure in such a manner as to require or permit a contractor, employer, employment agency, grantee or labor organization to establish goals, quotas, timetables, ratios or any other numerical objective for any person or persons on the bases of race, color, religion, national origin or sex." 125 *Congressional Record* 2 (March 7, 1979)

If enacted the "Freedom From Quotas Act of 1979" will extermi-nate fifteen years of affirmative action and leave Blacks with inadequate protection against the devastating effects of racial discrimination.

Illustrative of the slippage of affirmative action by the judiciary is reflected in *Uzell* v. *Friday*, decided by the United States Circuit Court of Appeals for the Fourth Circuit in March, 1979. In an *en banc* 4 to 3 decision that Court held that *Bakke* compelled the result that the affirmative action program at North Carolina University was unconstitutional.

SOCIETAL DISCRIMINATION—ONLY EFFECTIVE APPROACH

Equality of opportunity for Blacks in America cannot be ensured without affirmative action. Affirmative action requires that societal discrimination be the measure of requiring employers and public education institutions to take positive steps to include Blacks. To require a showing of individual discrimination in each case would not ensure equality of opportunity.

The EEOC takes the position that the lawfulness of remedial action is not dependent upon a finding that the individual, the company, or institution of public education taking affirmative action has violated a federal or state statute. The Commission is of the opinion that an individual act of discrimination need not be proven.[7] The Commission suggests that a showing of underrepresentation of Blacks when compared with the number available in the relevant workforce, constitutes a *prima facie* case of race discrimination. This can be rebutted by a showing by the alleged discriminator that the underrepresentation resulted from non-discriminatory causes.[8]

The use of affirmative measures to prevent an evil is not a foreign concept. In the field of health, consumer affairs, environmental law and others, government regulations require the regulatees to take affirmative actions of a preventive nature. In many instances to react to violations on a case-by-case basis would not be in the best interest of the public. Once a pattern is established, positive steps are ordered to minimize the chances of recurrence.

There is clearly a pattern of excluding Blacks from public educational institutions and meaningful employment opportunities.

---

[7] National Urban League, Inc.: The State of Black America, 1979. January 17, 1979, p. 170.
[8] *Ibid.*

Blacks have systematically been excluded from desirable positions in the labor force and in public educational institutions. Blacks have suffered these dehumanizing effects of racism since the inception of this nation, and continue to suffer. For, though the chains and whips have been discarded, more sophisticated methods and institutional practices are used today to perpetuate the effects of racism.[9]

Today an inordinately high percentage of the Black population is poor. This poverty is a direct consequence of their history of unemployment. Poor Blacks are also less educated than Whites. It hardly merits argument to say that there is a correlation between their poverty and their ignorance. For example, on January 10, 1979, when the State of North Carolina announced the results of the state-wide Competency Test, state officials explained that the test results showed that school systems with the higher than average failure rates had two key characteristics in common: relatively low family income and relatively low levels of adult education attainment.[10] It is submitted that these two conditions reinforce each other, thereby creating a vicious cycle out of which the Black and the poor may never break, without some form of preferential treatment. And this preferential treatment merely fosters the ideal of equality, a concept articulated in the Constitution. Failing this preferential treatment, these poor will forever remain trapped in this vision of a "second hell."

In political philosophy the concept of equality has been given eloquent treatment. Aristotle noted the utter significance of this concept to the "political man" when he stated that "justice is equality as all men believe it to be, quite apart from any argument." Thus, he distinguished two principles of justice: "rectificatory" justice (involving strict or "arithmetic" equality) and distributive justice (involving proportional or "geometrical" equality, that is, a distribution in accordance with unequal merit). (Aristotle in Book V of the *Nicomachean Ethics* 11319013.)

The principle of numerical equality often considers those respects in which men are different as being irrelevant for the distribution of benefits and burdens among members of society. An obvious

---

[9] Myrdal, G.: *An American Dilemma* (New York, 1944); Ross and Hill, *Employment, Race and Poverty* (New York, 1976).

[10] Thompson, R.: Test Failures Linked to Low Family Income. *The News and Observer*, p. 1, January 11, 1979.

advantage of this principle is the ease of administration and the justification of inequalities in terms of social utility. It is submitted that this principle of numerical equality is inappropriate in the distribution of scarce goods, where this simplistic adherence to a kind of formal equality is, by definition, impossible (1974 Black L.J. 132, 151).

In contrast, the principle of proportional equality takes cognizance of differences among men and may require different treatment based on these differences ("Developments—Equal Protection," 82 *Harvard Law Review* 1160, 1165). These may be differences of merit or differences of need. The question is whether these differences give rise to any moral claims as a predicate for differential treatment among those who must share the scarce benefits. The reason articulated to justify unequal treatment is all-important; for arguments about equality are, in fact, arguments about criteria of relevance.

Professor Ronald Dworkin has contributed much to our understanding of this rather complex concept. In his major work, *Taking Rights Seriously,* (Harvard University Press, Cambridge, Mass. 1977), he has delineated two principles that take equality to be a political ideal. The first requires that the government treat all those in its charge as equals, that is, as entitled to its equal concern and respect. The second principle requires that the government treat all those in its charge equally in the distribution of some resource or opportunity, or at least work to secure the state of affairs in which they all are equal or more nearly equal in that respect.

The first principle is taken to be fundamental because it purports to recognize the inherent equality of all men. It is conceded that, sometimes, treating people equally is the only way to treat them as equals. But this is not always the case. Take the instance of a mother with two children whom she loves equally. One child is gravely ill; the other is slightly so. The mother, having a very limited supply of medicine, may decide to give half to each child. But, to do this is to ignore the very special need of the child who is gravely ill. In this instance, the mother cannot be said to have treated the children as equals by giving them equal treatment. To treat them as equals she has to take into consideration any special circumstances making for unequal or differential treatment; thus giving to the child who is gravely ill, either all or most of the medicine. This does not say that she has no concern or respect for the child who receives less. Rather, it suggests her concern and respect; and, if the situation were reversed, then, according to the principle upon which the unequal distribution is made, the child who now receives less would receive more. This example is to make the rather significant point that to treat people as equals is fundamental, and to accord them equal treatment is derivative of this more fundamental principle.

The question remains: When is it justified to treat people differently—more specifically, when is it justified to treat Blacks differently from Whites? The fact of being Black is not, *ipso facto*, a predicate of a moral claim. But the fact of Blackness, in correlation with certain other considerations, may give rise to a moral claim for differential treatment.[11]

Earlier on, we noted that differences among men may be based on need or merit, and in certain circumstances, either of the two may be the basis for differential treatment. But we argue that distribution according to merit operates on principles too closely akin to those at work in the competitive context of the private sector of this society. By making an individual's merit the relevant criterion for determining his proper allocation of burdens and benefits, the State purports to measure—and to reward accordingly—the individual's perceived value to society for some particular purpose. (82 *Harvard Law Review, supra* at 1166.) It harmonizes well with the concept of a free market economy and justifies its use on principles of utility.

This principle, in certain contexts, harbors grave dangers for Blacks, because it ignores the historic reason for their unequal circumstance. The instance of the *Weber* case is instructive, if merit—work experience—is taken to be the only relevant basis for the distribution of the scarce benefits. Thus, in the case of merit, one cannot properly speak of the distribution of a certain good without taking into consideration the distribution of the opportunity of achieving that good (see Williams, *Ibid.*). Therefore, in order to treat all persons equally, to provide genuine equality of opportunity, society must give more attention to those with fewer native assets and to those born into the less favorable positions.

The idea is to redress the bias of contingencies in the direction of equality.[12] Witness Professor Dworkin's thoughtful and impassioned plea for the proper use of preferential treatment.

---

[11] Williams, B.: The Ideal of Equality. In Bedau, H. (ed.): *Justice and Equality* (1971), p. 127.

[12] Rawls, J.: *A Theory of Justice*, (1971) p. 100.

We are all rightly suspicious of racial classifications. They have been used to deny, rather than to respect, the right of equality, and we are all conscious of the consequent injustice. But if we misunderstand the nature of that injustice because we do not make the simple distinctions that are necessary to understand it, then we are in danger of more injustice still. It may be that preferential admissions programs will not, in fact, make a more equal society, because they may not have the effects the advocates believe they will. That strategic question should be at the center of the debate about these programs. But we must not corrupt the debate by supposing that these programs are unfair even if they do work. We must take care not to use the Equal Protection Clause to cheat ourselves of equality. Ronald Dworkin, *supra* at 239.

In *Bakke, supra,* at page 2782, in the opinion by Justice Brennan, joined in by Justices White, Marshall and Blackmun, it was observed:

The assertion of human equality is closely associated with the proposition that differences in color or creed, birth or status, are neither significant nor relevant to the way in which persons should be treated. Nonetheless, the positions that such factors must be "(c)onstitutionally an irrelevance," *Edwards* v. *California,* 314 U.S. 160, 185, 62 S.Ct. 164, 172, 86 L.Ed. 119 (1941) (Jackson, J., concurring), summed up by the shorthand phrase. "(O)ur Constitution is colorblind," *Plessy* v. *Ferguson,* 163 U.S. 537, 559, 16 S.Ct. 1138, 1146, 41 L.Ed. 256 (1896) (Harlan, J., dissenting), has never been adopted by this Court as the proper meaning of the Equal Protection Clause. Indeed, we have expressly rejected this proposition on a number of occasions.

And Justice Marshall in the same case, *Bakke, supra,* at page 2803, noted:

In light of the sorry history of discrimination and its devastating impact on the lives of Negroes, bringing the Negro into the mainstream of American life should be a state interest of the highest order. To fail to do so is to ensure that America will forever remain a divided society. . . .
I do not believe that the Fourteenth Amendment requires us to accept that fate. Neither its history nor our past cases lend any support to the conclusion that a University may not remedy the cumulative effects of society's discrimination by giving consideration to race in an effort to increase the number and percentage of Negro doctors.

And Justice Blackmun:

> I suspect that it would be impossible to arrange an affirmative
> action program in a racially neutral way and have it successful. To
> ask that this be so is to demand the impossible. In order to get
> beyond racism, we must first take account of race. There is no
> other way. And in order to treat some persons equally, we must
> treat them differently. We cannot—we dare not—let the Equal
> protection Clause perpetuate racial supremacy. *Bakke, supra* at
> 2808.

Four Justices (Brennan, White, Marshall, and Blackmun) agreed
that:

> In order to achieve minority participation in previously segregated
> areas of public life, Congress may require or authorize preferential
> treatment for those likely disadvantaged by societal racial dis-
> crimination. Such legislation has been sustained even without a
> requirement of findings of intentional racial discrimination by
> those required or authorized to accord preferential treatment, or a
> case-by-case determination that those to be benefitted suffered
> from racial discrimination. These decisions compel the conclusion
> that States also may adopt race-conscious programs designed to
> overcome substantial, chronic minority underrepresentation
> where there is reason to believe that the evil addressed is a product
> of past discrimination (*Regents of the University of California* v.
> *Bakke,*—U.S. ,98 S.Ct. 2733, 2787.)

The growing emphasis on a finding of prior discrimination by the
Courts and experts in the field represents another instance where
Anglo-American jurisprudence is interpreted and applied in the
field of race relations to buttress and support a social order designed
to keep Blacks at the bottom of the social order. In applying the
more restrictive test of prior discrimination, the Courts are saying
that the evil object must be obtained before judicial relief will be
afforded. That in this area of the law we must wait for the antisocial
result to occur before the Courts will act.

Why have the Courts rejected in this field the jurisprudence of
prevention which has been a part of law in other fields for
generations?

Historically, equity developed affirmative relief before the event
as required on the law side. Equity would enjoin the parties to avoid
an antisocial result before it occurred. This equitable remedy of
prevention was engrafted in the labor law field and is the basis of the

National Labor Relations Act and all of the regulatory law in the labor field. Likewise, in the field of Government regulations of business, prevention has been a key factor. Section 4 of the Sherman Antitrust Act provides:

> Jurisdiction of courts; duty of district attorneys; procedure. The several district courts of the United States are invested with jurisdiction to prevent and restrain violations of sections 1 to 7, inclusive, or section 15 of this chapter . . . and it shall be the duty of the several district attorneys of the United States, in their respective districts, under the Attorney General, to institute proceedings in equity to prevent and restrain such violations.

In the field of administrative law, the law is expounding the use and importance of preventive action through inspections. (See *Frank* v. *Maryland,* 359 U.S. 360 (1959); *Camara* v. *Municipal Court,* 387 U.S. 523 (1967); *See* v. *Seattle,* 387 U.S. 541 (1967).) See also *Wyman* v. *James,* 400 U.S. 309 (1971) upholding home inspections as a prerequisite to receiving welfare payments.

This jurisprudence of prevention is being ignored in the affirmative action field. Why? Is it because the Court is seeking ways to nullify affirmative action rather than legal ways to promote the only meaningful programs to prevent second class citizenship in perpetuity?

The future of affirmative action may rest upon the Courts, legislature or the executive, in the first instance. The real future of affirmative action will rest ultimately upon the people and their commitment to justice and equity as a concept of equality.

CHAPTER 22

The Role of Foundations in Promoting Participation of Minorities in Medical Education

Christine Grant

Private foundations have been important stimuli of efforts to support all higher education of minorities, especially Black Americans, and of women since the early 1900's. More recently, the same institutions have been very important sources of support for programs for minorities in premedical and medical education.[1] Those individuals trying to obtain support for their own efforts to further increase the number of disadvantaged students in medicine should learn the history of foundation involvement in the area. If they take cues from what has transpired in the past between foundations, professional associations, medical schools, and colleges, they are more likely to come up with more effective strategies of fund raising and can develop programs which reflect the experiences of those who tried before them.

Christine Grant is Program Officer of The Robert Wood Johnson Foundation, Princeton, N.J.

[1] Further details of programs supported by private philanthropy during the 1900's can be found in *Negroes and Medicine*, Dietrich Reitzes, Harvard University Press, 1958; *Blacks, Medical Schools, and Society* by James L. Curtis, University of Michigan Press, 1971.

PRIVATE FOUNDATIONS AND HEALTH EXPENDITURES

There are some 26,000 private foundations operating in the United States. They have diverse program interests, boards and staff. Their styles of grantmaking vary widely. A few of the large nationally oriented foundations are devoted primarily to health care and medical education. Most local community trusts and regional foundations spread their funding more broadly among the arts, education, health, and social services. A 1976 report of the Commission on Philanthropy, *Giving in America,* and background papers prepared for that Commission, traced philanthropic giving in the area of health since the early 1930's.[2]

Table 1 illustrates the significant contribution private philanthropy has made relative to federal expenditures in health since the 1930's.[3] However, it also shows the declining share of philanthropic expenditures in the health field as a percentage of federal and other government and health expenditures (Column A) and philanthropic expenditures for medical research and health facilities construction as a percentage of federal, state, and local government expenditures during the same period (Column B).

Not only have philanthropic expenditures declined significantly compared to federal expenditures, but their decline has been more dramatic when considered as a percentage of total health expenditures in the United States since the 1930's. According to the American Fundraising Council, only about $4 billion or 4.2 percent of the total 1973 health expenditures were contributed by private philanthropy. Of this 4 percent, only 14 percent came from private foundations. What data are available indicate the same declining share of total expenditures by philanthropies relative to total educational expenditures during the same period. It is particularly significant, therefore, that the interest of private philanthropy in the area of increasing opportunities for minorities in medical education was vigorous and sustained during the 1960's and early 1970's for specific areas of medical education while its proportional share of support for other health-related and educational activities was steadily declining.

---

[2] Commission on Private Philanthropy and Public Needs: *Giving in America—Toward a Stronger Voluntary Sector.* Washington, D.C., Commission on Private Philanthropy and Public Needs, 1975.

[3] Blendon, R.: The Changing Role of Private Philanthropy in Health Affairs. *N Eng J Med.,* 292:946-950, 1975.

Table 1.   Philanthropic Expenditures in the Health Field as a Percentage of Federal Government Health Expenditures (Column A), and Philanthropic Expenditures for Medical Research and Health-Facilities Construction as a Percentage of Federal, State, and Local Government Expenditures (Column B).

YEAR	A	B
1929	90	97
1950	39	42
1973	16	28

Reprinted by permission from *The New England Journal of Medicine*, Vol. 292(18):947.

Philanthropic Support From 1930 to 1960

During the 1930's, 40's, and 50's there were a few American foundations which supported the preparation of minorities for higher education. Most of this support was in the form of funding for predominantly Black undergraduate schools and Meharry Medical College. The United Negro College Fund was an important organizing force for obtaining philanthropic support and in the late 40's, the National Medical Fellowships, Inc. began fund-raising in the philanthropic community. The Rockefeller Foundation, the Commonwealth Fund, the Julius Rosenwald Fund, the Josiah Macy, Jr. Foundation, and the Alfred P. Sloan Foundation all acted very early on the need for more minority physicians.

Philanthropic Support During the 1960's

The first stirrings of what was to become a pervasive interest by foundations in the preparations of minority students for medical careers began during the 1960's. For the first time, foundation funds were used to support public discussions and pilot programs to determine what could be done to increase minority representation in medical school.

Beginning in 1966, the Josiah Macy, Jr. Foundation financially supported the Post-Baccalaureate Premedical Fellowship program.

During its five years of operation, this visible and ambitious program enabled 72 Black college graduates to spend an additional academic year at Haverford, Bryn Mawr, Swarthmore, Oberlin, Knox, Kalamazoo, or Pomona Colleges taking regular courses intended to strengthen their academic preparation for medical school. Ninety percent of these students subsequently matriculated at medical school.[4] The Macy Foundation and the Alfred P. Sloan Foundation supported several conferences and task forces on the subject of increasing minority representation in medical school during 1967, 1968, and 1969. One of these groups, the Association of American Medical Colleges (AAMC) Task Force produced the landmark report, "Expanding Educational Opportunities in Medicine for Blacks and Other Minority Students."

By late 1969, a few medical schools, including Cornell, Harvard, and Tulane, as well as a group of predominantly Black colleges working through The United Negro College Fund, obtained small grants from several different foundations to begin pilot summer programs to strengthen the academic preparation of Black under-graduate students. These efforts were launched before federal funds became available through the Office of Economic Opportunity and later through the Public Health Service. During just a few years, the number of small foundations which funded these efforts increased significantly.

Philanthropic Support During the 1970's

The AAMC Task Force Report, mentioned above, was released in the spring of 1970. It was the harbinger of what was to become the largest concentrated private effort to increase the number of minority physicians in the United States. This report was submitted to the Inter-Association Committee representing the American Medical Association, the National Medical Association, the American Hospital Association, and the AAMC. It provided a rationale for public and private decision-makers to think about specific strategies which might be taken to increase opportunities for minority students in medicine. It proposed a short-term goal that medical

---

[4] Bleich, M.: Funding of Minority Programs from the Private Sector: A Perspective from the Josiah Macy, Jr. Foundation. *J.A.M.A.*: 234:1339, 1975.

schools increase the representation of minorities in the first year of medical school classes to 1800 or 11.9 percent by 1975-76. This number was based on enrollment projections which turned out later to be understated and notions of the available applicant pool of minority college students with premedical preparation which turned out to be overstated. In retrospect, members of the Task Force which released the report offered a challenge and a goal which turned out to be much more difficult to achieve than probably even they had imagined. The closest approach to the goal was 10.1 percent in 1974-75; the next year, when the figure was 9.1 percent, the goal had receded still further.*

A follow-up report of the AAMC Task Force was released in October, 1978, eight years after the first.[5] The more recent report documented that the country has not met the gaols set for it, although enormous personal efforts and millions of dollars had been spent along the way. Of course, dramatic increases did occur; 200 minority students were admitted in 1967. Ten years later, almost 1,400 were admitted.

The important issue to understand is the high level of complexity of the problem, as well as the slowness of the natural course of human events. This means that money may be necessary but is surely an insufficient condition for sustained change in this area.

Within a year after the release of the first AAMC Task Force Report, other activities began. The Grant Foundation provided money which was later supplemented by federal funds to enable medical schools to run numerous national and regional workshops in order to design specific programs to identify, recruit, select, educate, and retain minority students.

In this chapter, figures on foundation expenditures for minorities refer mainly to the underrepresented groups as follows: American Blacks, mainland Puerto Ricans, Mexican-Americans, and American Indians. The amount spent to date exclusively for women who are the other group still generally considered to be somewhat underrepresented is a very small fraction of the total expenditures.

Many other foundations followed with individual grants made directly to medical schools, undergraduate schools, professional

---

* See Table I, Chapter 17, for data from the AAMC on first-year minority enrollment.

[5] Report of the Association of American Medical Colleges Task Force on Minority Student Opportunities in Medicine. October, 1978.

associations, or community-based organizations. It was on the basis of the pilot Foundation support that a number of schools successfully qualified for the much larger federal grants as they became available during the early 70's. By 1976, at least one third of U.S. medical schools had received some philanthropic support for this type of activity. A large number of undergraduate schools were also involved.

Philanthropic expenditures for the purpose of supporting the recruitment and preparation of minority health professionals were highest during the 1970's. Table 2 reflects the magnitude of giving during this period: $46,054,000 was given by foundations for the support of minority health professional student aid; minority health professional recruitment progams; minority health professional institutional support; and other minority health professional support between 1970 and 1977. Grants peaked at $9,607,500 in 1972, declined in 1973-75, rose to $6,058,700 in 1976, but declined sharply in 1977 to $1,272,200, to the lowest level during the eight years.*

Most of the funding during the 1960's and early 70's was targeted toward Black students. More recently, Hispanics and American Indians have been specifically included in grants in more significant numbers. There are two probable reasons why this has been so. First, Black Americans have historically and currently still do form the largest racial minority in the United States. Secondly, predominantly Black undergraduate schools were the first to initiate contact with private philanthropies to request assistance to prepare more of their students for application to previously all-White medical schools.

Few undergraduate schools or community-based organizations have coalesced around the issues of minority recruitment for Hispanics or American Indians in comparison with the number of Black-oriented schools. An exception to this has been ASPIRA of America, Inc. Headquartered in New York with affiliates in Illinois, New York, New Jersey, Pennsylvania, and Puerto Rico, this group is Puerto Rican oriented. However, numerous young people in the program have South or Central American, Caribbean, or Mexican-American backgrounds. ASPIRA has high school and college level programs for students, and a few undergraduate programs in the Southwest for Mexican-American students.

---

* The figures refer to the years when the grants were made. Expenditures from the grants in some cases were spread over several years.

Table 2. Minority Health Professional Support by Private Foundations: Reported Grants, 1970-1977 (in Dollars)

	1970	1971	1972	1973	1974	1975	1976	1977
Minority Health Professional Student Aid	330,000	1,596,500	9,395,500	2,863,400	1,887,800	1,227,600	3,288,500	607,400
Minority Health Professional Recruitment	1,640,300	1,086,600	135,000	658,700	1,907,400	689,500	2,755,200	628,800
Minority Health Professional Institutional Support	320,000	3,721,000	5,000,000	923,400	100,000	2,104,800	10,000	2,525,000
Other Minority Health Professional Support	27,000	115,900	77,000	205,100	71,800	168,800	5,000	11,000
TOTAL	2,317,300	6,520,000	14,607,500	4,650,600	3,967,000	4,190,700	6,058,700	3,772,200

Source: The Foundation Center *Grants Index*, 1970-1978. The *Grants Index* lists grants in excess of $10,000 which are voluntarily reported by member foundations. The index is believed to reflect at least 70 percent of the dollar volume of grants made.

Table 2 was prepared for the author by John Craig, et al at the Health Policy Research Group, Georgetown University School of Medicine.

Women, who now form more than a quarter of entering medical school classes, never put together an organized lobby to raise foundation support. As a group, however, they achieved dramatic increases in enrollment since 1969 when they constituted less than 9 percent of medical school enrollment. The most recent studies of women medical students' problems indicate that they are not related to difficulty in obtaining admission to medical school due to inadequate secondary or undergraduate preparation or due to an insufficient applicant pool, but rather are related to the need for emotional support and counseling during and subsequent to medical school years.[6] Private philanthropy has not provided much support for women's premedical or medical education programs to date. What support there has been for women's premedical or medical education programs has come from very few foundations.[7]

Therefore, although this chapter may seem to stress philanthropic efforts in increasing Black representation in medical school, it is not a result of the lack of foundations' interest for other groups' education, but rather reflects their longer history of involvement with Black education in the country.

FINANCIAL AID FOR MINORITY MEDICAL STUDENTS

Since 1970, more than $21,196,700 of financial aid has been provided by private foundations to minority medical students. The most prominent national scholarship organization for minority medical students is the National Medical Fellowships, Inc., based in New York City. Organized in 1946, this group has itself distributed more than $16,000,000 (only some of which is reflected in the figure $21,196,700 because NMF support comes from other than just foundations), to more than 4,000 young physicians in training over 32 years. The organization has traditionally raised funds from private philanthropy. More recently they have obtained funds from corporate giving, as well as from individual minority alumni who themselves had been NMF scholarship recipients during their medical school years. The funds are distributed directly to students

---

[6] Grant, C.: Women's Programs Aren't for Women Only. *Foundation News* 17:15-24, March/April 1976.
[7] *Ibid.*

on the basis of need. Over the years, more than 200 private foundations around the country have contributed money to NMF for scholarships and loans.

Within the past five years, NMF has moved much more aggressively to secure corporate support as well as support from past scholarship recipients. This move, by the most sophisticated fund-raising group in this field, is in part due to the recognition of the difficulty of maintaining sustained support from individual private foundations for this type of activity. It also reflects the decline of direct foundation support for financial aid for minority students as was shown in Table 2.

The largest single program of financial aid for minority students occurred in 1972 when The Robert Wood Johnson Foundation awarded $14 million to the nation's schools of medicine ($10 million), dentistry and osteopathy ($4 million) for use as scholarships and/or loan support for students from rural backgrounds, from racial minority groups, or for women. Although this program was the largest student aid effort ever funded by a private philanthropy, the approximately $3.5 million provided each year over the four-year program, constituted less than five percent of the total student aid funds available during the same period.[8] An additional $2,500,000 was granted to the schools in 1976.

The evaluation of this program documented that "disadvantaged, particularly minority students received larger average awards than did other recipients, and awards to disadvantaged students were more likely to be made as scholarships than as loans during the student's first two years. Moreover, at least 30 percent of all minority students in medical, dentistry, and osteopathy schools during this period (1973-1977) received a loan or scholarship from this source."[9]

In 1977, the same foundation announced a different program—a Guaranteed Student Aid Program for all students. The shift from a student aid program run through the medical schools, to one which leverages private lenders' dollars, occurred as part of the recognition that private philanthropy alone could not fill the student aid gap during the coming decade. The move of this foundation occurred in parallel with skyrocketing tuitions and the federal government's

[8] Craig, J.: Georgetown University School of Medicine Monograph, February, 1979.

[9] Interim Communication from John Craig. Health Policy Research Group, Department of Community and Family Medicine, Georgetown University, 1979.

expansion of its own programs through the National Health Service Corps (Public Health Service), and Armed Forces Scholarships.

The RWJF program is designed to provide money of last resort. It is expensive money to borrow. The hope of the program, however, is that no student will be unable to matriculate at medical, dental, or osteopathy school due to lack of funds. An evaluation of the first year of the program indicates that minority students are using this source of funding in larger numbers than their proportional representation in medical school.

A review of U.S. medical school catalogues distributed during the 1970's disclosed that many medical schools have had particular scholarship and/or aid programs for disadvantaged students. The guidebook, entitled *Medical School Admission Requirements* and distributed annually by the Association of American Medical Colleges, is the "Bible" of premedical students. This directory has since 1973, included a section directed to minority medical students advising them about the availability of scholarship aid from private as well as public sources.

It is clear that private foundations made available significant amounts of student aid for minority medical students during the critical period when the doors were beginning to open and when their numbers were increasing rapidly. It is unclear, however, as to the extent that private philanthropy will continue to contribute a level of funding for scholarships and/or loans which can keep pace with the tuitions of medical schools which are rising much more rapidly than tuitions of any other schools of higher education.

PREMEDICAL PROGRAMS FOR MINORITY STUDENTS

There are common elements to most of the programs funded by private foundations during the 1970's. Either these efforts tended to be sponsored by community groups, such as the American Foundation for Negro Affairs, ASPIRA of America, Inc., La Raza, or, more typically, medical schools developed programs independently or in concert with one or more undergraduate schools. The efforts by community groups concentrated on the identification of high school students interested in health careers and the subsequent counseling of such students concerning appropriate academic courses of study and concerning the process of applying to medical school.

Programs involving medical schools and colleges have been of two general types. The first type has been summer recruitment and intensive science and study habit programs sponsored by individual medical schools alone. In these programs, the medical school typically enrolls minority undergraduate students already conditionally accepted or students appearing to be academically promising candidates. During the summer preceding entry or application to medical school, the students take review courses in biology, biochemistry and perhaps a first year medical school course such as anatomy. The goal of these programs is to insure the student's successful completion of the first year of medical school and to improve the school's ability to enroll those students it most wants to enroll.

The second program typically links the resources of medical schools and undergraduate schools. The programs include summer and academic year activities and are for post-freshman, sophomore, and junior students. The summer component may consist of intensive academic preparation in reading, writing, biological sciences, and test-taking skills. Financial aid information and counseling about the application process are also provided. Thirty to 50 students are usually in the summer programs which also have year-round recruitment activities which include premeds at each of the undergraduate schools in the consortium. Students who are eligible to apply are those who believe themselves to be educationally disadvantaged by virtue of their racial, ethnic, or economic background. Some white students also participate in these programs. The academic year activities include periodic seminars to reinforce what occurs in the summer and hopefully, strengthening of the science curricula at the participating undergraduate schools and continued counseling. Detailed accounts of these activities appear in other chapters of the book. Some medical schools have also developed outreach programs for high school students.

IMPACT OF FOUNDATION SUPPORT OF MINORITY MEDICAL EDUCATION

What has been learned from the minority recruitment programs during the 1970's from an educational point of view? Certainly, some efforts have been successful. The minority applicant pool increased from about 400 in 1967 to 3,300 in 1977. The number of entering minority medical students increased from 200 to 1,400 during the same period. Students who have participated in such programs appear to have improved chances of acceptance over the general minority population. For example, the Post-Baccalaureate Program described earlier in this chapter saw 90 percent of its 72 participants enter medical school. One Macy-sponsored survey suggested that 40 percent of minority acceptees had attended one or more summer programs and found them helpful. There is some evidence that medical schools that have such programs have better retention rates for the disadvantaged student than schools that do not. Descriptions of programs for undergraduates at Tulane, the University of Texas at Galveston, The College of Medicine and Dentistry of New Jersey, and the PREP Programs in New York City, report that substantially higher percentages of their participants were accepted to medical school than were accepted from the general minority applicant pool during each of the last several years.

However, despite such fragmentary evidence, it is disappointing that only a paltry amount of solid analysis has appeared in the literature as to why the applicant pool remains so low and to what extent the educational interventions funded have made a difference. Over 40 medical schools and a growing number of undergraduate schools have run programs for disadvantaged and minority students, yet fewer than 12 papers have been published in the *Journal of Medical Education*. Most of these were descriptive—not analytical studies. Studies of the pre- and post-academic performance of participants in these programs and the batting average of admissions per program are needed.

Foundation staffs and their boards of trustees faced with allocating limited resources to this particular area of medical education have inadequate information as to which particular elements of a program are most important to achieving the ultimate goals of increasing the total applicant pool of minority students who are academically and emotionally prepared to be accepted to medical school. They need to know if it is the counseling, the study skills sources, or MCAT reviews which make the difference. It appears that the counseling, laboratory work, and study skill sessions are important, but there is insufficient evidence as to which is more important. In the absence of such information, it should not be surprising that foundations are reluctant to invest an increasing amount of dollars in these efforts. They are more likely to maintain at best a steady-state level of funding.

In addition to increasing and strengthening the applicant pool, foundation funding has supported the development of a cadre of people who are most knowledgeable on the issues related to minority recruitment. A review of the members of the 1969 AAMC Task Force, the Committee which redesigned the MCAT, the most recent AAMC Task Force, and the NIH study groups read like a Who's Who of people who received private foundation support during the critical years when they were struggling to establish themselves and their institutional bases. These people were ahead of their colleagues in the establishment of premedical and medical school programs. The dilemma for the 80's for these individuals, as well as for private sources which may continue to support them, will be how best to utilize the specific skills they have developed during this period. How can their experience best be communicated to other people in other institutions who wish to develop programs, but who should not be encouraged to "reinvent the wheel"? Privately supported technical assistance by the most experienced people to the newer groups could be working better than it is. Advisors and undergraduate faculty have not implemented even simple modifications in counseling techniques or curricula although successful examples are all around them and do not need much money to implement. The nature of the proposals still being submitted to private foundations and HEW for support of what are represented as "new ideas" suggests that existing programs should be educating others about what they have learned. Perhaps this book will help to disseminate some of these ideas.

In the area of financial aid for minority medical students, as distinct from the remedial efforts, foundation support has been of mixed value. Financial aid officers and minority organizations believed that private support for financial aid was critically important to increased enrollment. However, a 1977 National Planning Association analysis of the total medical school financial aid situation 1972-76, offered as one of its findings that, during the years 1972-76, private foundations' contribution of student aid for minority students was not a *major* cause of the increase in the number of minority medical students. Indeed, the most dramatic percentage increases took place in 1968-72. If foundations' support of financial aid were very important we would have expected to see even larger increases than what occurred 1968-72 when foundation funding was low in this area. Rather, the private foundations' support in some cases during 1972-76 permitted individual schools to compete with each other for the most desirable minority candidates available at that time rather than increase the total number who were accepted. The applicant pool did not increase as much as would be expected either. In retrospect, it appears there was a student aid surplus during that period. However, the pendulum has swung to the other extreme. By 1977, there was again a large student aid gap. It was caused by large shifts in the federal scholarship and loan program funds and in skyrocketing tuitions. Medical schools quickly were without unrestricted scholarship monies for minority and very poor students. However, at the same time, the largest single private scholarship and loan program terminated and an abrupt decline of other foundation support for financial aid also occurred. (See Table 2 and discussion of NMF.) Thus, private philanthropy's timing of an infusion of scholarship support appears in retrospect to have been premature and money will be needed greatly during the foreseeable future if schools are to be able to continue to attract financially disadvantaged minority students.

Private philanthropy has traditionally provided support for the capital, faculty, tuition, and operational deficits of Meharry Medical Center. Numerous articles have appeared describing the particularly complex dilemmas facing that institution and will not be repeated here. Clearly, however, private philanthropic support alone cannot stabilize that institution's financial plight. State and federal public funds and the optimization of their third-party reimbursement for services provided are required. Howard Medical School receives primarily public funds and has not had the level of private support that Meharry has traditionally had although foundations have contributed to that institution.

Although it is too early to analyze private philanthropy's role in supporting the new medical school at Morehouse in Atlanta, early indications are that more public funds have been contributed than private support in the two areas of medical school costs which private foundations usually fund in institutional settings, capital development, and program development. It will be several more years before the extent to which private foundations fund the development of the nation's third predominantly Black medical school currently operating is known. That Morehouse may not be attracting large amounts of private funding is not surprising given the general climate with respect to medical school funding today. Public dollars are more in evidence than ever in private institutions across the country.

THOUGHTS ON FUTURE FOUNDATION SUPPORT
FOR MINORITY RECRUITMENT PROGRAMS
IN THE 1980's

As described, private philanthropy provided substantial support for minority premedical and medical students during the 1970's. The most significant contributions were in the areas of student financial aid, and premedical counseling and remedial programs sponsored by medical schools and undergraduate schools. What will the role of philanthropies be during the 1980's? It is impossible to predict precisely what will happen. A large new foundation could emerge with an interest in the area overshadowing what other foundations have done. Existing foundations may shift their foci. There are, however, some early indications of what may happen and individuals looking for foundation support should be alert to these factors as they plan for the future.

In general, the largest foundations' staff and boards are aware of what the various trends in society are and respond or initiate programs accordingly. Several of the more important sets of events are the changing financial situations in medical schools, and the social attitudes concerning minority recruitment.

This author believes that the climate is shifting within the field of medical education. The optimism and enthusiasm to admit minority and other disadvantaged students which characterized the years 1967-77 in medical education is now being tempered by several factors. The first is the deceleration in the number of new medical schools and students. Both the number of new medical schools and students increased dramatically during the years 1967-77. The number of medical students doubled during that period. The number of minority students increased more than fivefold during the same period. An increase of this magnitude won't recur. There will be fewer new medical schools and students during the 1980's. This means that unless total applications continue to decline, as they have done for two years consecutively, while minority applications increase, which is not occurring, minority students will continue to be at a competitive disadvantage in the application process. It is encouraging to note that while medical schools realize they can't solve the minority enrollment problem alone, they have maintained an open mind and interest in continuing to work for increased enrollment.

Not only has the rate of growth of new schools declined, but existing schools are facing unprecedented requirements to control costs. This means that tuitions will continue to rise and more and more students from all backgrounds will have to assume debts and service commitments. For the first time, medical schools may have to talk openly about the relationship between a student's financial needs and the likelihood of admission. This will mean that although private foundations will not be able to take on the full cost of tuition for minority students, they might be in a particular position to close the gap between available public money for loans and the total cost of a medical education so no low-income student feels unable to apply.

Society's attitudes will also have some impact on philanthropic behavior as regard to assistance to minority premedical students. The recent, much publicized, Bakke decision reflected rather than initiated the public's interest in questioning how much and at what cost had minority enrollment been increased. It appears that foundations will continue to be sensitive to the importance of encouraging low-income or otherwise disadvantaged White students as well as disadvantaged minority students who are seeking admission to medical school. Most of the better and longer-established minority recruitment programs have already been working with both groups. They would not be adversely affected by foundations moving more in this direction.

Mention of these factors does not mean that private philanthropy won't continue to provide strong sustained support for actions designed to increase the qualified minority applicant pool for medical, dental, and other health professional schools. On the contrary, several of the larger foundations appear to have made solid commitments for the next few years. However, the nature of the support may change.

The first order of business will definitely be the preparation of a sufficiently large pool of qualified applicants. There are more than 400,000 minority students in undergraduate schools. The number of minority applications has hovered around 3,300 for several years, and 38 to 40 percent of these applicants have been accepted during this period. Therefore, if just one percent more of all minority undergraduate students could be adequately prepared for medical school applications, the number of applicants would be doubled to more than 6,000, and a sufficiently large pool of qualified applicants would be achieved.

Foundations may be expected, therefore, to concentrate support for those programs which can demonstate their ability to expand the total applicant pool and to get a high percentage of their program participants admitted. It will be especially important and could be of great benefit if the number of minority applications increased while the general number of applications are decreasing.

There will probably be a continued shift from scholarship support to loan guarantees. Rather than supporting directly large amounts of student aid for disadvantaged students, foundations may look for ways to maintain a floor of financing for low-income students of all backgrounds. The goal would be to pick up the final dollars of financing needed to make sure that students can matriculate. Because premedical students need counseling about financial aid to assist them in making a decision to apply, foundations could play an important role in the next few years in publicizing ways in which students can finance their education.

Finally, as increasing numbers of minority physicians enter practice and academic careers, there may be some philanthropic interest in supporting such individuals. The goal of such support would be to develop a group of highly qualified faculty and research physicians and dentists as well as physicians in practice who would assume leadership positions in medicine and in turn, serve as role models to young premedical and medical students. Such role models continue to be very important.

STRATEGIES FOR FINANCING MINORITY RECRUITMENT AND ENROLLMENT PROGRAMS

The societal and economic factors and the recent behavior of foundations suggests that program directors should employ several strategies in securing support for their programs in this author's view. First, programs should be structured to emphasize the basic techniques of academic remediation, test-taking skills, and financial and emotional counseling, which earlier chapters in this book described in detail. Programs should be realistic and truly aimed to enlarge the qualified applicant pool. Evaluation data about a program's success in monitoring and assisting students through the college years, through the application process and into medical school are a very critical factor in identifying a program's potential.

Program directors should be able to supply such information to foundations to whom they apply.

Because funding for new programs or duplicative programs will not be easy to obtain, undergraduate schools and medical schools will have to swallow hard and work much more closely with each other. If they share resources, they can achieve a consolidation of costs and information and can bring greater stability to their programs.

As described earlier, there are only a few national foundations interested in the area of minority recruitment at the present time. Therefore, program directors should try to fundraise from local or regional foundations and be prepared for the hard, difficult task of packaging several different sources of funds to run a program. Program directors have to recognize that most philanthropic support is short term. To remain in operation, they should plan early on to fold as much program activity into existing budget lines as possible. Most colleges can't afford to run duplicative student support services. This integration of recruitment and remediation activity is also a sure sign of a program's value to the student body.

In summary, the future of philanthropic support for minority recruitment and retention programs should be viewed with optimism. There will be a continued, and difficult burden on the program director or dean to fund-raise and maintain support. That, however, is increasingly so for all charitable activities and is not unique to this area. It is also true that program directors will have to be even more conscientious in documenting their program's impact and describing articulately what they expect to accomplish. The goal of increasing and maintaining a qualified applicant pool for medical school is so important and there has been so much ground work done in the last decade that those working in this field have an important role to play and can provide a very valuable service by keeping at the job.

Subject Index

Table Index